Over 650 titles from "Abbott & Costello Meet Frankenstein" to "Zombie." Plus:

■ ALTERNATE TITLES ■ YEAR OF RELEASE ■ COLOR OR B&W ■ DIRECTOR ■ LEADING PLAYERS ■ RUNNING TIME ■ PLOT SUMMARY/ BRIEF REVIEW ■ RATING ■ VIDEO FORMAT (VHS, BETA, CED DISC OR LV DISC) ■ VIDEO SOURCE OR SOURCES ■ OVER 120 ILLUSTRATIONS

With added information covering:

■ VIDEO EQUIPMENT ■ MAIL ORDER & VIDEO SWAPPING ■ RENTING TAPES OR DISCS VS. BUYING THEM ■ VIDEO SPECIALTY MAGAZINES ■ ADDRESSES FOR ALL SOURCES MENTIONED ■ CARE & FEEDING OF YOUR VIDEOTAPES & DISCS ■ DIRECTORS & THEIR FILMS (AN EXTENSIVE INDEX)

Everything you need to know and more about the most popular films now in release on home video. Use it for reference. Use it for fun. The 1983 edition of VIDEO SCREAMS is your official sourcebook for horror, science fiction, fantasy and related films on videocassette and disc.

VIDEO SCREAMS™ 1983

The official sourcebook to horror, science fiction, fantasy and related films on videocassette and disc.

by
John McCarty

Other books by John McCarty:

You're on Open Line: Inside the Wacky World of Late-Night Talk Radio

Splatter Movies: Breaking the Last Taboo

The Amazing Herschell Gordon Lewis and His World of Exploitation Films
(with Daniel Krogh)

ISBN 0-938782-02-9

Published by: FantaCo Enterprises, Inc.
21 Central Avenue
Albany, New York 12210

Typography & Design: Unicomp
Cover Design: Spence Raggio, Tom Skulan, Mary Clare
Type for alphabetical listings chapter headings designed by Jean Larcher, from "Fantastic Alphabets," published by Dover Publications, Inc.

Printed in the United States of America
First printing: January 1983

FOR RAB

Who puts up with it all

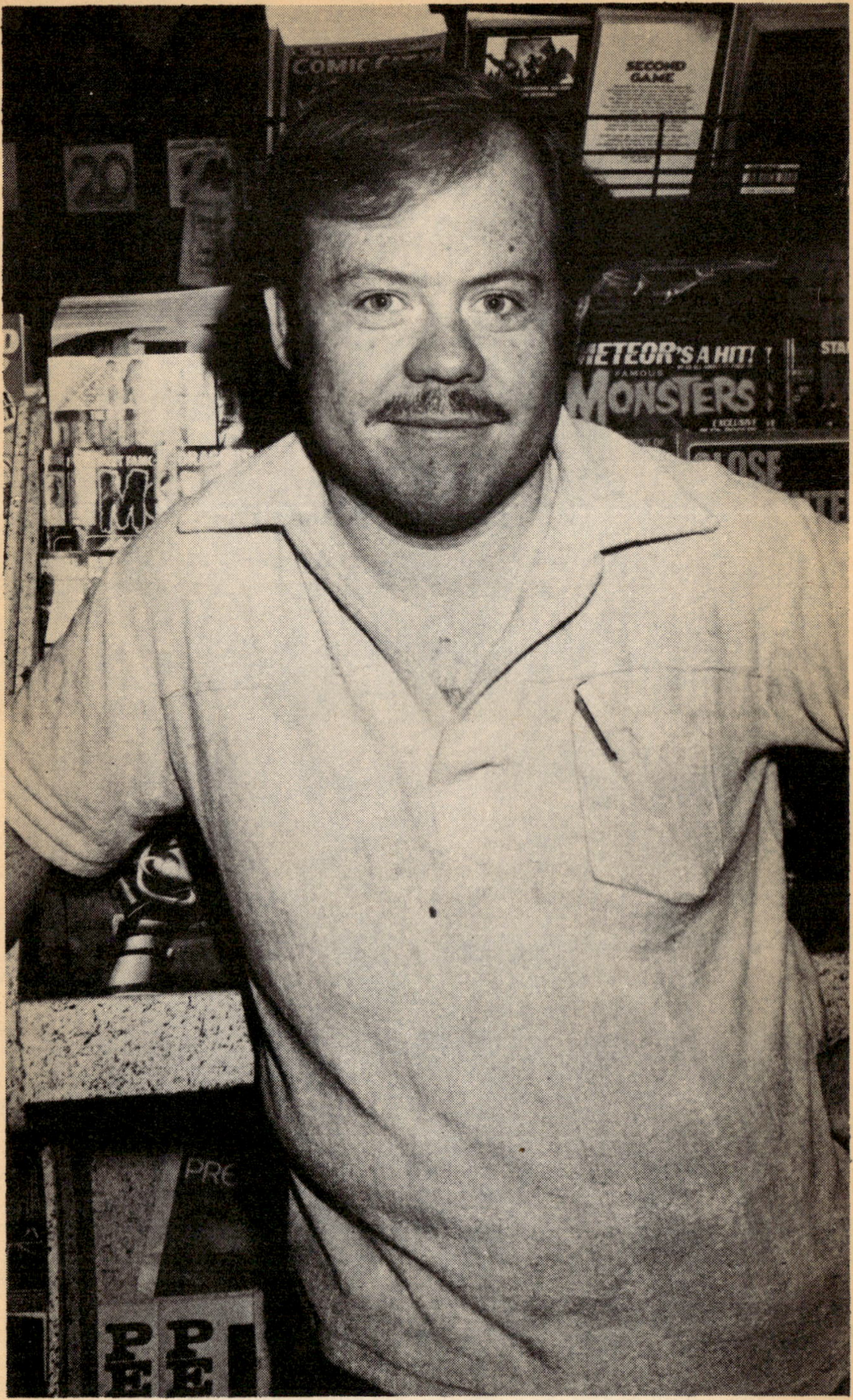
COMIC
SECOND GAME
FAMOUS
MONSTERS

About the Author

John McCarty has been a fan of horror, science fiction and fantasy films since the age of five. His private collection of genre and other type films numbers in the hundreds.

A graduate of Boston University's film school, he has, over the years, contributed articles and reviews to film magazines as diverse as *Cinefantastique, Filmaker's Newsletter, Classic Images, Take One,* and *Today's Filmmaker.*

His other books include *You're on Open Line: Inside the Wacky World of Late-Night Talk Radio,* the cult favorite *Splatter Movies: Breaking the Last Taboo,* which *Fangoria* magazine has termed, ". . .the definitive history of the gore film, and likely to remain as such," and (with Daniel Krogh) *The Amazing Herschell Gordon Lewis (And His World of Exploitation Films).*

Table of Contents

Welcome to *Video Screams '83*

The United States and other "high tech" societies around the world are today experiencing an unprecedented home entertainment explosion. At the forefront of the boom is home video itself, that wonder of modern electronics which allows us to transform our TV sets into movie screens and our living rooms into picture palaces. Thanks to the invention of the home videocassette recorder (VCR) and videodisc player, we movie fans no longer have to put up with annoying commercials or any unnecessary scissoring by our networks and local stations when we view a film in the privacy of our homes. We simply pop in the cassette or disc and watch the film uncut and uninterrupted—just as its makers intended it to be shown. Who knows, without all the traditional interruptions we've come to expect from home screen fare, we Americans may once again regain our attention spans.

Thanks to home video also, movie fans can take in the latest big budget releases as well as the more obscure films from Hollywood and abroad without having to move from their armchairs. Sure the screen is a lot smaller, but who cares? In the future, that will change too. Meanwhile, we armchair moviegoers are fully compensated by not having to suffer the indignities of crowds, uncomfortable theatre seats, rotten projection, and audiences that can't sit or keep still.

No doubt about it, home video has the potential to make moviegoing fun again. And cheaper too. A family of four, for example, can rent a tape of *Star Wars* for anywhere from $2.50 to $5 whereas seeing it at the theatre would cost between $8 and $16—plus an outrageous $1.25 apiece for a *small* box of popcorn. By renting tapes of movies rather than laying down big bucks at the box office to see them, our family of four can thus afford to see more movies per year, providing a shot in the arm for the film industry that should make moviemakers everywhere jump for joy. In addition to renting tapes, of course, fans and collectors can buy them—though at present the prices are a little steep, thereby adding certain cherished films to their home libraries for repeated viewings for years to come. Yes, folks, home video is like a dream come true. And more and more people are waking up to it each and every year.

Publications like *Video Review* and *Home Video* as well as the advertising industry's own marketing bible, *Advertising Age,* report that an estimated 5 million VCRs had found their way into American homes by the close of 1982. Though in its infancy compared to tape, over 200,000 videodisc players have already been purchased for home use as well. And sales of both machines are steadily climbing. The message is clear. Home video is here to stay. In fact, it's proving to be even more popular than television was when it first appeared.

There's another message that's coming through loud and clear also. Research conducted by many of these same publications as well as my own informal canvassing of various video retailers and mail order houses around the country indicates that the single most popular films being rented and/or purchased for home consumption belong to the horror, science fiction, and fantasy film category. X-rated tapes come in a distant second. It seems that while most home video addicts invariably have a copy of *Citizen Kane* on their shelves and will stand in line along with everyone else to rent the latest Oscar-winner like *Chariots of Fire* as soon as it becomes available on tape, the films they *really* want to see and have are not mainstream movies, but genre hits like *Star Wars* and *Star Trek II,* stop motion classics like *King Kong* and *The 7th Voyage of Sinbad,* cult nail-biters like *Night of the Living Dead* and *The Texas Chainsaw Massacre,* and special effects extravaganzas like *The Exorcist* and *Poltergeist.* It's at this vast audience of genre film lovers and collectors that *Video Screams, the* guide to horror, science fiction, fantasy and related films on videocassette and disc, is aimed.

Included in this '83 edition are over 600 currently available titles ranging from well-known and popular video screamers like *Alien* and *Close Encounters of the 3rd Kind* to some of the more obscure entries in scream film history, like *The Driller Killer, The Flesh and Blood Show* and *Dr. Heckyl and Mr. Hype.* Listed alphabetically, each title is followed by its year of release, whether it's in color or black & white, its running time, the name of its director, its principal stars, a brief plot summary and other comments, plus the name of its manufacturer as well as the video format(s) it's available in. VC stands for videocassette (both VHS and Beta); LV for LaserVision Optical Disc; and CED for Capacitance Electronic Disc—today's three most common modes of home entertainment equipment.

If you're just now entering the fabulous world of home video and are struggling to decide whether to go tape or disc, you should know that at present the number of films—genre or otherwise—being released on tape far outweighs the number of releases on either Laser or CED disc. This situation may change in the not too distant future, however, as the popularity of videodisc hardware continues to grow. The fact that one can record with a VCR but not with a videodisc player gives the VCR a decided advantage. On the other hand, movies on videodisc are presently much cheaper to buy than pre-recorded movies on videocassette, enablng you to add more movies to your collection more quickly for roughly the same amount of money. This too is a factor that should be weighed before making your final buying decision.

There are other factors as well, but it is not within the scope of this book to go into them. A good way to find out whatever you want to know about what kind of home video equipment to buy is to consult your local video retail store. But there are also a number of very helpful books on the market that you might consider consulting as well. These include: *The Complete Home Video Handbook* by Mark Dunton and David Owen (Random House, 224 pages, $19.95); *The Video Primer* by Richard Robinson (Quick Fox, 400 pages, $8.95); *The Home Video Handbook* by Charles Benginger (Scribners, 304 pages, $9.95); *Home Video* by Marvin Grosswirth (Doubleday/Dolphin, 160 pages, $7.95); and *The Complete Home Video Recorder Book* by Len Buckwalter (Bantam, 377 pages, $2.95).

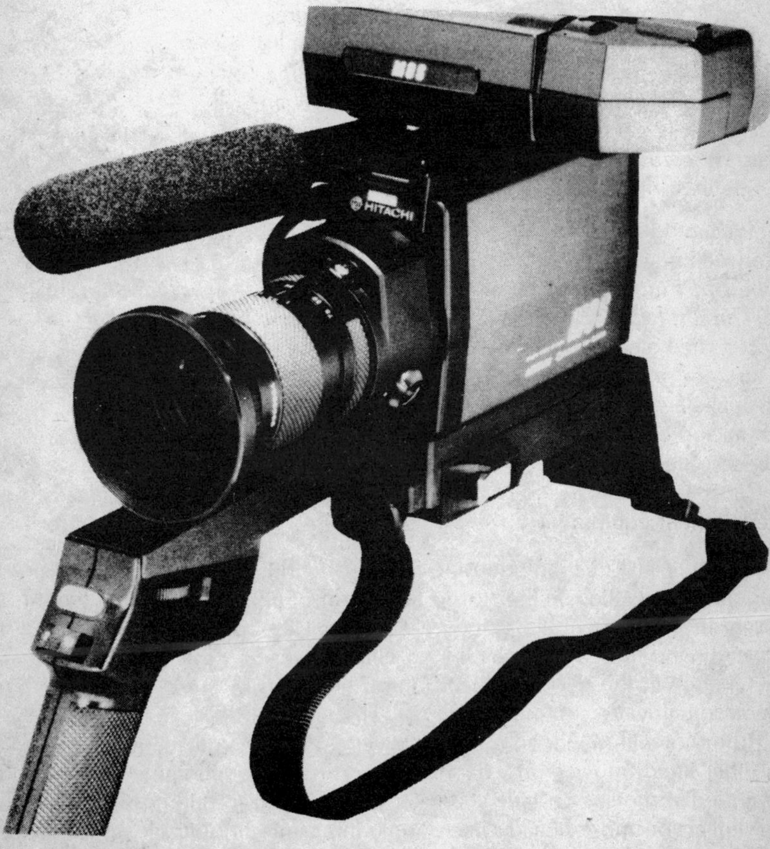

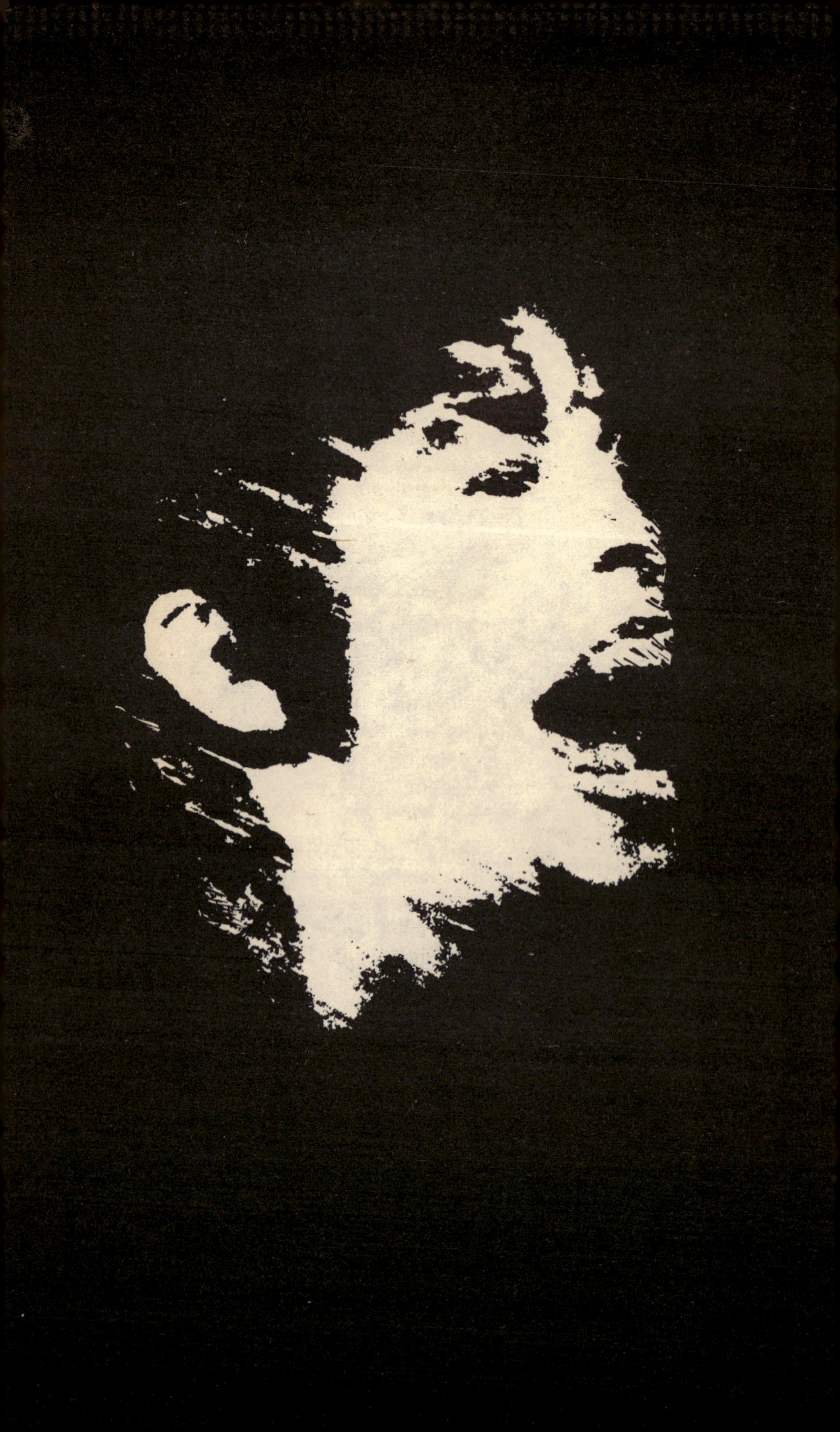

The *Video Screams* Screaming Head Rating System

Included also in this book for easy reference is a handy *Video Screams* Screaming Head rating system which shows you at a glance which films are the real screamers in the crowd (i.e., worth shouting about) and which are just plain mute. Here's how it works:

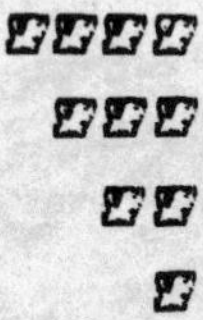

Excellent
Good
Fair
Poor

Of the 650-plus films listed here, I have seen roughly two-thirds. My rating of them is therefore based on first-hand knowledge and reflects my own personal judgment. Ratings for films I have not seen were arrived at by averaging the critical evaluations of them that have appeared in such diverse film journals as *Cinefantastique* and *Variety.* The reader is, of course, invited to disagree with all of us and form his or her own opinion.

I also admit to having taken a rather broad view of the genre in making my selection of films which do appear. For example, *Sherlock Holmes and the Secret Weapon* is not strictly speaking either a horror, science fiction or a fantasy film. And yet the character of Sherlock Holmes has become such a recognized figure of fantasy over the years that I feel any checklist of genre films would be incomplete without the inclusion of most if not all of Holmes' cinematic adventures. Thus the words in the book's subtitle referring to "related films."

Also, because *Video Screams* is devoted exclusively to cataloging only feature length genre films that are currently available on tape and disc, serials like *Zombies of the Stratosphere*, collections of old TV programs like *Space Patrol*, and cartoon compilations like *The Best of Tom and Jerry* are not included. An additional checklist of obscure titles about which little or nothing is known follows in Appendix I.

A directory of videocassette and disc manufacturers whose titles appear in the book plus information on how to contact them follows the A to Z checklist in Appendix II. The final Appendix consists of a cross-indexing of directors and their films.

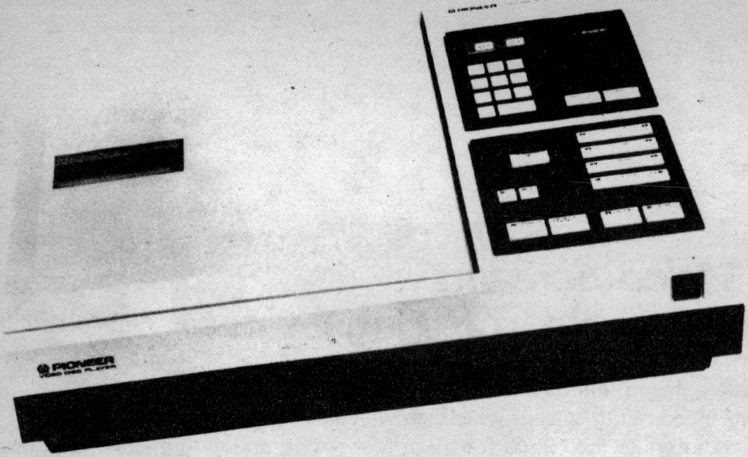

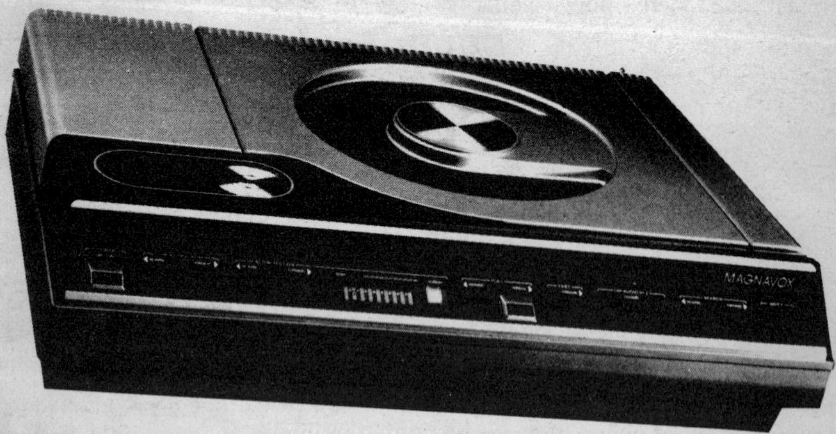

Rent vs. Buy

The biggest problem any video enthusiast faces in trying to build up his home collection of favorite movies is, of course, cost. After spending anywhere from $300 to $1,000 for your videodisc player or VCR, coming up with an extra $20 to $35 for each desired videodisc or $50 to $100 for the prerecorded videocassettes you want may be a bit prohibitive.

Video retailers have long recognized the fact that most people would rather rent than buy films, so most of them have established rental plans whereby you take home the films you'd like to see for a modest rental fee, return them after a brief period, then take out additional titles as you choose. The advantage of renting is, of course, that it allows you to screen many different films for the price of purchasing just one of them. The disadvantage is that you can't keep them.

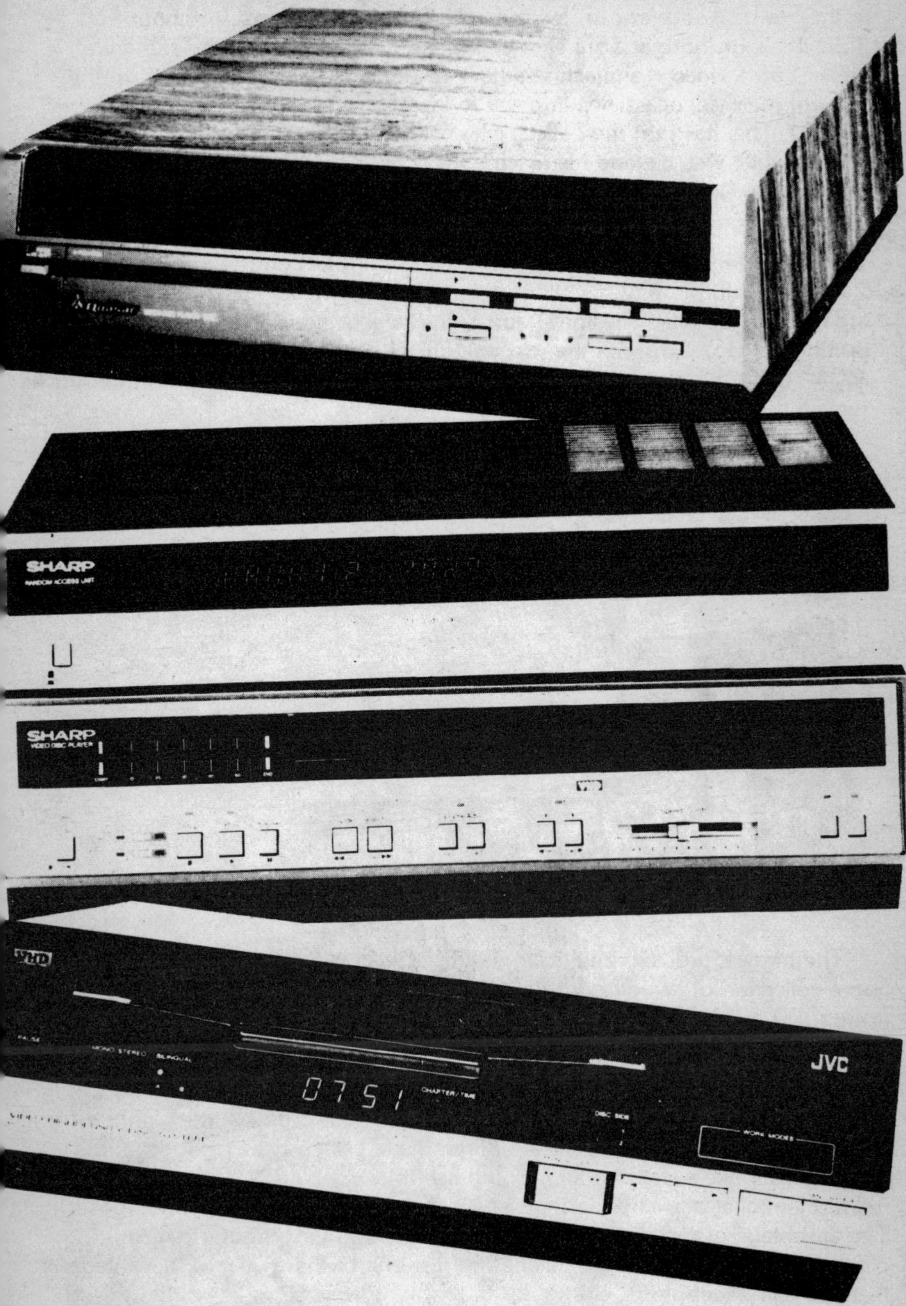
SHARP
RANDOM ACCESS UNIT
SHARP
VIDEO DISC PLAYER
VHD
MONO STEREO
BILINGUAL
0751
CHAPTER/TIME
JVC
DISC SIDE
WORK MODES

Many of the big name video manufacturers have objected to the practice of renting because it tends to put more profits in the pockets of retailers than in their own. A retailer can, for example, buy a tape at cost for about $60, rent it 30 times or more at $5 a shot and make back its cost several hundred times. Some video manufacturers have responded to this by jacking up the price of their videocassettes in order to increase their profit margins with retailers. This has hurt the collector by placing the cost of the average videocassette well beyond his reach. Discs, on the other hand, have remained relatively low in price due to the fact that most retailers prefer to sell rather than rent them.

A number of video manufacturers like MGM/UA and Warner Home Video flirted for time with setting up cumbersome rental plans of their own, but the experiment failed abysmally due to the reluctance of video retailers and distributors to put up with the vast amount of paperwork involved. And so MGM/UA and Warner have gone back to selling their product, but their prices remain very high.

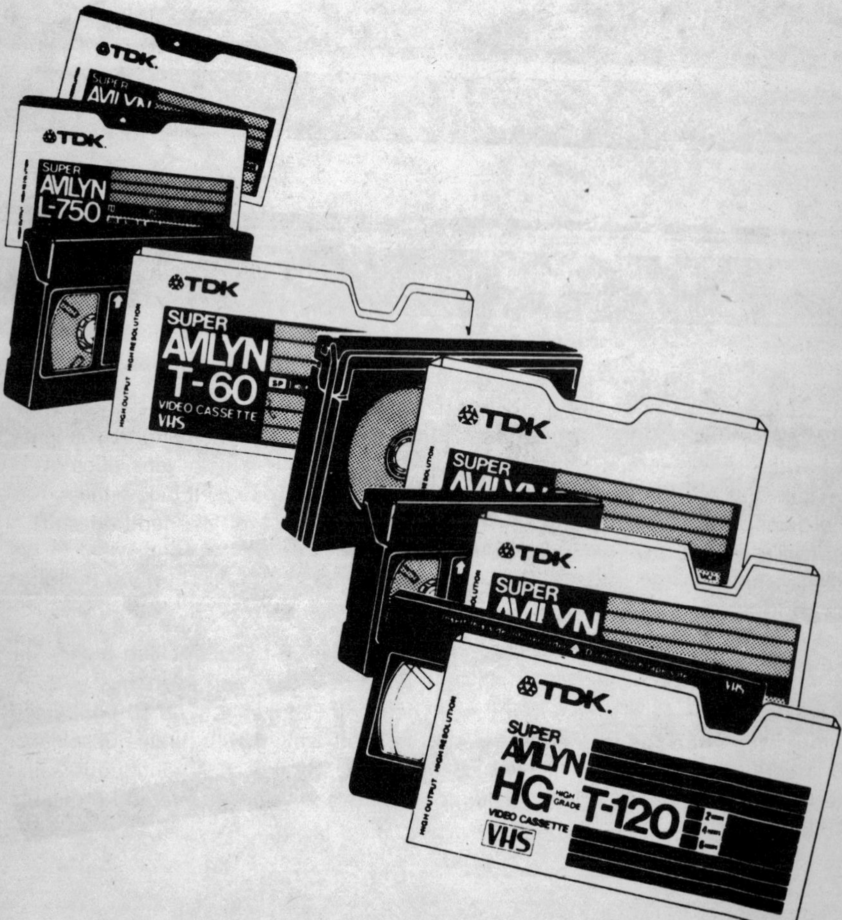

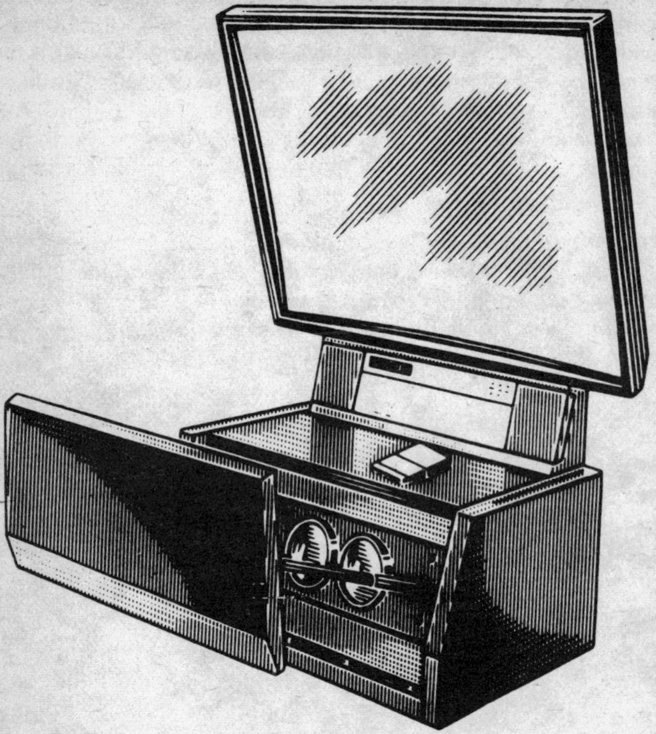

The chief result of all this price and rental warfare has been the creation of a very profitable market for videotape piracy. The video pirate can shoot a film right off a movie screen with a home video camera, then make tape dubs of the film and sell them to enthusiastic collectors for a price well below that charged by the legitimate manufacturer. The quality of a pirated tape doesn't approach that of a professionally duped pre-recorded tape, of course, but to the collector this disadvantage is far outweighed by his being able to get a desired title at a more affordable price.

Piracy is a totally illegal activity and if the pirate is caught selling his ill-gotten material, he faces stiff penalties in the form of fines or even imprisonment. But let's face it, the FBI can't be everywhere. And so until video manufacturers decide to render the advantage of dealing with pirates obsolete by lowering the price of their own videocassettes, pirates shall continue to sail the high seas of home video providing customers with a valuable and profitable service.

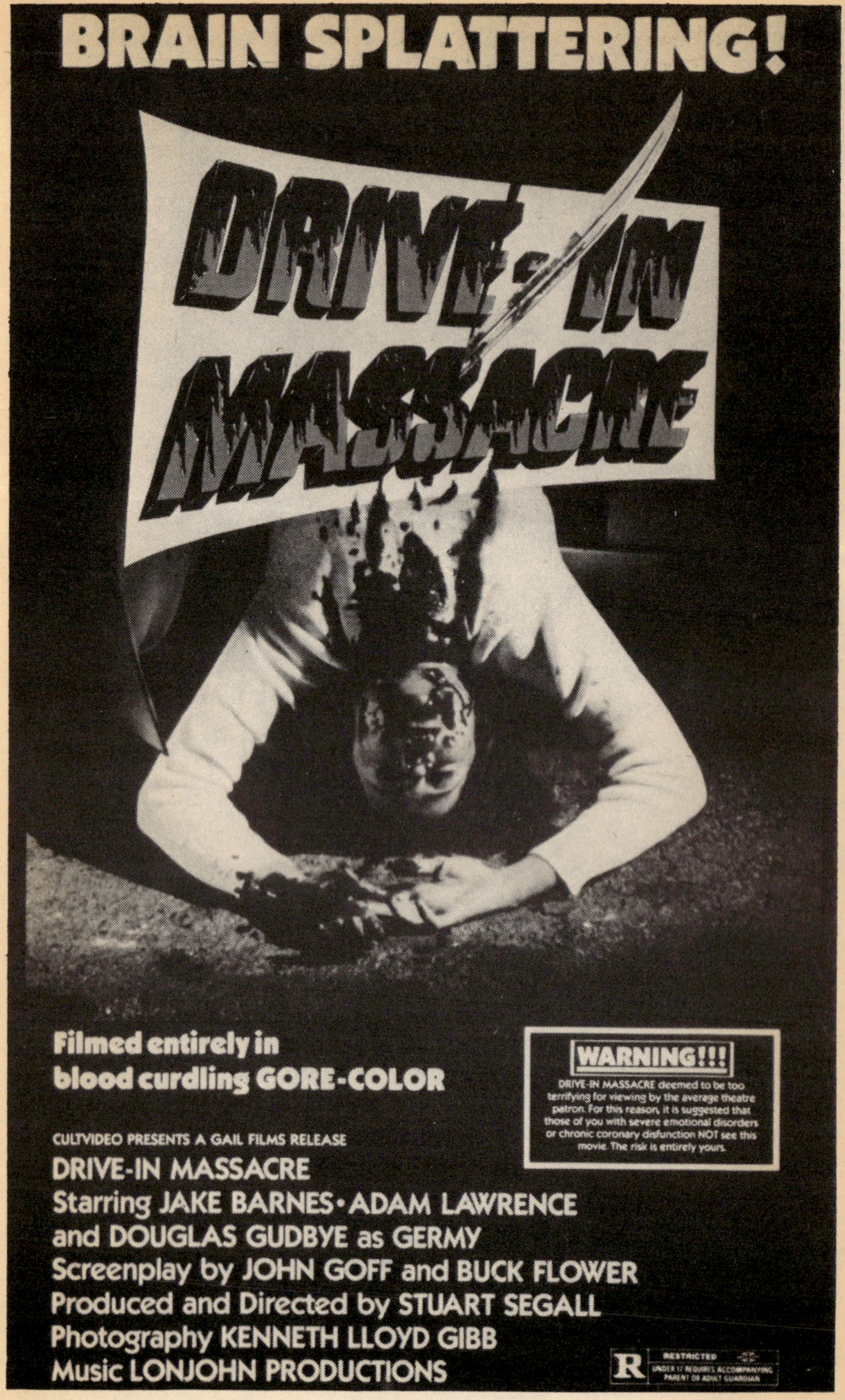

Drive-In Massacre (1976)

In a bold move to diminish piracy and reclaim the frustrated buyer's market for pre-recorded videocassettes, Paramount Home Video announced the release of its blockbuster film *Star Trek II: The Wrath of Khan* in August '82 at the attractive price of $39.95. Within two months of the announcement, orders for over 70,000 copies of the film had been placed by retailers and consumers around the country. About the same time, MCA Videocassette inaugurated its own "Reel Deal" by reducing the price of a number of its older cassettes from around $60 to $39.95. It's way too soon to tell whether this indicates a coming trend throughout the industry. But the fact does remain that the prices of many pre-recorded videocassettes (and discs) are coming down. Slowly. And so the prospect of building that cherished home library of your favorite video screams on high quality pre-recorded videocassettes and discs without having to sell the wife and kiddies to do so currently appears to be quite optimistic. Time alone will tell.

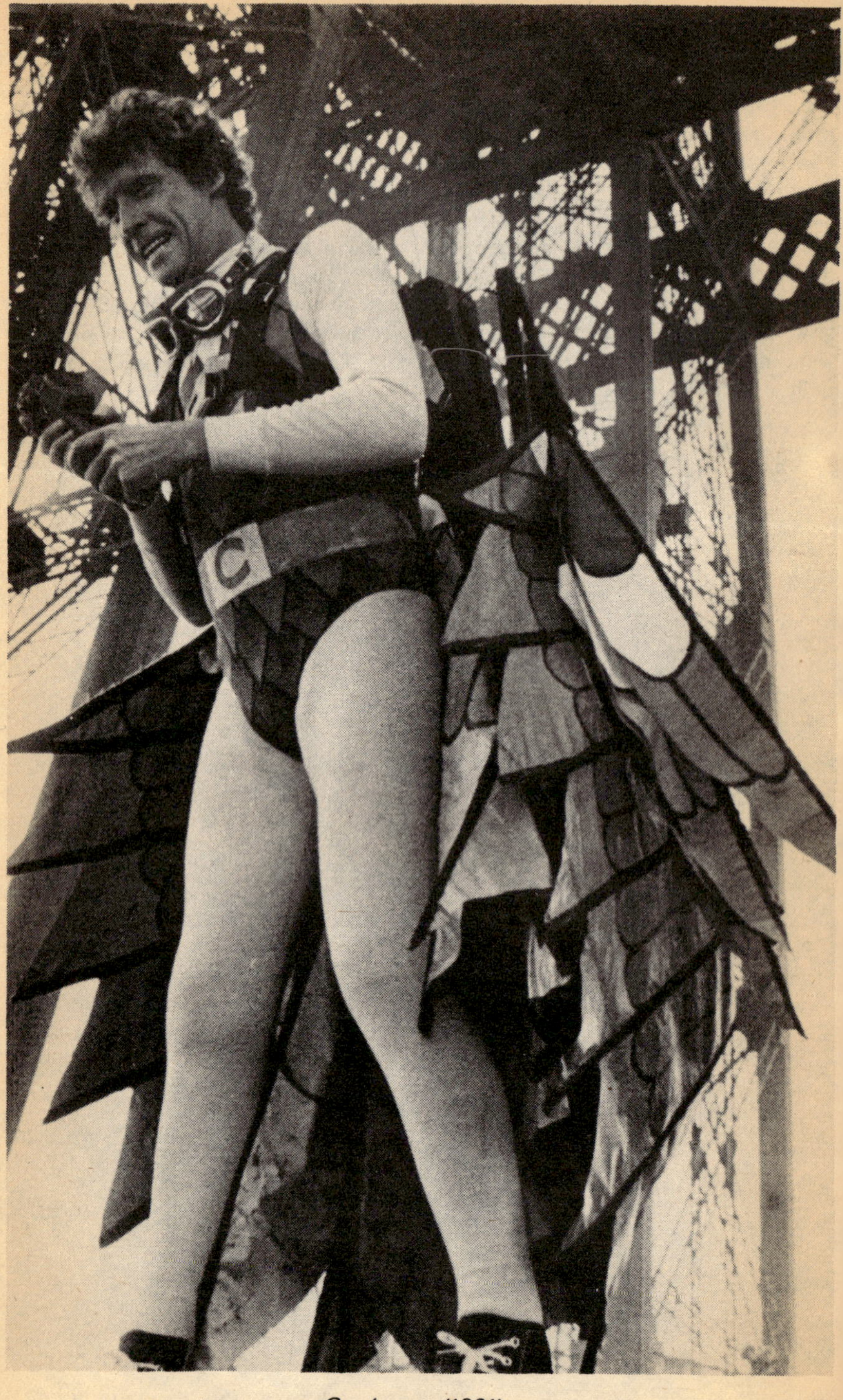

Condorman (1981)

Mail Order and Video Swapping

One way of coping with the current high cost of most pre-recorded videocassettes is to shop around for the best price you can get. Many mail order houses sell videocassettes at prices well below their suggested retail cost plus a small shipping fee. Almost all of them offer catalogues absolutely bulging with titles from every major manufacturer. Many of these titles—including a lot that appear in this book—you will rarely see on the shelves of your local video retailer (unless you live in a big city like New York) because he simply can't afford to stock every available tape to suit every customer's individual taste.

Mail order houses don't usually stock a large inventory of pre-recorded tapes either, but because they buy from their distributors in bulk, they can generally offer customers better deals as well as fill special orders for hard-to-find titles a lot faster.

Some mail order houses will send you their catalogue for free on request. Others charge a small fee of $1 or $2 which is then refunded upon receipt of your first order. Unless an item must be back-ordered from the distributor, delivery (via UPS) is prompt and hassle-free. Reputable mail order films also guarantee their merchandise. If any tape or disc you receive from them is defective in any way, they'll replace it or offer you a full refund or a credit on your next purchase, whichever you wish.

If you do decide to go the movies-by-mail route, there are a lot of good mail order houses to choose from. Four of the biggest who offer a large selection of titles on both tape and disc at good prices coupled with top-notch service are:

Blackhawk
Box 3990
Davenport, Iowa 52808
1-319-323-9736

Movies Unlimited
6736 Castor Avenue
Philadelphia, Pennsylvania 19149
1-215-722-8298

Red Fox Enterprises
Route 209, East
Elizabethville, Pennsylvania 17023
1-717-362-3391
1-800-233-7514

The Video Connection
3240 Sylvania Avenue
Toledo, Ohio 43613
1-419-472-7727

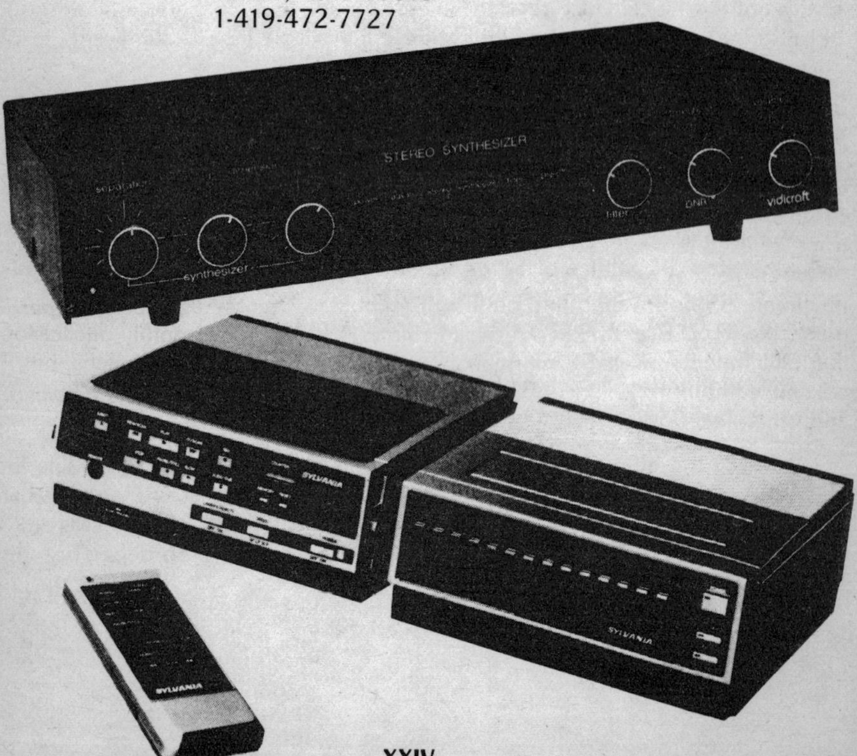

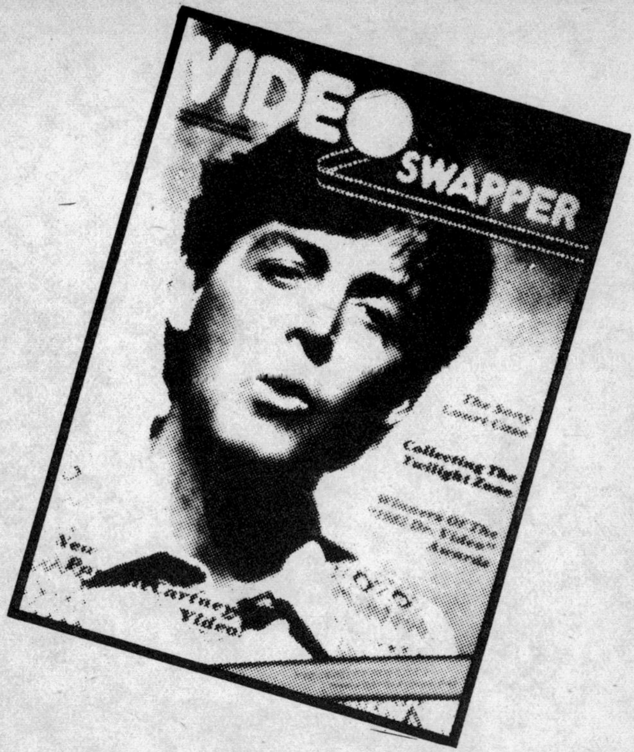

Video swapping is another viable alternative open to the cost conscious home video enthusiast. Video exchange clubs are currently sprouting up in various cities around the country that allow you to swap tapes you no longer want for used tapes you'd prefer to have with other club members. Membership fees vary from club to club as do the ways in which each club functions. A good way to find out about them is to check out *Video Swapper* magazine (P.O. Box 309-V, Fraser, Michigan 48026), a bi-monthly publication that offers plenty of useful information not only on video exchange clubs, but on new equipment advances, industry trends, the latest releases in home video and other items of interest.

If you're not interested in belonging to a club, but would like to be able to offer your used tapes up for sale or trade to other collectors as well as see what other collectors have that you might be interested in, *Video Swapper* sells ad space to its readers at inexpensive rates for just this purpose. So does *The Video Gazette* (P.O. Box 541, Gilmer, TX 75644).

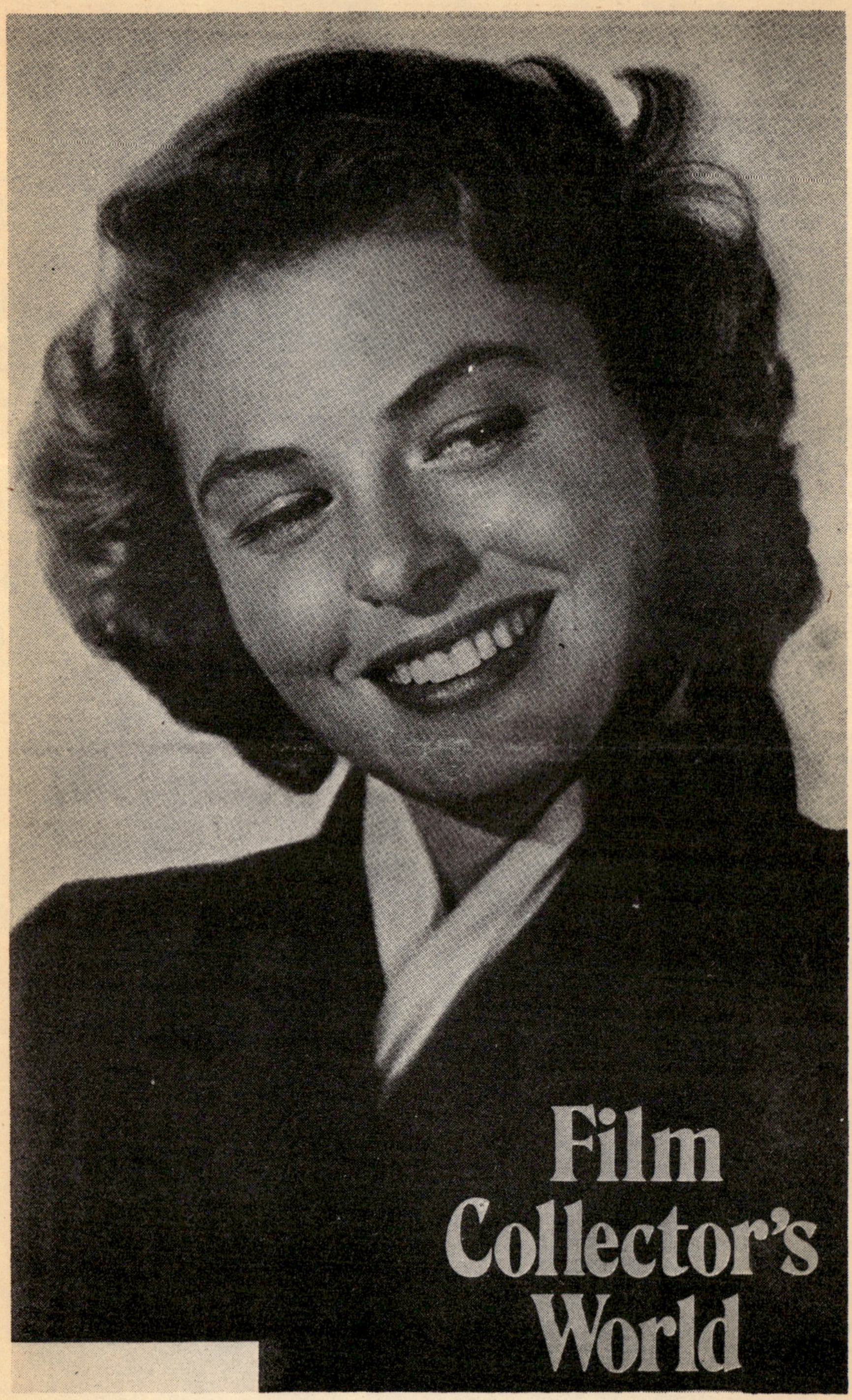
Film
Collector's
World

Oriented more towards the collector of motion pictures on film rather than tape, but possessing a certain amount of intriguing video collectors' ads sprinkled throughout their pages as well, are two other monthly tabloid-size publications that are also worth looking into for video swapping and/or bargain spotting purposes:

> *Film Collector's World*
> P.O. Box 248
> Rapids City, Illinois 61278
>
> *The Big Reel*
> Drawer B
> Summerfield, North Carolina 27358

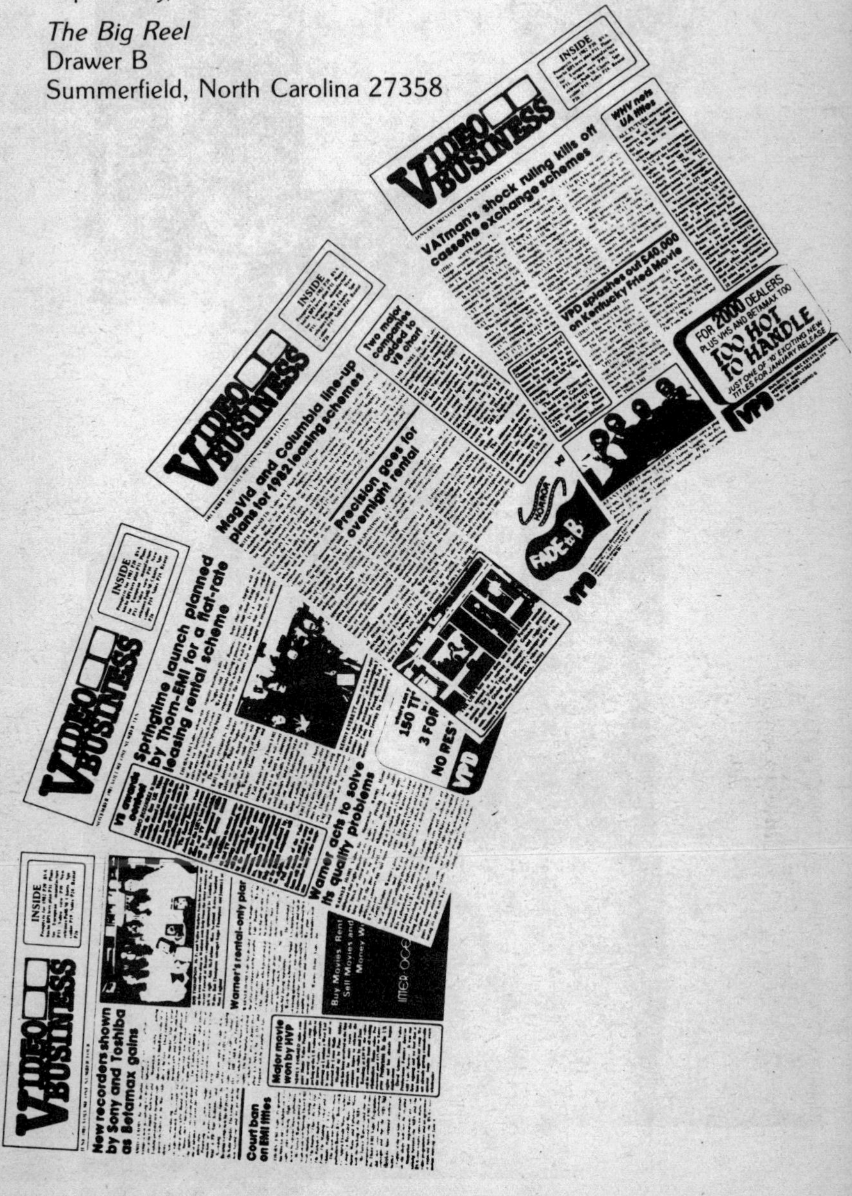

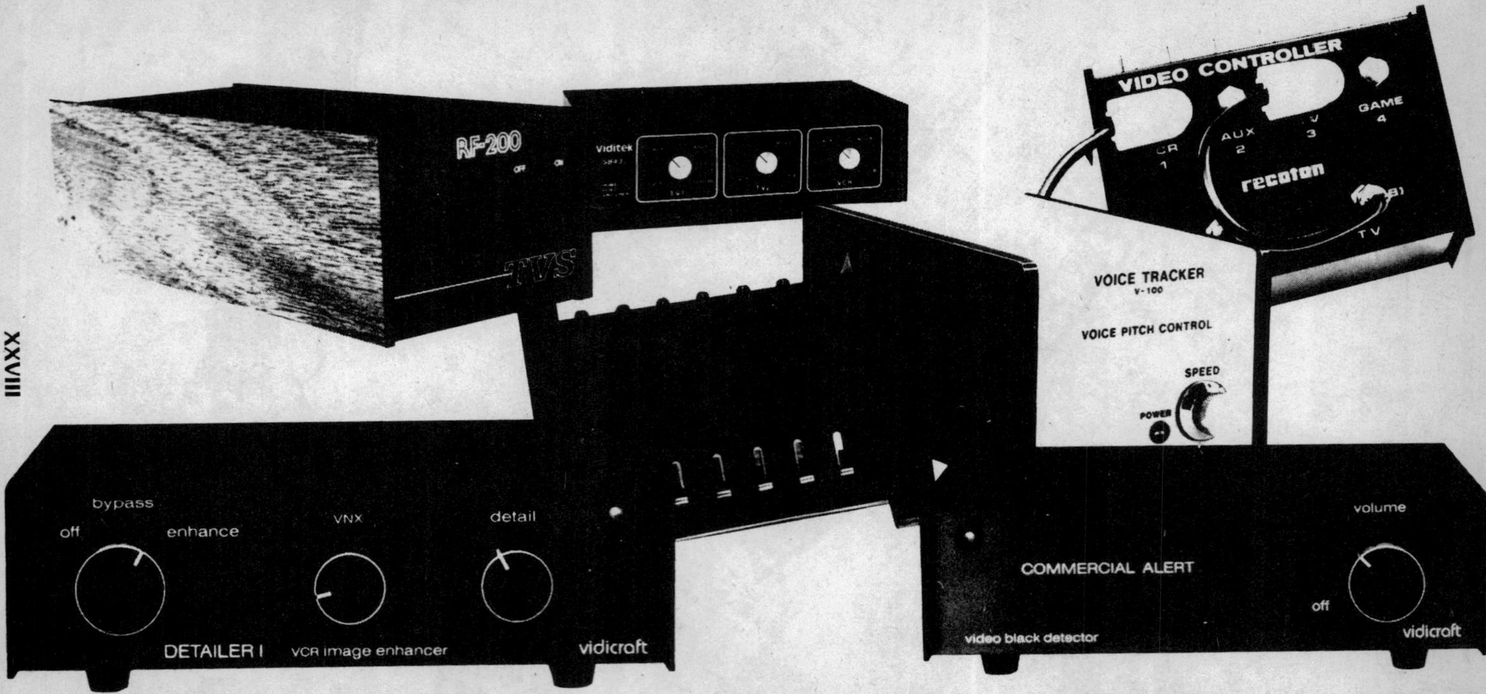
RF-200
OFF
ON
TVS
Viditek
VIDEO CONTROLLER
CR
1
AUX
2
V
3
GAME
4
recoton
TV
VOICE TRACKER
V-100
VOICE PITCH CONTROL
SPEED
POWER
off
bypass
enhance
VNX
detail
DETAILER I
VCR image enhancer
vidicraft
COMMERCIAL ALERT
volume
off
video black detector
vidicraft

Both pubs are chock full of ads from private collectors with many rare and desirable films for sale or trade. Ads are inexpensive and tend to get results. The only real shortcoming of both these publications is that most of the ads you see in them are for 16mm, Super 8 and Standard 8mm films and film memorabilia rather than tapes and discs. *The Big Reel* is particularly heavy in its emphasis on film over tape and disc. But I'm sure this situation will change as more collectors of films on film start going video. In the meantime, both *Film Collector's World* and *The Big Reel* are well worth subscribing to for the occasional video bargains which do show up in their pages as well as for the abundance of video mail order ads and news of upcoming releases on tape and disc which regularly appear in each issue.

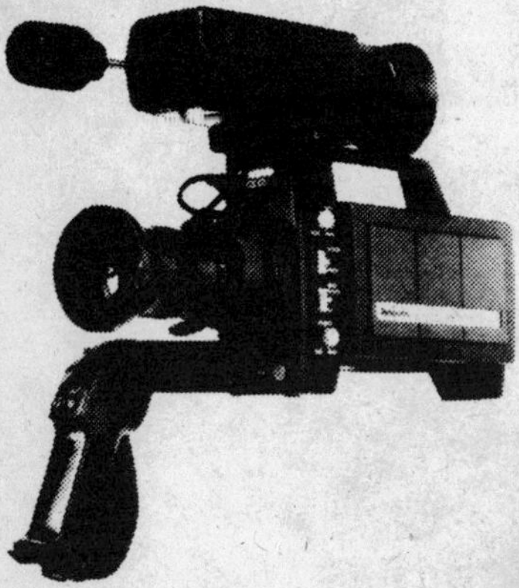

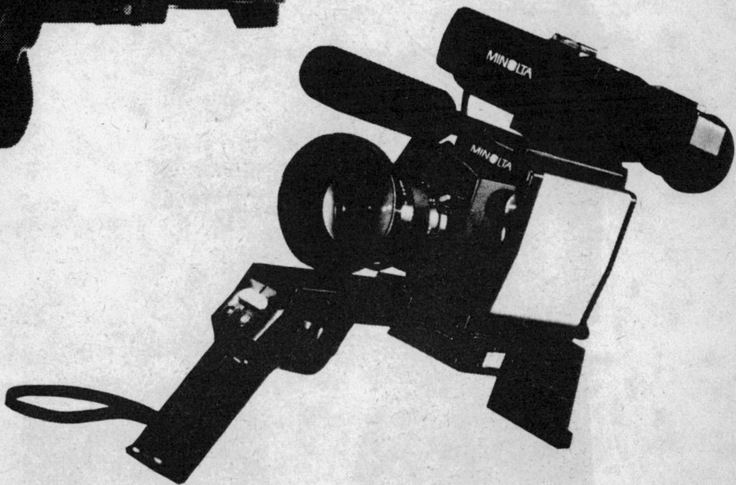

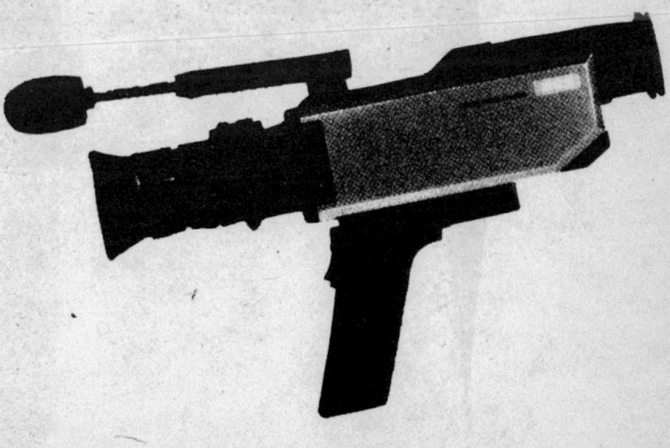

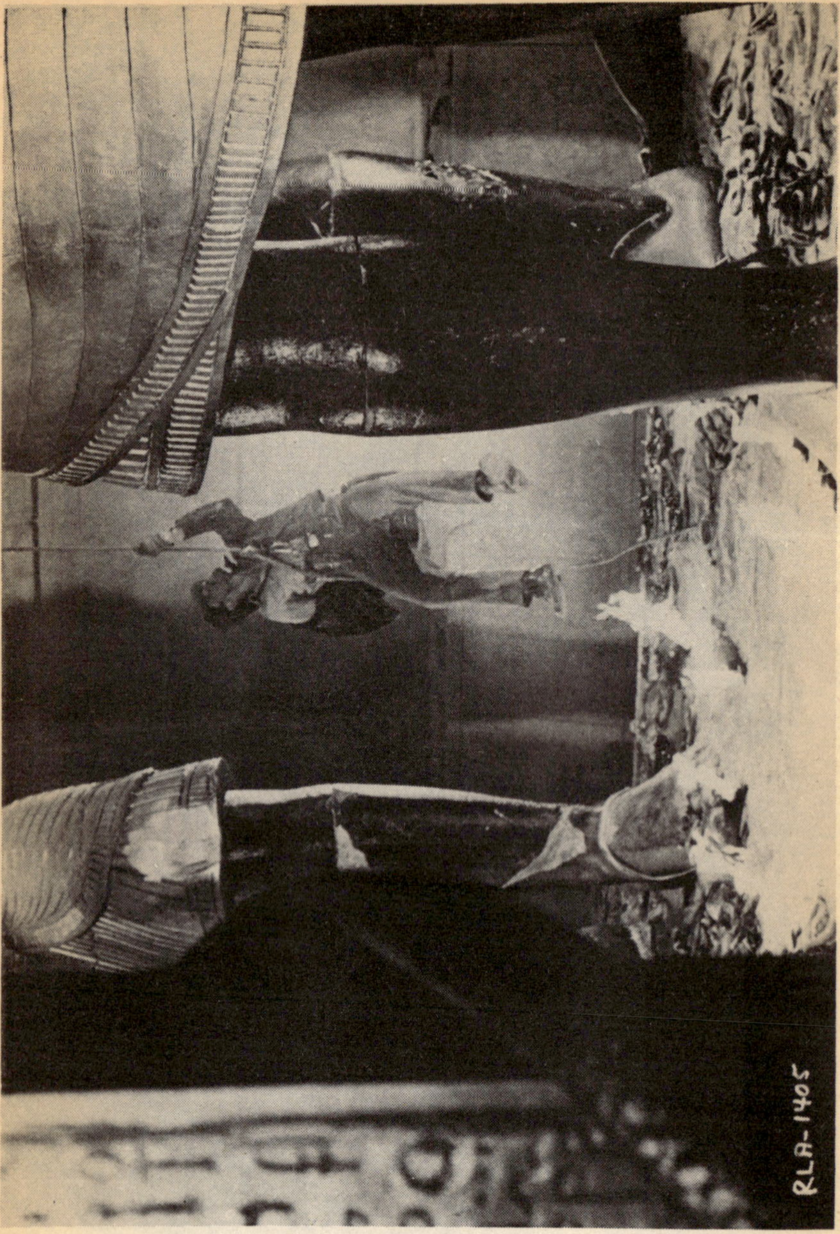

The Great Movie Stunts/The Making of Raiders of the Lost Ark (1981)

New Releases

Home video is such a rapidly growing industry that the 40-plus tape and disc manufacturers listed in Appendix II of this book are issuing new titles all the time. In fact, releases of brand new films like John Carpenter's *The Thing*, for example, are occurring an average of 90 days after their first-run theatrical debuts.

Unless you are on these manufacturers' mailing lists, you can't possibly keep tabs on everything that is being or has been released each month. And even mailings can't keep you informed sufficiently because they are frequently in need of updating the moment you receive them. You can always ask your local video store for help, of course, but retailers are likely to be just as at sea as you are in that they are usually so swamped with printed material from manufacturers and distributors each day about everything that's going on in the field of home video that they can't possibly hope to answer all your questions.

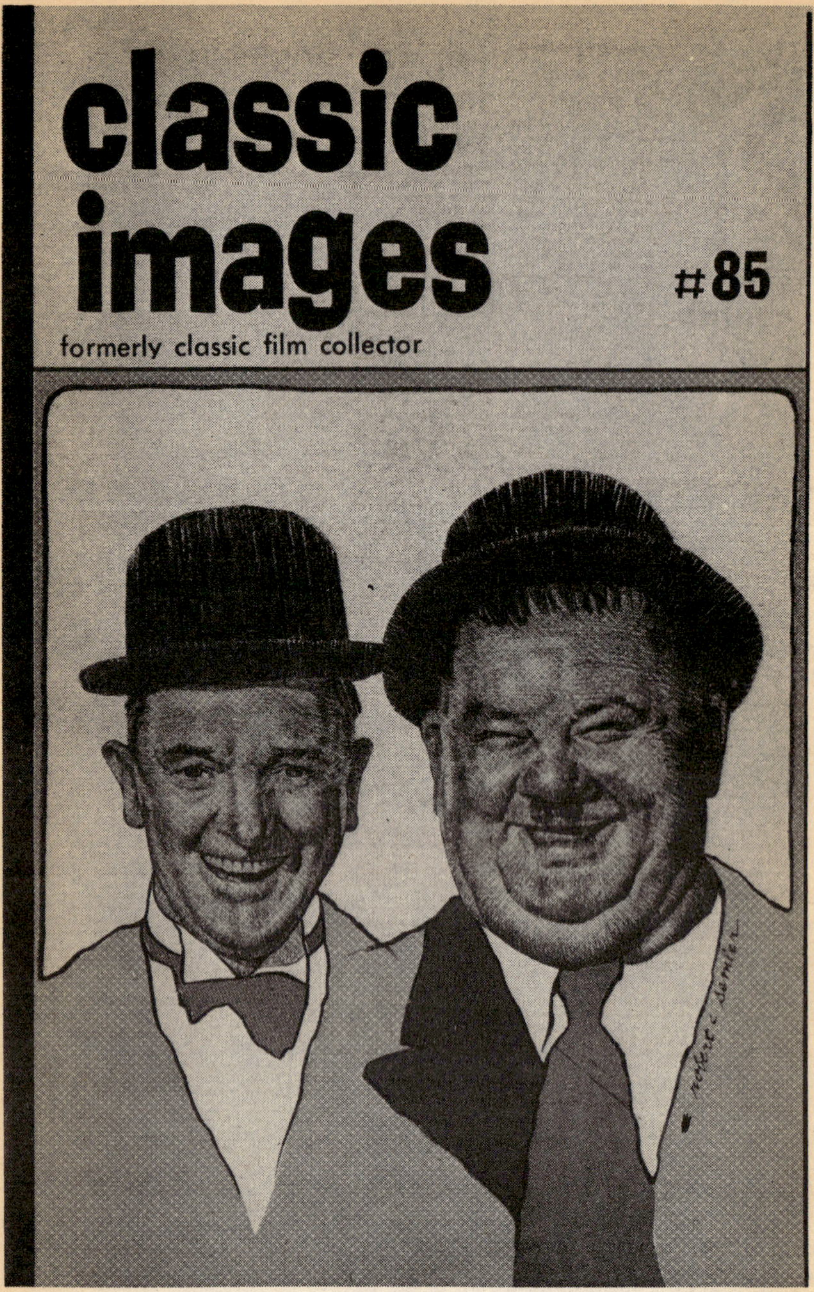
classic images
#85
formerly classic film collector

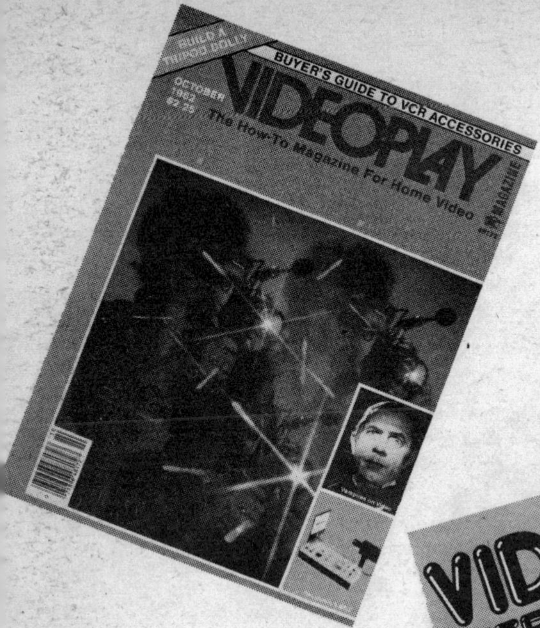

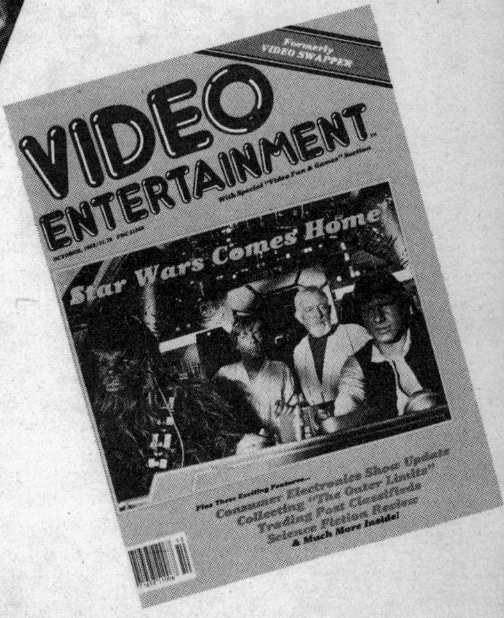

One of the best, though by no means complete, sources of current information on the latest video releases are the so-called video specialty magazines. Many of them provide reviews of the latest films in release on tape and disc plus a wealth of other information and product reviews on new equipment and accessories. Most of them are published monthly—they have to be just to keep reasonably up-to-date—and cost between $1.50 and $2 at your local newsstand. If you're interested in subscribing, however, here are the addresses:

Classic Images
P.O Box 809
Muscatine, Iowa 52761

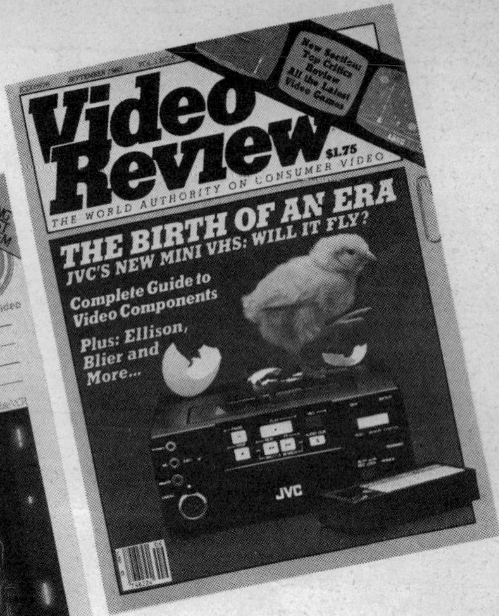

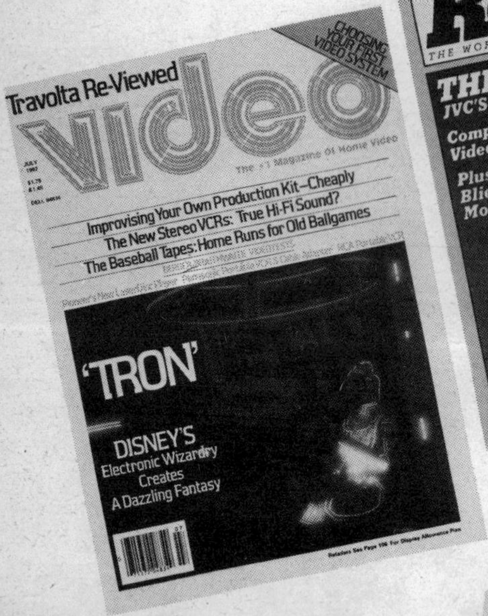

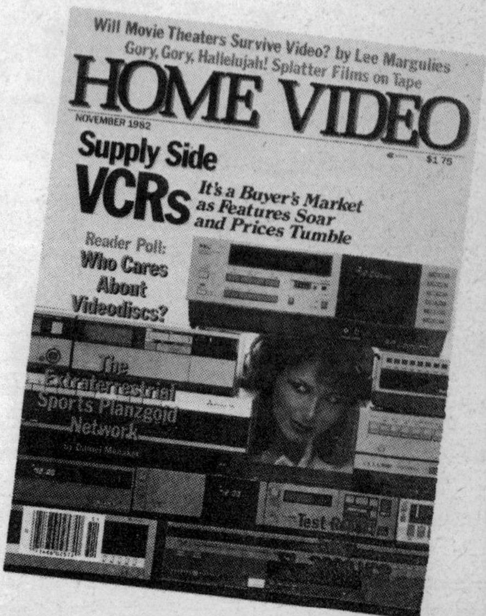

Home Video
P.O. Box 2651
Boulder, Colorado 80321

Video Action
21 West Elm Street
Chicago, Illinois 60610

Video Magazine
P.O. Box 1118
Dover, New Jersey 07801

Video Review
P.O. Box 919
Farmingdale, New York 1173

Videoplay
51 Sugar Hollow Road
Danbury, Connecticut 06810

In this and subsequent editions of *Video Screams*, of course, I will attempt to bring you the most comprehensive information available on *all* the horror, science fiction and fantasy films in release, as well as where to find them.

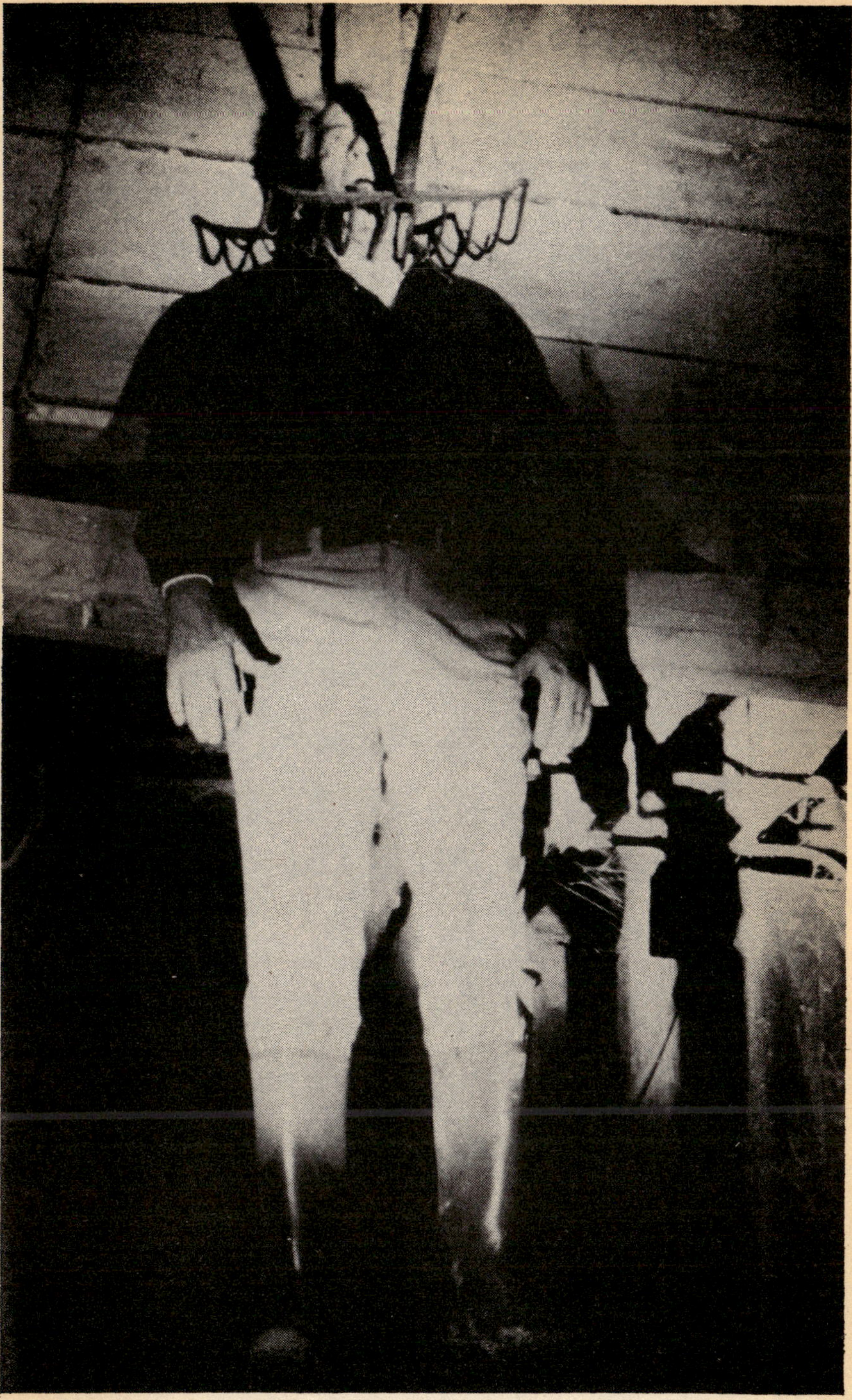

The Boogey Man (1980)

The Care and Feeding of Your Video Screams

To make sure you continue to get the best performance possible out of your VCR or videodisc player, carefully follow the maintenance instructions that come along with it. As for the discs themselves, LaserDiscs are fairly indestructible because they are vinyl coated. Laser machines do not use a stylus, so groove wear is avoided. CED discs come carefully protected in plastic cases that can only be removed by inserting the disc into the disc player. Your "greasy" fingers, therefore, never come into contact with the disc itself. As with regular stereo LPs, however, you should avoid placing your Laser of CED discs on or near any source of excessive heat. Otherwise melt-down will occur. Discs should also be stored upright when not in use.

Pre-recorded tapes on the other hand are a bit trickier to take care of. For one thing, you should always avoid playing them immediately after receiving them in the mail or bringing them home from the video store if it's cold outside as moisture may condense on the tape if the cassette is brought into a warm room from the cold outdoors. The tape may be damaged when used in a moistened condition, so before using it, wait until the cassette has warmed up to room temperature and moisture condensation has been eliminated.

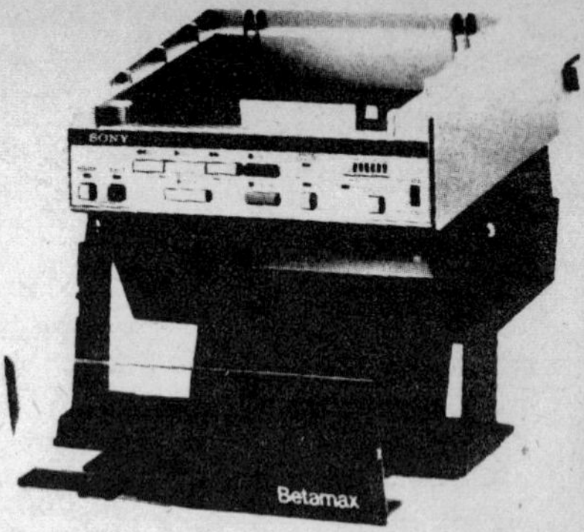
SONY
Betamax

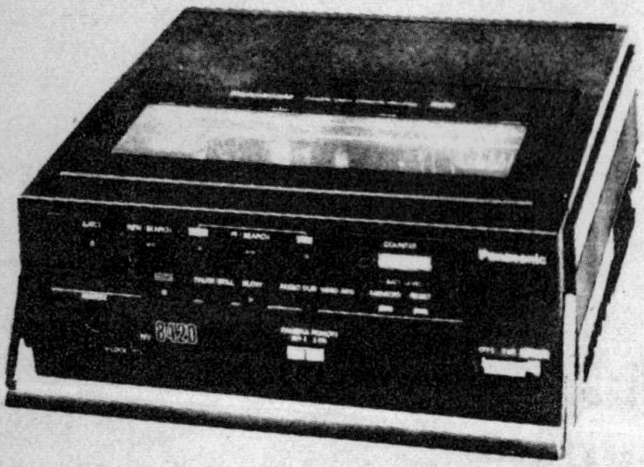
Panasonic

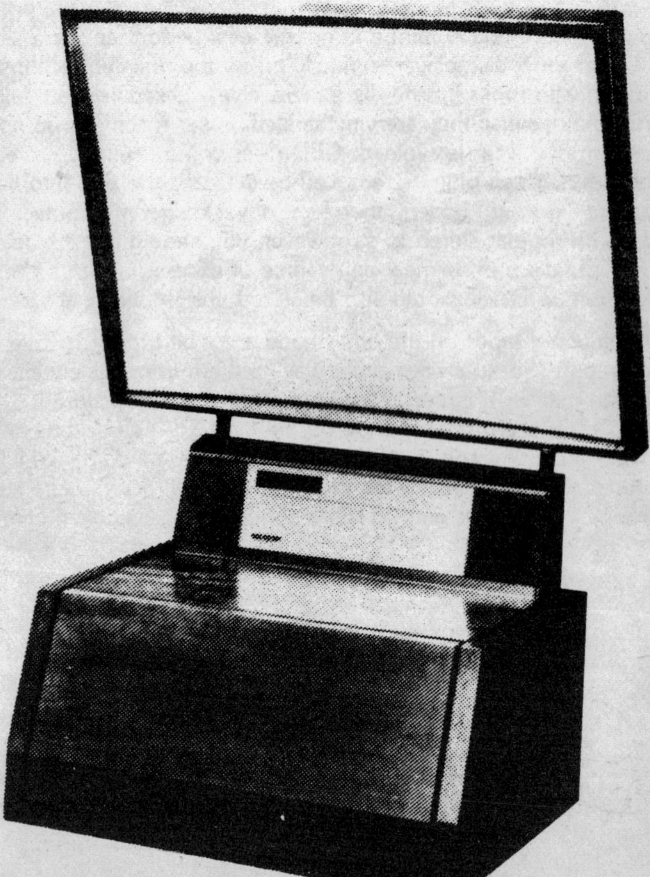

The tape may also be damaged if stored in an irregularly wound condition. Always rewind the tape completely and evenly after use, then insert it into its storage case or sleeve and keep the cassette standing upright when not in use. Also, avoid storing your video screams in any of the following places:

1. Where they will be exposed to high temperature.
2. Where they will be exposed to direct sunlight or any adjacent heating equipment. Especially do not place your videocassettes inside the dashboard of your car or over the rear window shelf.
3. In the vicinity of a strong magnetic field such as near a motor, transformer, or magnet.
4. Under high humidity.
5. Where they will be exposed to dust or dirt.

When your video recorder's head is soiled, noise or streaks may appear on your TV screen during playback. To remove the oxide or dirt build-up, use a convenient video head cleaning cassette. Allsop, Maxell and other manufacturers make them for both VHS and Beta VCRs; you can pick them up at your local video store.

And now on to the films themselves. Good luck in finding that special video scream you've been looking for. And happy viewing forever after.

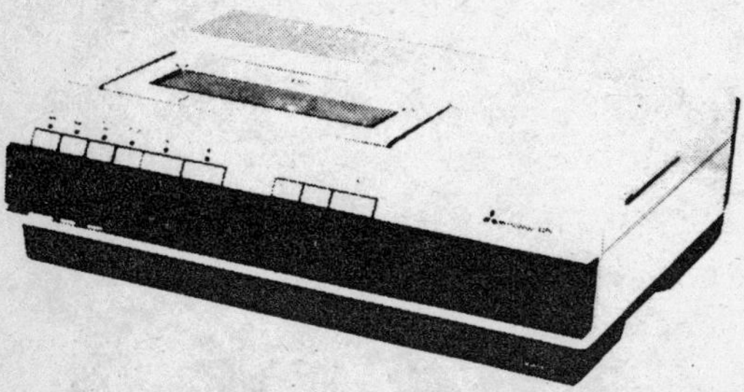

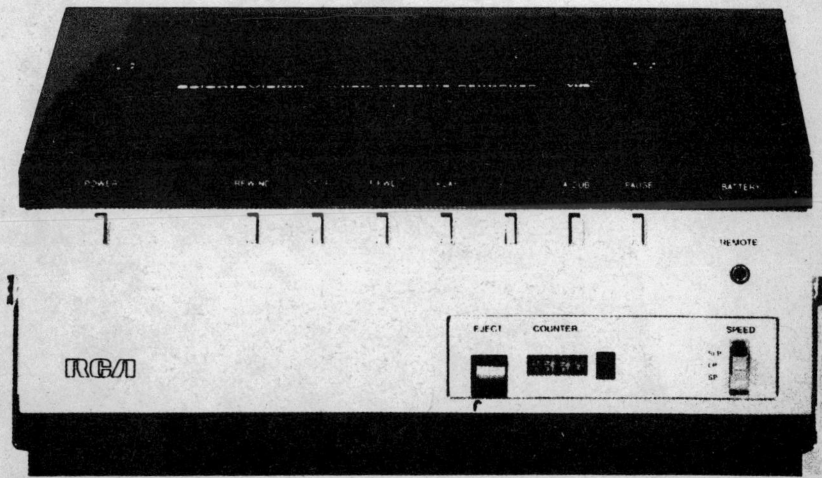

VIDEO SCREAMS™

A to Z

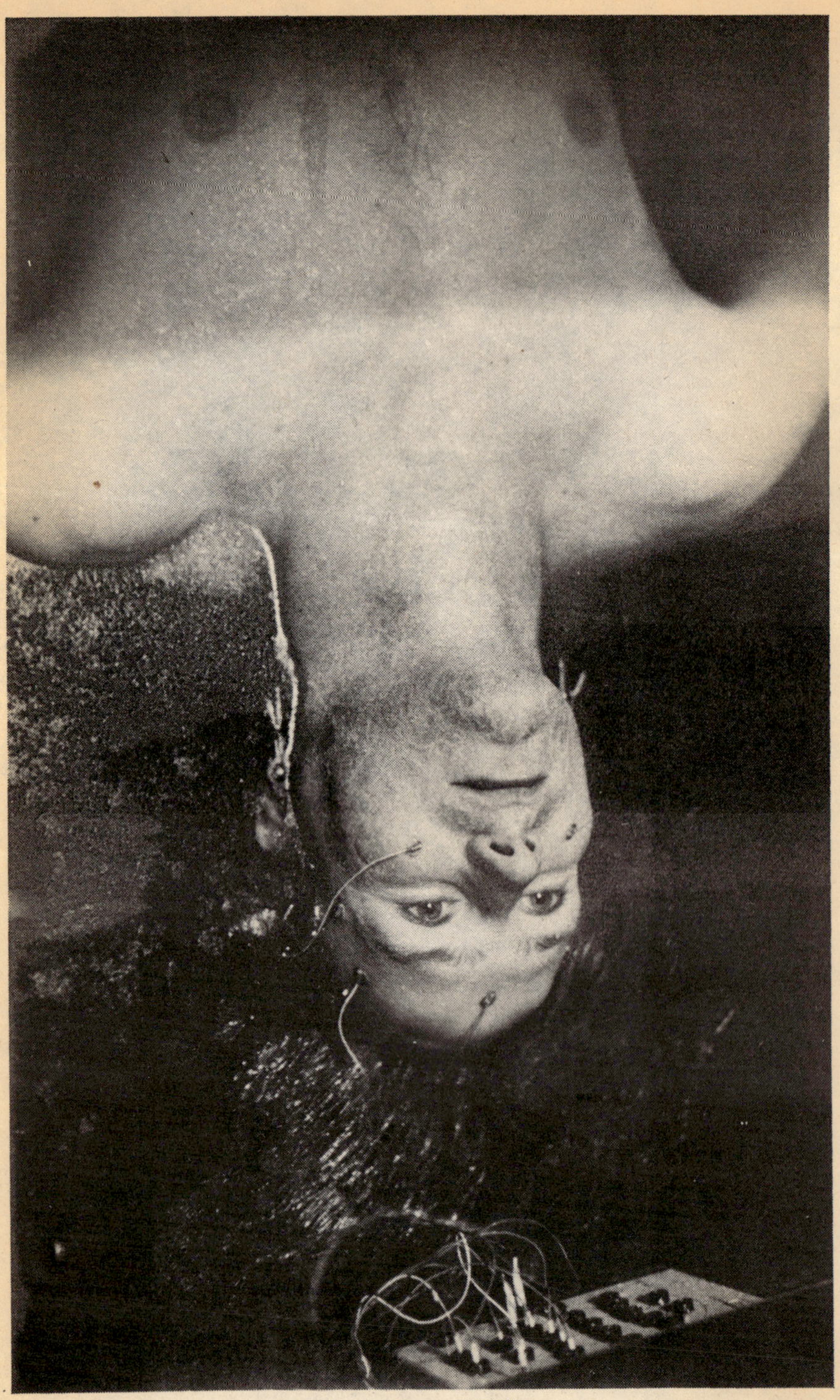

Altered States (1980)

2

Abbott & Costello Meet Frankenstein

(1948) B&W, 90 min. Director: Charles Barton.

Bud Abbott, Lou Costello, Bela Lugosi, Lon Chaney, Jr., Glenn Strange, Lenore Aubert, Jane Randolph, Frank Ferguson, Vincent Price. The film that sealed the doom of Universal's famed horror stock company by turning them into comic characters. A&C don't exactly meet Frankenstein, but they do meet his creature, as well as the Wolf Man, Dracula and even the Invisible Man (well, his voice anyway). Sophomoric parody of horror films, but very, very funny. A&C's best.

(MCA Videocassette) VC

Absent-Minded Professor, The ½

(1961) B&W, 97 min. Director: Robert Stevenson.

Fred MacMurray, Nancy Olson, Tommy Kirk, Keenan Wynn. MacMurray discovers an amazing anti-gravity concoction which he proceeds to call "flubber" (flying rubber), using it to make his Model-T fly. Wynn is the bad guy out to steal the formula. Vintage Disney, with nice special effects.

(Walt Disney Home Video, RCA VideoDisc) VC, CED

Adventure of Sherlock Holmes' Smarter Brother, The ½

(1975) Color, 91 min. Director: Gene Wilder.

Gene Wilder, Marty Feldman, Madeline Kahn, Dom DeLuise. Tripling as writer, director and star, Wilder tries to pass himself off as Mel Brooks' smarter brother by stealing most of Brooks' stock company as well as much of his bathroom humor to tell this lame story of Sherlock's younger brother, Sigerson (Wilder), and his involvement with a mysterious musical hall artiste (Kahn). Some nice atmosphere, but totally sophomoric.

(CBS/Fox Video) VC

Adventures of Robin Hood, The ½

(1938) Color, 106 min. Directors: Michael Curtiz, William Keighley.

Errol Flynn, Olivia de Havilland, Basil Rathbone, Claude Rains. Spectacular Warner Brothers treatment of this classic Howard Pyle tale, with a great score by Erich Wolfgang Korngold and a rousing swordfight between Flynn and Rathbone.

(CBS/Fox Video, RCA VideoDisc) VC, LV, CED

Adventures of Sherlock Holmes, The

(1939) B&W, 85 min. Director: Alfred Werker.

Basil Rathbone, Nigel Bruce, Ida Lupino, George Zucco. The redoubtable master sleuth of Baker Street takes on his arch nemesis, Professor Moriarty, who is out to steal the crown jewels, in this first entry in the long running Rathbone/Bruce series, and one of the few to be done in period.

(MGM/UA Home Video) VC

Albino

(1979) Color, 85 min. Director: Jurgen Goslar.
Christopher Lee, James Faulkner, Trevor Howard, Sybil Danning. A police officer in charge of a district in Africa confronts a gang of black terrorists that is trying to drive the white settlers out. The gang's ringleader is a knife-wielding albino. Standard action-exploitation melodrama with political overtones. The locale of the story lends the film some interest.
(Media Home Entertainment) VC

Alice in Wonderland ½

(1951) Color, 75 min. Directors: Clyde Geronimi, Hamilton Luske, Wilfred Jackson.
Voices of Ed Wynn, Jerry Colonna, Sterling Holloway, Kathryn Beaumont. Classic Walt Disney animated feature based on the stories of Lewis Carroll. Though never as popular or highly touted as Disney's *Snow White, Bambi, Fantasia,* etc., it's really just as good and just as superlatively animated. It's also quite funny.
(Walt Disney Home Video) VC

Alice, Sweet Alice ½

(1977) Color, 108 min. Director: Alfred Sole.
Paula Sheppard, Linda Miller, Mildred Clinton, Brooke Shields, Lillian Roth, Alphonso DeNoble. Shields (who was around 10 when she debuted in this film) is murdered by her evil sister, who then proceeds to knife a disgustingly obese tenant in her apartment building as well as anyone else who attempts to tie her into the original killing. Turns out to be a ruse, however, and sis isn't really the bad seed she appears to be. Confusing thriller that strives for seriousness by setting the action within a religious milieu. Sole may be a director to watch, but not on the basis of this film. A.k.a. *Holy Terror.*
(Discount Video, King of Video) VC

Alien

(1979) Color, 124 min. Director: Ridley Scott.
Sigourney Weaver, Tom Skerritt, John Hurt. Scott and his scriptwriters lifted the wildest elements from a whole range of B-movies, from *It, the Terror From Beyond Space* to *They Came from Within,* to tell this story of a malevolent creature that is brought on board a space age garbage scow, the *Nostromo,* upon which it immediately starts slaughtering off the crew. Atmospheric and genuinely shocking, with a fine score by Jerry Goldsmith and a nice performance by Weaver as the put-upon but resourceful heroine.
(CBS/Fox Video) VC, LV

Alien Contamination ½

(1980) Color, 89 min. Director: Luigi Cozzi.
Alien eggs are brought back to earth by a team of astronauts, the eggs hatch and the gore begins. Uninspired, Italian-made rip-off of *Alien.*
(Paragon Video) VC

Aliens from Spaceship Earth ½

(1977) Color, 107 min. Director: (?)
Donovan, Lynda Day George. Low budget documentary which poses the question: are strange, cosmic forces invading our universe? Doesn't answer it, just poses it. And uses dramatized scenes to recreate supposedly recorded incidents of visitations from alien beings to confuse things all the more.
(Video Gems) VC

Alphaville ½

(1965) B&W, 100 min. Director: Jean-Luc Godard.
Eddie Constantine, Anna Karina, Akim Tamiroff. Photographer Raoul Coutard's striking shots of a futuristic city that is actually Paris save this early example of Godardian pretentiousness from being a total bore. The plot is about a Bogart-like private eye named Lemmie Caution (Constantine) who battles robots and a giant electronic brain to rescue an important scientist. Unexciting is the word.
(Vintage Video) VC

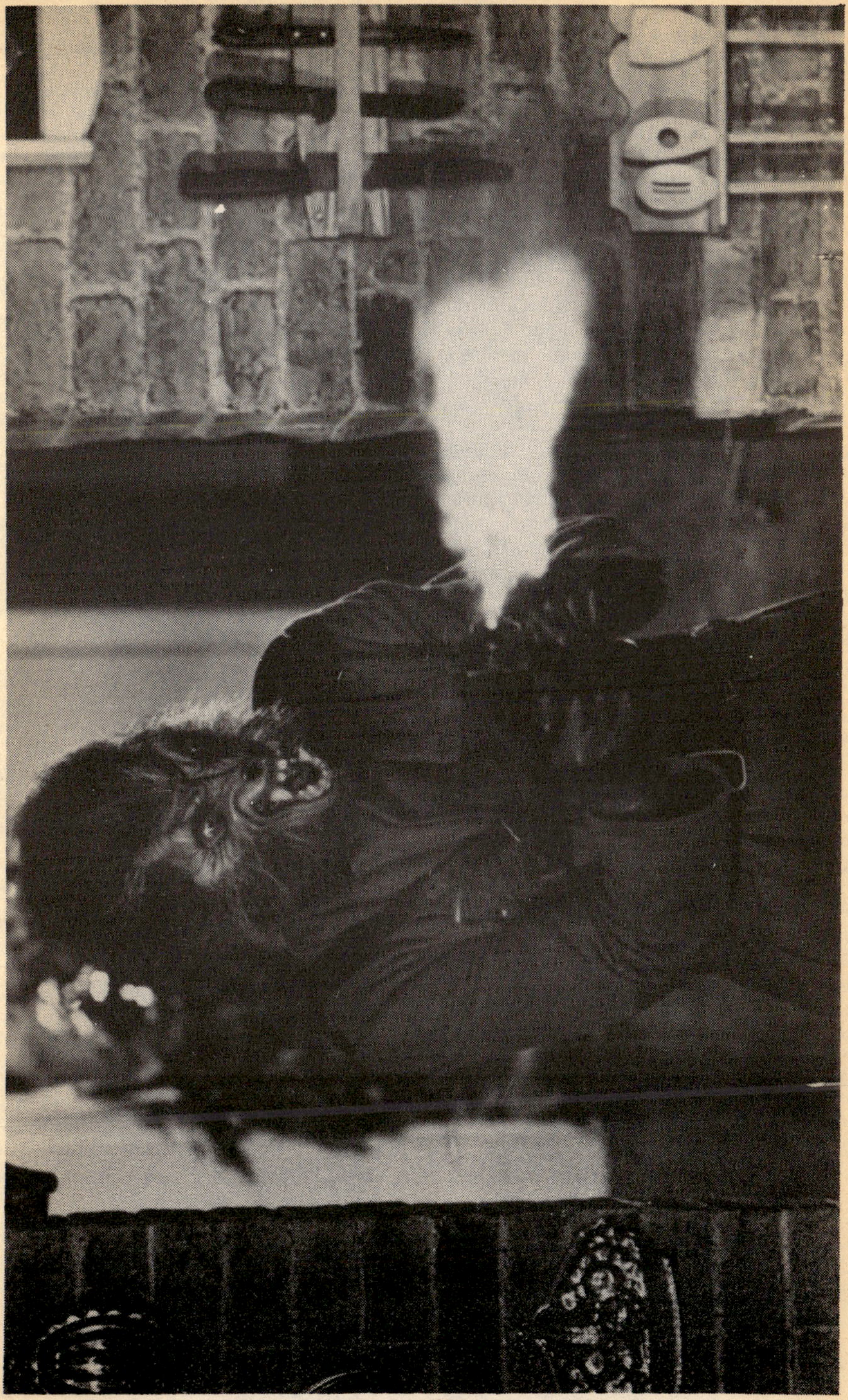

An American Werewolf in London (1981)

Altered States

(1980) Color, 103 min. Director: Ken Russell.
William Hurt, Blair Brown, Charles Haid. A young research scientist (Hurt) submits to a series of sensory deprivation experiments in an effort to uncover some ultimate truths about the human mind and its capacity to achieve alternate states of consciousness. A fascinating, pyrotechnical display of sound and fury that has everything but a good story.
(Warner Home Video) VC

Amazing Spiderman, The ½

(1977) Color, 92 min. Director: E.W. Swackheimer.
Nicholas Hammond, Lisa Eilbacher, Michael Pataki, Jeff Donnell. A bite from a radioactive spider turns newspaper reporter/photographer Hammond into a crime-fighting superhero with the ability to crawl up large buildings and spin deadly webs for catching villains. Enjoyable made-for-TV movie, pilot for the short-lived series, based on the Marvel comic book character.
(CBS/Fox Video) VC

Amazing Transplant, The ½

(1970) Color, 80 min. Director: Louis Silverman.
A man murders his girlfriend and is relentlessly pursued by a detective, who also happens to be his uncle. At the root of the whole mess is a terrible secret involving a very bizarre transplant. An exercise in total brainlessness.
(Electric Video) VC

Amazing World of Psychic Phenomena ½

(?) Color, 91 min.
Narrated by Raymond Burr. An in-depth (hah!) look at parapsychology and other occult mysteries.
(VidAmerica) VC

American Werewolf in London, An ½

(1981) Color, 97 min. Director: John Landis.
David Naughton, Jenny Agutter. Despite some marvelous werewolf transformation effects by make-up wiz Rick Baker (for which he received an Oscar), this schizoid mixture of humor, horror, and rock 'n roll is little more than a grade B exploitation film dressed up in a $10 million budget. Some of the scares work; some of the jokes work, but overall, the film is hollow, pointless, and sleazy.
(MCA Videocassete, RCA VideoDisc) VC, CED

Amityville Horror, The ½

(1979) Color, 117 min. Director: Stuart Rosenberg.
James Brolin, Margot Kidder, Rod Steiger. A young couple, the Lutzes, move into an expensive Long Island home, where six people had been murdered six years before, and come face to face with something even more monstrous than their first mortgage payment. The house, you see, is possessed. After a month of enduring attacks by flies, slime, and phantom pigs, the pair decides this is no place like home and splits, leaving all its "possessions" behind. Resolutely unscary.
(Warner Home Video, RCA VideoDisc) VC, CED

Andy Warhol's Dracula ½

(1974) Color, 106 min. Director: Paul Morrissey.
Udo Kier, Vittorio de Sica, Joe Dallesandro, Roman Polanski (unbilled). In this X-rated farce of camp sex and violence, the Count (Kier) can only dine on virgin's blood, otherwise he throws up. So he heads for Roman Catholic Italy where virgins are supposed to be in good supply, but is done in at the climax by a lascivious handyman who always seems to be one step (or one virgin) ahead of the starving vampire.
(Video Gems) VC

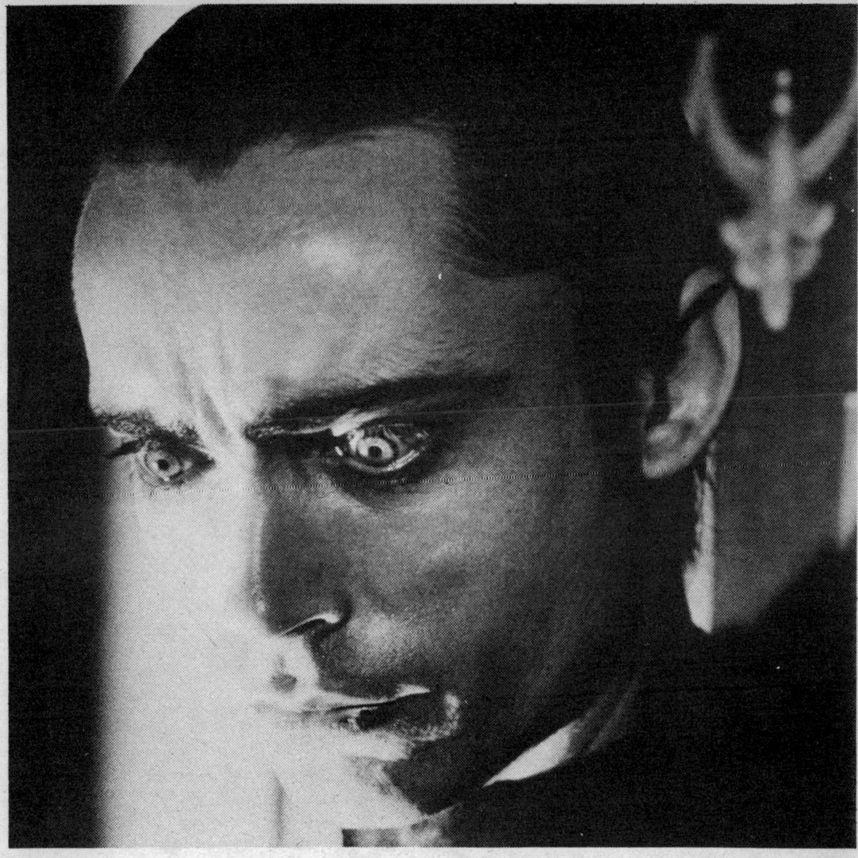

Andy Warhol's Dracula (1974)

". . .X-rated farce of camp sex and violence. . ."

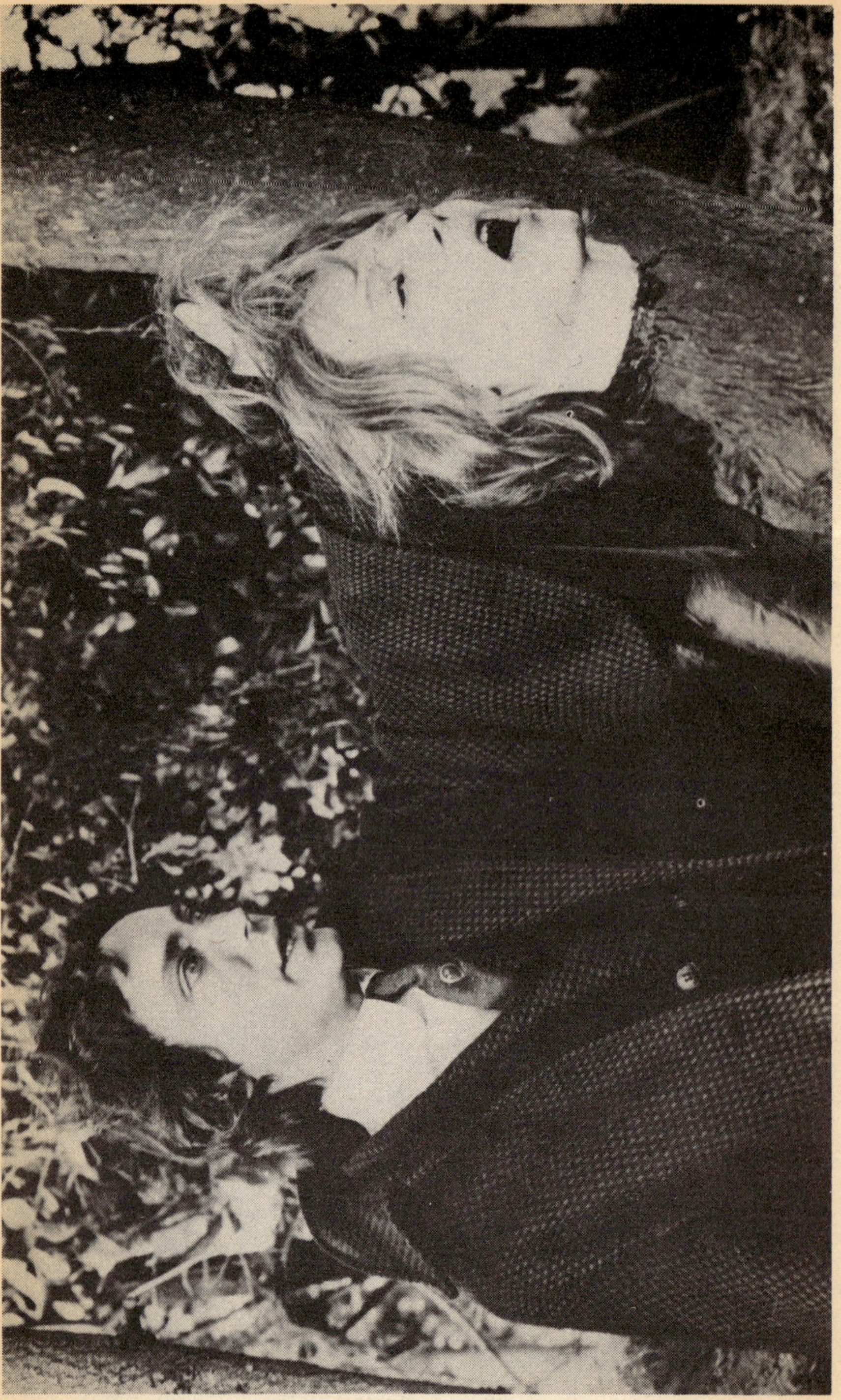

Andy Warhol's Frankenstein (1972)

Andy Warhol's Frankenstein

(1972) Color, 95 min. Director: Paul Morrissey.
Udo Kier, Monique Van Vooren, Joe Dallesandro. In this outrageously gruesome spoof of the viler implications of the Frankenstein legend, the Baron (Kier) is a pervert whose main obsession is not just to build a creature, but to paw, grope, and fondle every internal organ the human body contains. My favorite line, spoken by the mad Dr. F to his dim-witted assistant: "To know death, Otto, you must first f--- life in the gall bladder."
(Video Gems) VC

And Now the Screaming Starts

(1973) Color, 91 min. Director: Roy Ward Baker.
Peter Cushing, Herbert Lom, Stephanie Beacham, Patrick Magee. A young bride moves into a large manor house and is welcomed by all manner of unsociable things, including a fleet-fingered severed hand and bloody faces that appear regularly at her window. Stylish, but not altogether very frightening or exciting.
(Nostalgia Merchant) VC

Andromeda Strain, The ½

(1971) Color, 130 min. Director: Robert Wise.
Arthur Hill, James Olson, Kate Reid. Colorful adaptation of Michael Crichton's novel about a killer virus from outer space. Full of flashing lights and noisy computers, but little suspense or excitement. Overlong.
(MCA Videocassette) VC

Animal Farm

(1954) Color, 75 min. Directors: John Halas, Joy Batchelor.
Animated version of George Orwell's sharp satire of socialism in particular and government in general. Not a party film for the kids.
(Media Home Entertainment) VC

Annie ½

(1982) Color, 128 min. Director: John Huston.
Carol Burnett, Albert Finney, Aileen Quinn, Bernadette Peters, Tim Curry, Ann Reinking. Elephantine movie musical based on the hit Broadway musical based on the popular *Little Orphan Annie* comic strip. Burnett and Reinking shine. Finney is an odd choice for the role of Daddy Warbucks, but he pulls it off. Quinn exudes terminal cuteness in the title role.
(Columbia Pictures Home Entertainment) VC

Ape Man, The ½

(1943) B&W, 64 min. Director: William Beaudine.
Bela Lugosi, Wallace Ford. A mad scientist (Lugosi) injects himself with a curious serum in order to make contact with his simian heritage, but turns into murderous ape instead. Tepid.
(Cable Films) VC

Assault ½

(1970) Color, 89 min. Director: Sidney Hayers.
Lesley-Anne Down, Suzy Kendall, Frank Finlay, James Laurenson, Tony Beckley. Violent sex murders in a girl's school. Inquiries lead to three suspects: a local doctor, the schoolmistress' husband, and a newspaper reporter. Art teacher Kendall acts as bait to smoke the killer out and almost gets done in, but previous victim Down recovers from the trauma of her experience to put the finger on the killer and save the day. A.k.a. *In the Devil's Garden.*
(Embassy Home Entertainment) VC

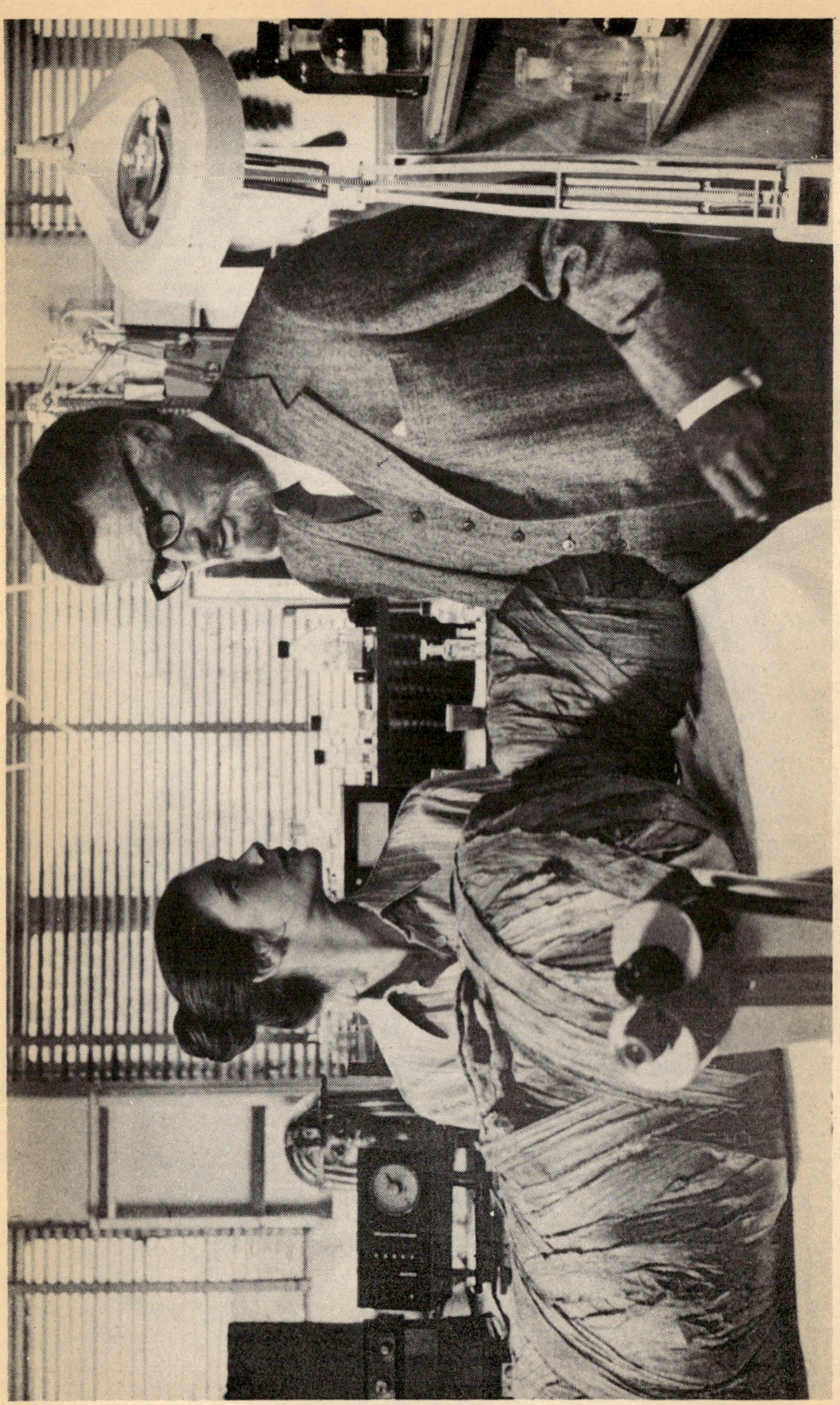

The Awakening (1980)

Assault on Precinct 13 ★★½

(1976) Color, 91 min. Director: John Carpenter.
Austin Stoker, Darwin Joston, Laurie Zimmer. Howard Hawk's *Rio Bravo* meets George Romero's *Night of the Living Dead* in this tense tale about a group of punks who lay seige to a soon-to-be-closed-down police station in the slums of Los Angeles. The acting is horrible, the character motivation negligible, but the film works anyway, thanks to Carpenter's sure hand at suspense.
(Media Home Entertainment) VC

Astro-Zombies ★

(1968) Color, 90 min. Director: Ted V. Mikels.
Wendell Corey, John Carradine, Rafael Campos. A real el-cheapo in which a scientist murders to get the organs he needs to build a creature. Now where do you suppose co-writers Mikels and Wayne Rogers (yes, *the* Wayne Rogers of *MASH* and *House Calls*) dug up that plot idea?
(Wizard Video) VC

Asylum ★★½

(1972) Color, 100 min. Director: Roy Ward Baker.
Peter Cushing, Herbert Lom, Britt Ekland, Robert Powell, Patrick Magee. The inmates finally take over the asylum in this quartet of terror tales from the pen of shockmaster Robert Bloch. Best episode is "Mannikins of Horror," involving Magee and a creepy little doll. Good fun.
(Nostalgia Merchant) VC

Attack of the Killer Tomatoes ★★

(1978) Color, 87 min. Director: John De Bello.
David Miller, George Wilson, Sharon Taylor. Mutant tomatoes become a red menace as they terrorize Los Angeles in this low-budget satire of every monster flick from *Jaws* to *Godzilla.* Some of the jokes are screamingly funny, but most of the others. . .*oh, brother!* And the songs are worse.
(Media Home Entertainment) VC

Avenging Conscience, The ★★½

(1914) B&W, 60 min. Director: D.W. Griffith.
Henry B. Walthall, Blanche Sweet, Mae Marsh, Spottiswoode Aiken. An early example of screen horror. . .or combination of horror and melodrama, based on Edgar Allen Poe's "The Tell-Tale Heart" and "Annabel Lee." A year later, Griffith went on to make *Birth of a Nation.* Well done.
(Video Yesteryear) VC

Awakening, The ★

(1980) Color, 101 min. Director: Mike Newell.
Charlton Heston, Susannah York, Stephanie Zimbalist. An Egyptologist defies a fearful curse and releases the imprisoned spirit of a monstrous queen to walk again among the living. Despite its title, a real sleeper—in the worst sense of the word. Based on Bram Stoker's *Jewel of the 7 Stars.*
(Warner Home Video) VC

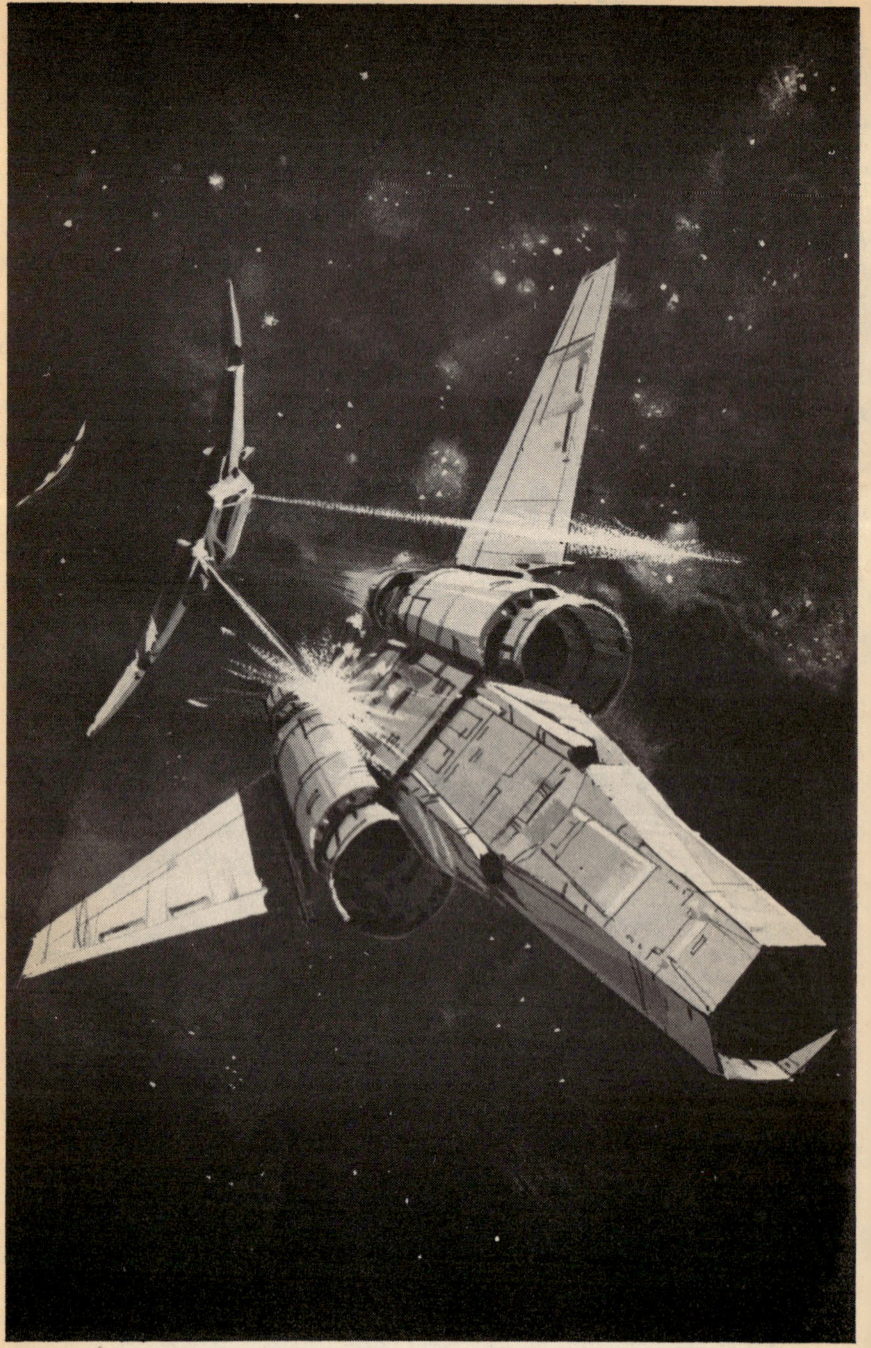

Battlestar Galactica (1978)

B

Babes in Toyland ★★½

(1961) Color, 105 min. Director: Jack Donohue.
Annette Funicello, Ray Bolger, Tommy Sands, Tommy Kirk, Ed Wynn. Disney version of the familiar Victor Herbert operetta abot a magical kingdom where toys come to life. Tuneful, but previous 1934 version with Laurel and Hardy is more entertaining.
(Walt Disney Home Video) VC

Baby, The ★★

(1973) Color, 86 min. Director: Ted Post.
Ruth Roman, Anjanette Comer, Marianna Hill, David Manzy. A social worker (Comer) attempts to free a retarded man-child from the suffocating over-protection of his mother and sisters, but winds up making matters quite a bit worse. Sleazy.
(King of Video) VC

Baffled ★★½

(1972) Color, 90 min. Director: Philip Leacock.
Leonard Nimoy, Susan Hampshire, Vera Miles, Rachel Roberts. Nimoy is a race car driver who is almost killed in a fiery crash, but survives to find himself possessing psychic powers. His visions tell him of other people who will soon be facing danger and he sets out to warn them. Originally made for television.
(CBS/Fox Video) VC

Barbarella ★½

(1968) Color, 98 min. Director: Roger Vadim.
Jane Fonda, John Philip Law, Terence Stamp, Marcel Marceau. Fonda stars as a sexually uninhibited, female version of Flash Gordon in this splashy, but not very erotic tone poem to the popular French comic strip by Jean Claude Forest. Best part is Jane's anti-gravity striptease under the opening credits.
(Paramount Home Video, RCA VideoDisc) VC, LV, CED

Battlestar Galactica ★★

(1978) Color, 152 min. Director: Richard A. Colla.
Lorne Greene, Richard Hatch, Dirk Benedict, Maren Jensen. Pilot for the short-lived series that strived to emulate *Star Wars* but lasted only one season. Film recounts the exploits of a massive battlecruiser in its efforts to defeat the warring Cylons, destroyers of the Galactica's home planet. Special effects by John Dykstra, who put in similar duty on *Star Wars.*
(MCS Videocassette and Disc) VC, LV

Beast Must Die, The ★★

(1974) Color, 93 min. Director: Paul Annett.

Calvin Lockhart, Peter Cushing, Charles Gray, Anton Diffring. Millionaire sportsman Lockhart invites a varied group of men and women to spend the night of the full moon at his isolated mansion, which is completely bugged for sight and sound. His purpose: to discover which of them is a werewolf. The film even gives us a chance to guess by providing us with a brief "werewolf break" at the climactic moment.

(Nostalgia Merchant) VC

Beast of the Yellow Night ★

(1971) Color, 87 min. Director: Eddie Romero.

John Ashley, Mary Wilcox, Eddie Garcia. Filipino-made horror film about a man who sells his soul to the devil to achieve eternal life, assumes the forms of a variety of evil men and ultimately turns into a monster. Sort of a tropical *Dorian Gray* with gore instead of wit.

(Cult Video) VC

Beauty and the Beast ★★★★

(1946) B&W, 90 min. Director: Jean Cocteau.

Josette Day, Jean Marais. Cocteau's surrealistic adaptation of the classic fable of the girl who falls in love with the hideous but spiritually fine beast is absolutely haunting. Done on a shoe-string, but with a wealth of cinematic imagination.

(Video Dimensions) VC

Bedazzled ★★★

(1967) Color, 107 min. Director: Stanley Donen.

Peter Cook, Dudley Moore, Eleanor Bron, Raquel Welch. Updated fantasy based on the Faust legend with Cook as the urbane Mephisto and Moore as the bumbling soul-seller. Welch puts in a memorable cameo as a voluptuous temptress. Sophisticated slapstick.

(CBS/Fox Video) VC

Bedknobs and Broomsticks ★★½

(1971) Color, 117 min. Director: Robert Stevenson.

Angela Lansbury, David Tomlinson, Roddy McDowall, Sam Jaffe. Disney musical fantasy with animation set in England during World War II. Lansbury is an amateur witch who, together with three abandoned charges, practices all manner of magic to stave off the Nazis. Oscar-winner for special effects.

(Walt Disney Home Video) VC

Bedlam ★★★

(1945) B&W, 79 min. Director: Mark Robson.

Boris Karloff, Anna Lee. Karloff stars as the sadistic warden of the infamous 18th century madhouse immortalized by the artist Hogarth, whose engravings inspired this visually elegant Val Lewton film. A bit talky at times, but occasionally chilling as well, and a class act throughout.

(Nostalgia Merchant) VC

Bees, The ★½

(1978) Color, 86 min. Director: Alfredo Zacharias.

John Saxon, Angel Tompkins. Man or insect: who will ultimately rule the world? is the cliche-ridden question raised by this, yet *another,* unimaginative entry in the seemingly unending parade of grade-B bee movies that moviemakers have persisted in foisting on horror fans over the years, *none* of which have been remotely scary. You'd think they would have learned their lesson by now: bee movies are for the birds.

(Warner Home Video) VC

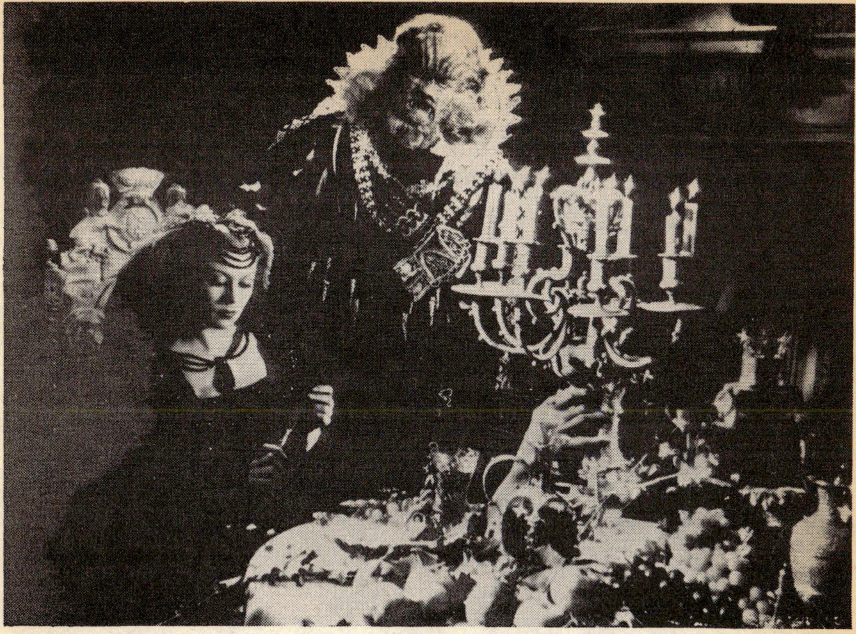

Beauty and the Beast (1946)

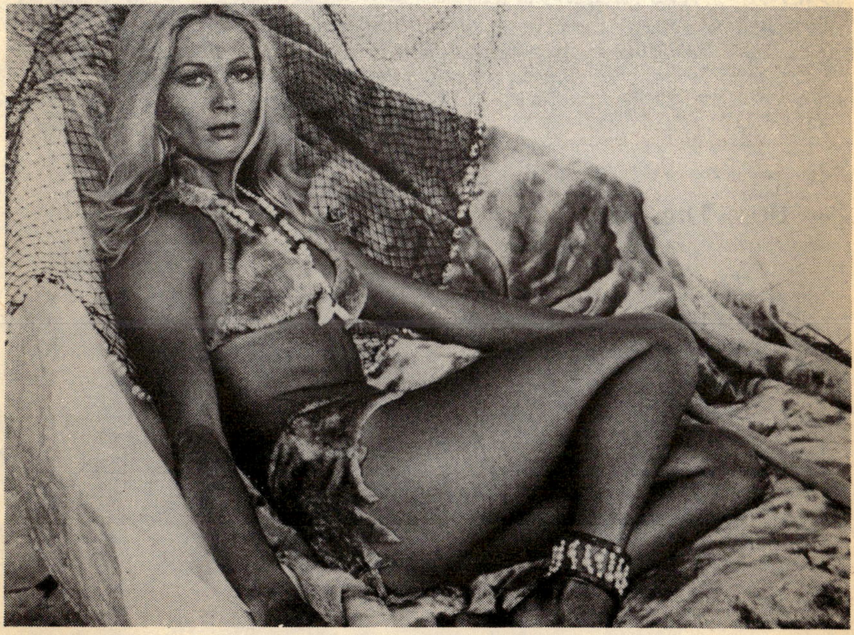

Beyond Atlantis (1973)

Bell, Book and Candle ☑☑½

(1958) Color, 103 min. Director: Richard Quine.
James Stewart, Kim Novak, Jack Lemmon, Ernie Kovacs. Amusing comedy laced with fantasy based on the successful Broadway play by John Van Druten about a soon-to-be-married publisher (Stewart) who is suddenly bewitched by. . .a witch (Novak).
(Columbia Pictures Home Entertainment) VC

Bermuda Triangle, The ☑☑

(1978) Color, 93 min. Director: Richard Friedenberg.
Narrated by Brad Crandall. Documentary based on the best-selling book by Charles Berlitz, which speculates that the loss of hundreds of ships, planes and people in the mysterious triangle off the coasts of Bermuda, Miami and Puerto Rico is the work of creatures from outer space. Far-fetched but provocative.
(VID America) VC

Beyond Atlantis ☑

(1973) Color, 89 min. Director: Eddie Romero.
Patrick Wayne, John Ashley, Sid Haig, George Nader. Archaeologists discover an island peopled by amphibious semi-humans, survivors of the long-destroyed Atlantis, who come up for air every now and then to mate with nubile island girls in order to perpetuate their race. Snore.
(Wizard Video) VC

Beyond the Door ☑

(1975) Color, 109 min. Director: Oliver Hellman (Sonia Assonitis).
Juliet Mills, Richard Johnson, David Colin, Jr. Italian made entry in the post-*Exorcist* sweepstakes involving attractive Mills who is suddenly possessed by the devil and turns into a revolting slob. A bomb.
(Media Home Entertainment) VC

Beyond the Valley of the Dolls ☑☑

(1970) Color, 109 min. Director: Russ Meyer.
Polly Read, Cynthia Myers, Marcia Broom, Michael Blodgett, Edy Williams, Erica Gavin. Sex and drugs and rock and roll rule the day as an all-girl rock combo struggles to stardom in Tinseltown. What makes it a horror movie—or, more precisely, a *splatter* movie—is the gruesome and graphic orgy of violence that climaxes the film in true Meyer fashion. Written by film critic and anti-splatter crusader Roger Ebert, who has publicly expressed much dismay over gory exploitation films like this one. But *not* this one. I wonder why?
(CBS/Fox Video) VC

Big Bus, The ☑☑

(1976) Color, 85 min. Director: James Frawley.
Joseph Bologna, Stockard Channing, Rene Auburjonois, Lynn Redgrave, Ruth Gordon. Pre-*Airplane* spoof of disaster movies about a nuclear-powered bus and the hell its passengers go through on a hair-raising trip cross-country. Does its best to torpedo all the cliches of the genre, but is only intermittently funny.
(Paramount Home Video) VC

Big Foot—Man or Beast ☑☑

(1975) Color, 92 min. Director: Lawrence Crowley.
A documentary about the legendary man-like creature that prowls the forests of the Pacific Northwest. Includes interviews with those who profess to have seen him (it?).
(Video Communications) VC

Bill and Coo

(1947) Color, 61 min. Director: Dean Riesner.
Oscar-winning live-action fantasy in which the entire cast—heroes, heroines and villains alike—is made up of trained birds. Unique to say the least. Produced and narrated by Ken Murray.
(Budget Video, Video Connection) VC

Birds, The

(1963) Color, 120 min. Director: Alfred Hitchcock.
Rod Taylor, Tippi Hedren, Jessica Tandy, Suzanne Pleshette. A reign of winged terror by our feathered friends descends upon an unsuspecting coastal village in this darkly ironic vision of Judgement Day by the screen's undisputed master of suspense. The first half of the film is literally a comedy of manners which reveals in telling detail the frivolousness and complacency of the main characters, setting them up as perfect foils for the struggle for survival that is to come. Hedren is a bit stiff, but then she's supposed to be. One of Hitch's best and most ingenious films.
(MCA Videocassette and Disc) VC, LV

Bird with the Crystal Plumage, The

(1969) Color, 98 min. Director: Dario Argento.
Tony Musante, Suzy Kendall, Eva Renzi, Mario Adorf. Violent psychodrama in which Musante, an American writer living in Rome, witnesses an attempted murder and is thereafter terrorized by the would-be assassin. Stylish, but somewhat overdone.
(Video Communications) VC

Blackenstein

(1972) Color, 87 min. Director: William A. Levey.
John Hart, Ivory Stone, Andrea King, Liz Renay. Low budget, ethnic reworking of the familiar Mary Shelley tale.
(Media Home Entertainment) VC

Black Hole, The ½

(1979) Color, 97 min. Director: Gary Nelson.
Maximillian Schell, Yvette Mimieux, Anthony Perkins, Ernest Borgnine, Joseph Bottoms, Robert Forster. A totally botched effort by Disney to capitalize on the success of *Star Wars*. It even includes a bevy of supposedly loveable robots; actually they're quite obnoxious. What's even worse, their wires show when they fly. But then the film's special effects on the whole (as well as *of* the hole) are consistently quite atrocious. Only the most fantasy-starved of toddlers are likely to be taken in by this one.
(Walt Disney Home Video) VC, LV

Black Magic

(1949) B&W, 105 min. Director: Gregory Ratoff.
Orson Welles, Akim Tamiroff, Nancy Guild, Raymond Burr. Welles stars as the evil magician Cagliostro in this stagey but atmospheric tale of power, corruption, and sorcery in 18th century Italy. He also overacts flamboyantly.
(Nostalgia Merchant) VC

Black Orpheus

(1960) Color, 98 min. Director: Marcel Camus.
Marpessa Dawn, Breno Mello, Lourdes De Oliveira, Lea Garcia. Remarkable updating of the Greek legend of Orpheus and Eurydice set in Rio against the backdrop of the Mardi Gras. Wild and colorful, beautifully acted and boasting a haunting score, the film weaves a magic spell. Won the Oscar as Best Foreign Film, and deserved it.
(MGM/UA Home Video) VC, CED

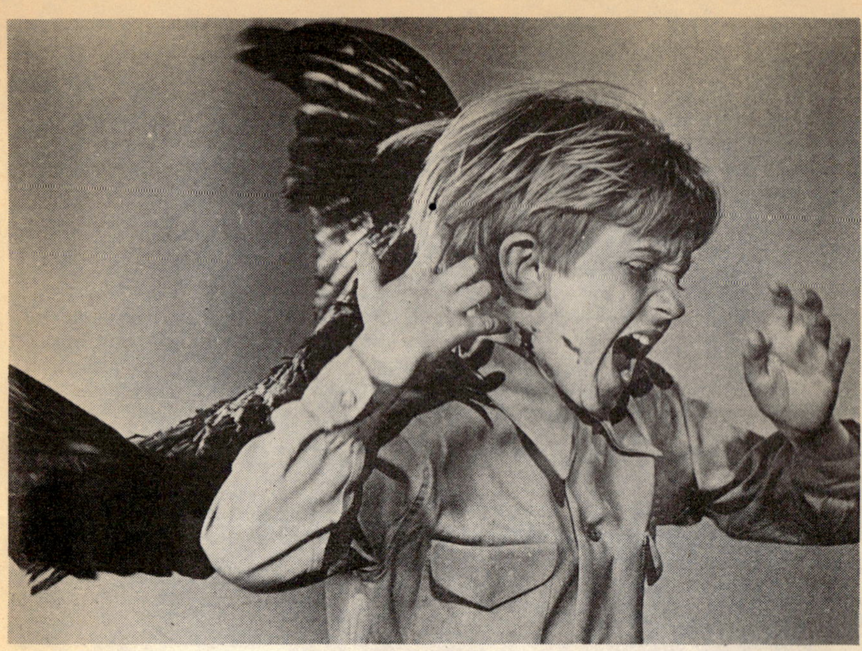

The Birds (1963)

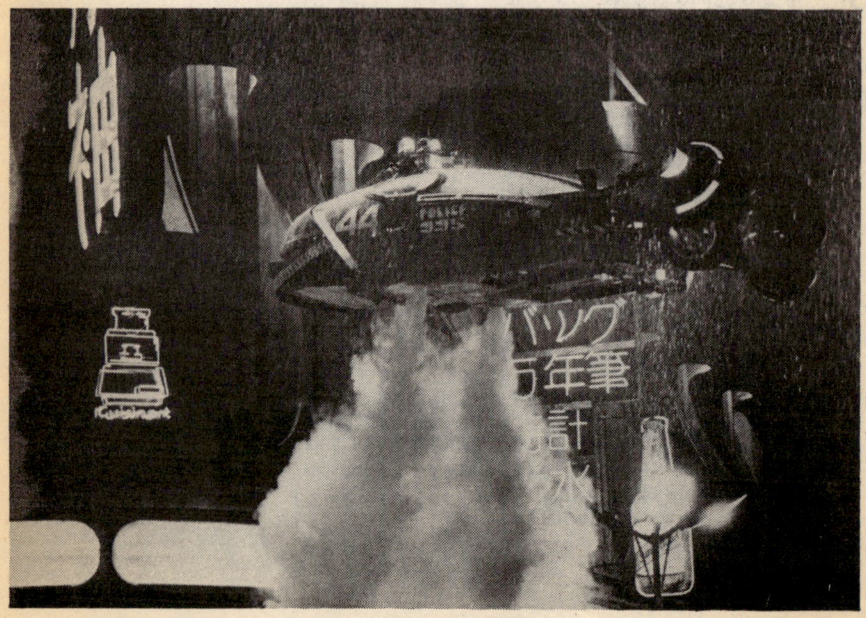

Blade Runner (1982)

Blackbeard's Ghost ⭐⭐⭐

(1968) Color, 107 min. Director: Robert Stevenson.

Dean Jones, Suzanne Pleshette, Peter Ustinov, Elsa Lanchester. Ghost of villainous pirate Blackbeard (Ustinov), condemned to walk the earth until he commits a good deed, returns to aid Jones in a fight against some racketeers. Entertaining Disney fantasy with Ustinov droll as ever.

(Walt Disney Home Video) VC

Blade Runner ⭐⭐⭐

(1982) Color, 114 min. Director: Ridley Scott.

Harrison Ford, Rutger Hauer, Sean Young. Futuristic hard-boiled detective yarn with Ford miscast as the world weary *film noir* hero whose job it is to smoke out replicants (androids) that have infiltrated the world of humans. Director Scott creates a powerful vision of Los Angeles circa 2019, but fails to provide any kind of a story to go along with it. Visually compelling but disappointing nonetheless. Based on a novel by Philip K. Dick.

(Embassy Home Entertainment) VC, LV

Blob, The ⭐⭐

(1958) Color, 85 min. Director: Irwin S. Yeaworth, Jr.

Steve McQueen, Aneta Corseaut, Earl Rowe, Olin Howlin. A fifties classic from cheapo producer Jack H. Harris and the film that marked the screen debut of superstar McQueen. Teenagers save the adults and the day when a marauding mass of gelatinous glop from outer space lands in a small California town and begins sucking people up right and left.

(Video Gems) VC

Blood Beach ⭐⭐

(1981) Color, 92 min. Director: Jeffrey Bloom.

David Huffman, Marianna Hill, John Saxon, Burt Young. A malevolent creature lurking beneath the sands of a crowded Southern California beach pulls unsuspecting sunbathers to their bloody doom in this half serious, half absurd parody of *Jaws*. My favorite line: "Just when you thought it was safe to go back in the water. . .you can't get to it."

(Media Home Entertainment) VC

Blood Feast ⭐

(1963) Color, 75 min. Director: Herschell Gordon Lewis.

Connie Mason, Thomas Wood, Mal Arnold, Lyn Bolton, Scott H. Hall. A weirdo who thinks he's sort of a modern Dr. Frankenstein attempts to revive the corpse of a long-dead Egyptian princess by replacing her moldy old parts with new ones—which he rips off of young girls (literally) while they're still quite alive and breathing. First of the gore films; overall, a crude, exploitative howler.

(Cult Video) VC

Blood Legacy ⭐

(1971) Color, 89 min. Director: Carl Monson.

Faith Domergue, John Russell, Marry Anders, Jeff Morrow, Rodolfo Acosta, John Carradine. An elderly millionaire fakes his own death to watch the in-fighting he knows will ensue among his heirs. The in-fighting soon turns to murder, however, as the heirs start killing each other off in all sorts of creatively grisly ways. Undistinguished except as an early example of the "creative death" form of splatter filmmaking. A.k.a. *Legacy of Blood.*

(Video Gems) VC

Blood Mania ⭐

(1970) Color, 90 min. Director: (?)

Low budget exploitation film in which the daughter of a retired surgeon, who hates her father dearly, decides to do him in in order to collect her inheritance early.

(Video Communications) VC

Blood of a Poet, The ½

(1930) B&W, 53 min. Director: Jean Cocteau.
Enrico Ribero, Lee Miller, Jean Desbordes. Cocteau's debut film is an adventure in total surrealism, filled with puzzling dream imagery built around the story of a poet who lives what he creates. Visually remarkable, but totally confounding.
(Thunderbird Films, Budget Video, Video Yesteryear) VC

Blood of Dracula's Castle ½

(1967) Color, 84 min. Directors: Al Adamson, Jean Hewitt.
John Carradine, Paula Raymond, Alex D'Arcy. A kinky Count and Countess Dracula way-lay young girls for their blood while a werewolf-type killer stalks the countryside. Never a dull moment! Photographed by ace cinematographer Laszlo Kovacs (under the name Leslie Kovacs) before he hit the big time with *Easy Rider.*
(Video Communications) VC

Bloodthirsty Butchers

(1970) Color, 79 min. Director: Andy Milligan.
John Miranda, Annabella Wood, Berwick Kaler. Low-budget saga of Sweeney Todd, the demon barber who killed people for their money and then disposed of their bodies by turning them into meat pies. Yum! Yum!
(Midnight Video) VC

Blow Out

(1981) Color, 107 min. Director: Brian De Palma.
John Travolta, Nancy Allen, John Lithgow, Dennis Franz. Movie sound effects man Travolta chance records the audio of a car crash while on location, then discovers the crash wasn't an accident at all, but a successfully carried out political assassination. Abruptly the film then turns into a typical De Palma-style mad slasher movie. The fact that this film, which represents the nadir of De Palma's career so far, is an outright rip-off of Michelangelo Antonioni's *Blow-Up* (even the titles are similar) as well as Francis Coppola's *The Conversation* is bad enough. But it is also badly written, horribly acted—pert Nancy Allen is again miscast as a hooker, just as she was in De Palma's *Dressed to Kill*—and full of alienating directorial flourishes. The pits.
(Warner Home Video, RCA VideoDisc) VC, CED

Body Snatcher, The

(1945) B&W, 77 min. Director: Robert Wise.
Boris Karloff, Henry Daniell, Russell Wade, Bela Lugosi. Karloff has one of his best roles as John Gray, the villainous cabdriver and graverobber who supplies corpses for "friend" Daniell's school of anatomy. Lugosi has a small role as one of Karloff's victims. Adapted by Philip MacDonald and Carlos Keith (Val Lewton) from Robert Louis Stevenson's short story.
(Nostalgia Merchant) VC

Boogey Man, The

(1980) Color, 86 min. Director: Ulli Lommel.
Suzanna Love, Ron James, John Carradine, Nicholas Love. A brother and sister, witnesses to a murder years before, relive their nightmare when the victim returns to haunt them. A psychological thriller with lots of gore from the German director of *Tenderness of the Wolves.*
(Wizard Video) VC

Boy and His Dog, A ½

(1975) Color, 89 min. Director: L.Q. Jones.
Don Johnson, Susanne Benton, Alvy Moore, Jason Robards. Muddled misogynistic sci-fi based on a novella by Harlan Ellison that takes place in the year 2024 following a nuclear war that has turned most of America into a landscape that resembles Death Valley—which is where most of the film was probably shot. Johnson and his telepathic dog, Blood, are the leads, struggling to survive against all odds. The ending is most distasteful, unless you're the ultimate dog lover.
(Media Home Entertainment) VC

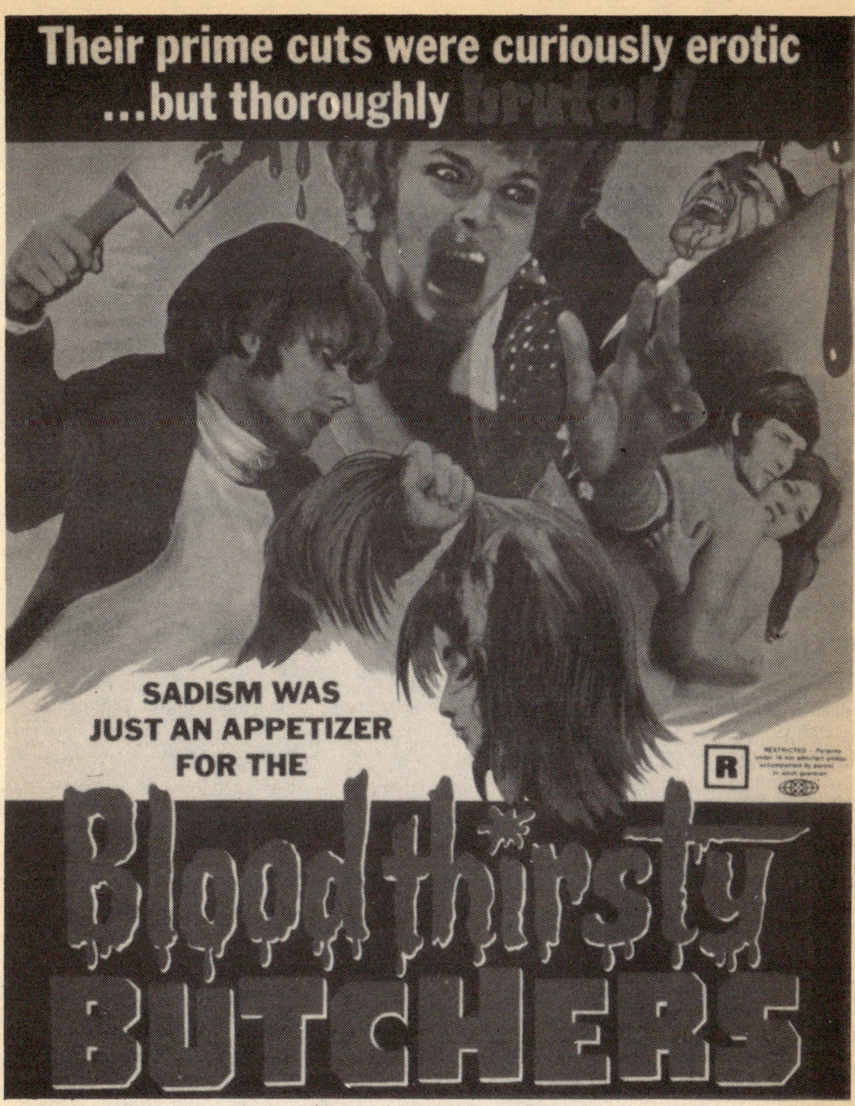
Their prime cuts were curiously erotic
...but thoroughly
SADISM WAS
JUST AN APPETIZER
FOR THE
R
Bloodthirsty
BUTCHERS

Bloodthirsty Butchers (1970)

"Low-budget saga of Sweeney Todd. . ."

Boys from Brazil, The ◪◪ ½

(1978) Color, 123 min. Director: Franklin J. Schaffner.

Gregory Peck, Sir Laurence Olivier, James Mason. Peck is the real-life Dr. Josef Mengele, whose bizarre experiments in genetics resulted in the deaths of countless innocent Jews at Auschwitz during the war, but who fled to Paraguay and avoided justice. Based on the best-selling thriller by Ira Levin, the film ponders what might have happened if Mengele had continued his experiments over the years with the mad object of cloning another Adolf Hitler—or a thousand clones! Olivier is the Simon Wiesenthal-like Nazi hunter who dogs Mengele's trail—at the conclusion, quite literally. Taut and well crafted, but aside from its nice alliteration, the title makes no sense.

(CBS/Fox Video, RCA VideoDisc) VC, CED, LV

Brainiac, The ◪

(1963) B&W, 77 min. Director: Chano Urueta.

Abel Salazar, Ariadna Welter, Mauricio Garces, German Robles. A brainiac is a maniac who kills people by sucking out their brains. Ouch! Dreary Mexican horror film.

(Budget Video) VC

Bride of the Monster ◪

(1956) B&W, 67 min. Director: Edward D. Wood, Jr.

Tor Johnson, Tony McCoy, Loretta King. A scientist invents a machine designed to prolong human life by giving people superhuman strength, but turns them into rubber octopuses instead. A camp classic from the incomparable director of *Plan 9 from Outer Space.* Yields plenty of laughs (all unintentional) provided you can summon enough superhuman strength to sit through it.

(Budget Video, Video Yesteryear) VC

Brigadoon ◪◪◪

(1954) Color, 108 min. Director: Vincente Minnelli.

Gene Kelly, Cyd Charisse, Van Johnson, Elaine Stewart. The story of a magical 18th century Scottish village that bounces to life once every 100 years. Kelly and Johnson are the American tourists who stumble upon it. Sprightly musical/fantasy based on the hit Broadway show by Lerner and Lowe.

(MGM/UA Home Video) VC, CED

Bug ◪

(1975) Color, 101 min. Director: Jeannot Szwarc.

Bradford Dillman, Joanna Miles, Jesse Vint, Patty McCormack. A Southern California earthquake unleashes a plague of incendiary cockroaches able to start fires by rubbing their legs together. Scientist Dillman is torn between reaching for a fire extinguisher and a can of Raid to stop them. A William Castle Production. Terrible.

(Paramount Home Video) VC

Bugs Bunny/Road Runner Movie, The ◪◪ ½

(1979) Color, 90 min. Director: Chuck Jones.

Bugs Bunny, Wile E. Coyote, Road Runner, Daffy Duck. Anthology of clips from some of Warner Brothers' funniest cartoons over the years, including *Duck Amuck* and *What's Opera, Doc?* Frequently hilarious, but the final Road Runner compilation is too repetitive.

(Warner Home Video, RCA VideoDisc) VC, CED

Buck Rogers Conquers the Universe ◪◪

(1953) B&W, 91 min. Directors: Ford Beebe, Saul A. Goodkind.

Buster Crabbe, Constance Moore, C. Montague Shaw, Henry Brandon, Jack Moran. Feature version of the 1939 Universal serial, extracted from the serial's original 12 parts and 24 reels. Offers all the same ingredients as *Star Wars,* but on a much less accomplished scale. Still, it offered them first. Based on the novels by Philip Nowlan and the comic strip by Nowlan and artist Dick Calkins.

(CBS/Fox Video) VC

Buck Rogers in the 25th Century ☐

(1979) Color, 89 min. Director: Daniel Haller.

Gil Gerard, Pamela Hensley, Henry Silva, Erin Gray. From the TV series of the same name—actually a cut down version of the pilot which was released to theatres before it was shown on TV. Gerard is a contemporary U.S. astronaut whose ship falls into a time warp and returns to earth five centuries hence. Confusion then reigns supreme as he is first rescued then taken prisoner by the voluptuous but nasty Princess Ardala (Hensley) and her evil co-hort, Kane (Silva). Film even has another of those cloying little robots on hand that makes you wish R2D2 had never been born—er, built.

(MCA Videocassette and Disc) VC, LV

Burning, The ☐☐

(1981) Color, 85 min. Director: Tony Maylam.

Brian Matthews, Leah Ayres, Brian Backer, Larry Joshua. Counselors at a lakeside summer camp are being done in by a vengeful masked psycho brandishing pruning shears. Splatter movie in the *Friday the 13th* mold with horrific special effects by Tom Savini. Music by Rick Wakeman.

(Thorn/EMI Video) VC

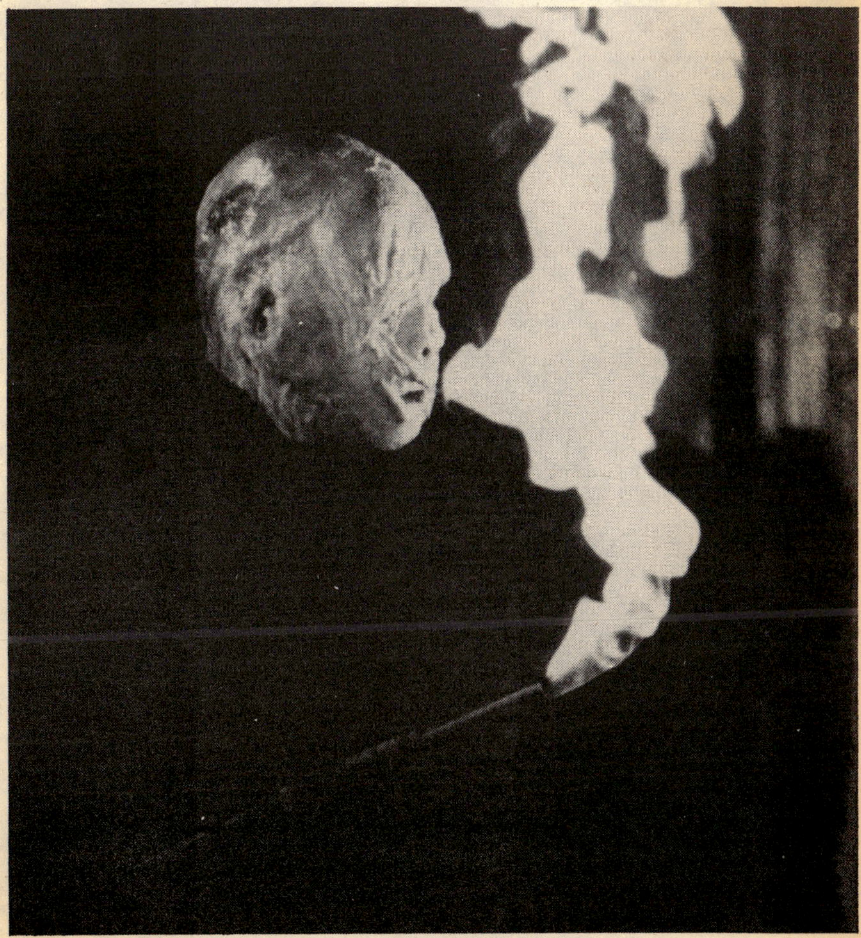

The Burning (1981)

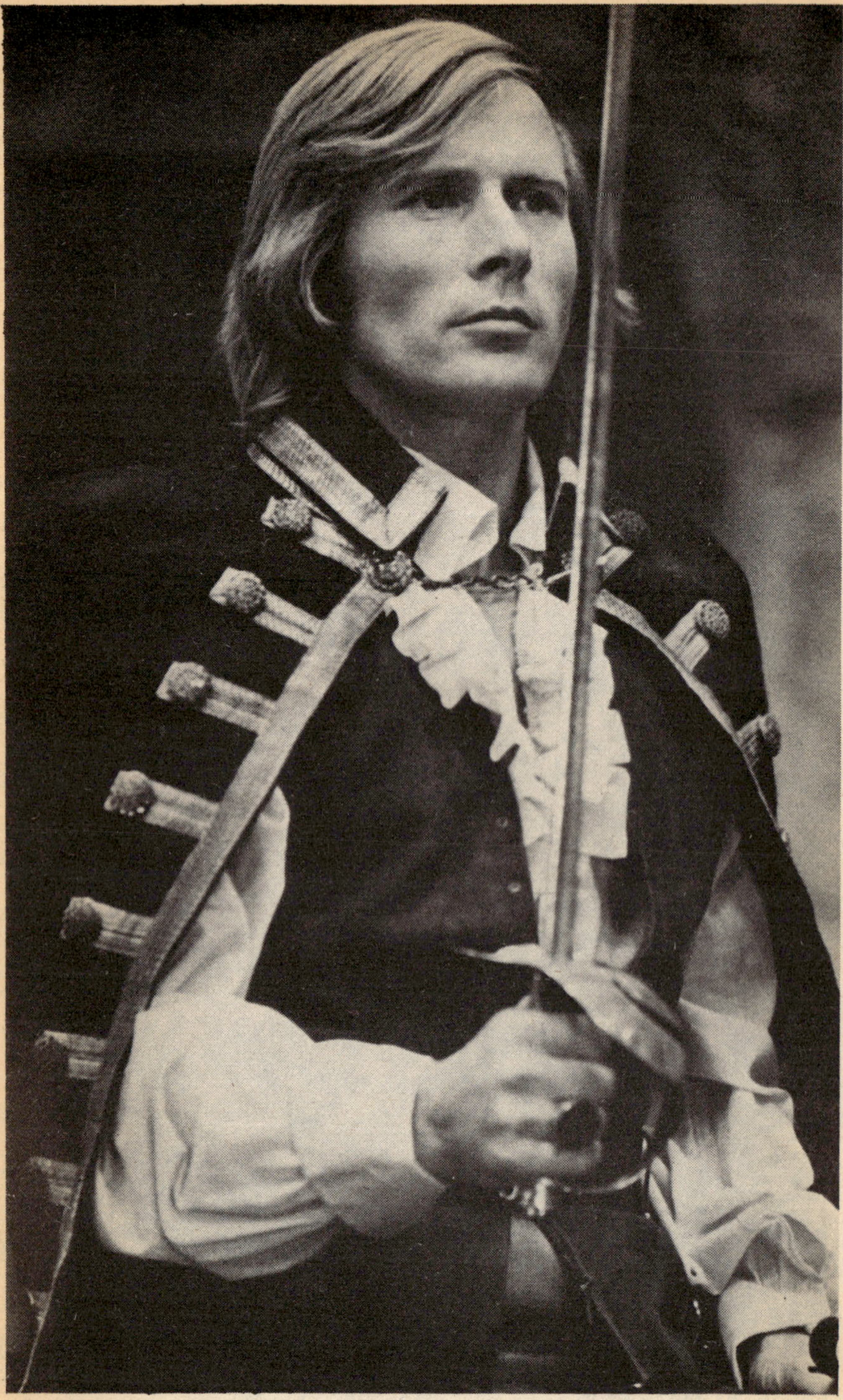

Captain Kronos: Vampire Hunter (1974)

Cabinet of Dr. Caligari, The

(1919) B&W, 69 min. Director: Robert Wiene.
Werner Krauss, Conradt Veidt, Lil Dagover. Influential silent film which launched the Expressionist movement in German cinema during the twenties. Caligari (Krauss) is a side-show magician who uses his somnabulist assistant (Veidt) to commit murder. Or does he? Slow moving but fascinating.
(Budget Video) VC

Camelot ½

(1967) Color, 150 min. Director: Joshua Logan.
Richard Harris, Vanessa Redgrave, Franco Nero. Long, long, long screen adaptation of the hit Broadway musical by Lerner and Lowe about the legendary triangle of King Arthur, Queen Guinevere and Sir Lancelot. Glistens with opulence, but exudes all the energy of a dead elephant.
(Warner Home Video) VC

Candleshoe

(1977) Color, 101 min. Director: Norman Tokar.
Jodie Foster, David Niven, Helen Hayes. Sinister happenings at a haunted English mansion. Unscary, unfunny, unimaginative and undistinguished.
(Walt Disney Home Video, RCA VideoDisc) VC, CED

Capricorn One

(1978) Color, 123 min. Director: Peter Hyams.
Elliot Gould, James Brolin, Brenda Vaccaro, Sam Waterston, Hal Holbrook. America's first manned spaceflight to Mars turns out to be a gigantic hoax. Gould is the reporter who discovers the cover-up. A post-Watergate popcorn movie. Very exciting.
(CBS/Fox Video) VC, LV

Captain Kronos: Vampire Hunter

(1974) Color, 91 min. Director: Brian Clemens.

Horst Janson, Caroline Munro, Shane Bryant, Ian Hendry, John Carson. When Kronos' (Janson) family is wiped out by vampires, he becomes a sort of Gothic Paladin ("Have Stake, Will Travel"), determined to bring an end to the toothy scourge wherever he goes. Friend Carson calls upon him and his hunchbacked side-kick, Professor Grost, for help, but things go excitingly awry when Carson himself becomes an undead. Writer-director Clemens, the creative force behind TV's *Avengers* series, stylishly combines elements from film genres as diverse as the horror film and the western to achieve a film that is alternately funny, scary and full of action. Produced by Hammer Films, *Kronos* was intended to be the first of a series, but when the film flopped at the box office, the idea was dropped. Too bad because this first installment is lively fun indeed. Munro is beautiful, but she can't act.

(Paramount Home Video) VC

Carnival of Blood ½

(1971) Color, 80 min. Director: Leonard Kirtman.

Burt Young, Earle Edgerton, Judith Resnick, Martin Barlosky, John Harris. Madman stalks the midway of a large amusement park, slaying the fun-seekers in all manner of grisly ways. A.k.a. *Death Rides a Carnival.*

(Wizard Video) VC

Carrie

(1976) Color, 97 min. Director: Brian De Palma.

Sissy Spacek, Piper Laurie, William Katt, John Travolta, Nancy Allen, Amy Irving. Vastly over-rated shocker based on the best seller by Stephen King. Spacek is the withdrawn, put-upon teenager of the title who lives under the shadow of her sexually repressed, religion-crazed mother (Laurie). A vicious prank played on her as she is crowned Queen of the senior prom unleashes her telekinetic powers in an orgy of destruction. Spacek is excellent, but De Palma's direction, a mixture of the exploitative, the derivative and the tedious—the most exciting scene in the film is made excruciatingly dull through languorous slow motion—sinks the entire film.

(CBS/Fox Video, RCA VideoDisc) VC, CED, LV

Cars That Eat People, The ½

(1977) Color, 76 min. Director: Peter Weir.

Terry Camilleri, Melissa Jaffa, John Meillon, Kevin Miles. Crazies who worship automobiles trap unsuspecting motorists passing through town at night. The cars are then stolen, the drivers reduced to vegetables through surgery, and the machines turned into supernatural death machines. Wacked-out Australian science-fiction film directed by the talented Peter Weir just prior to his big international success with *Picnic at Hanging Rock*. A.k.a. *The Cars That Ate Paris.*

(Cult Video) VC

Castle of Fu Manchu, The

(1968) Color, 92 min. Director: Jesus Franco.

Christopher Lee, Richard Greene, Maria Perschy, Howard Marion Crawford. Fu attempts to destroy the world through the use of a deadly potion. Lee's last film in the Fu Manchu series, and his worst.

(Electric Video) VC

Cat and the Canary, The

(1927) B&W, 70 min. Director: Paul Leni.

Laura LaPlante, Tully Marshall, Flora Finch, Creighton Hale. Filmed at the close of the silent film era, this is the prototype of every old dark house movie ever made, full of billowing curtains, skulking shadows, and slithering camera movements. Leni's direction is matchless.

(Budget Video, Video Yesteryear) VC

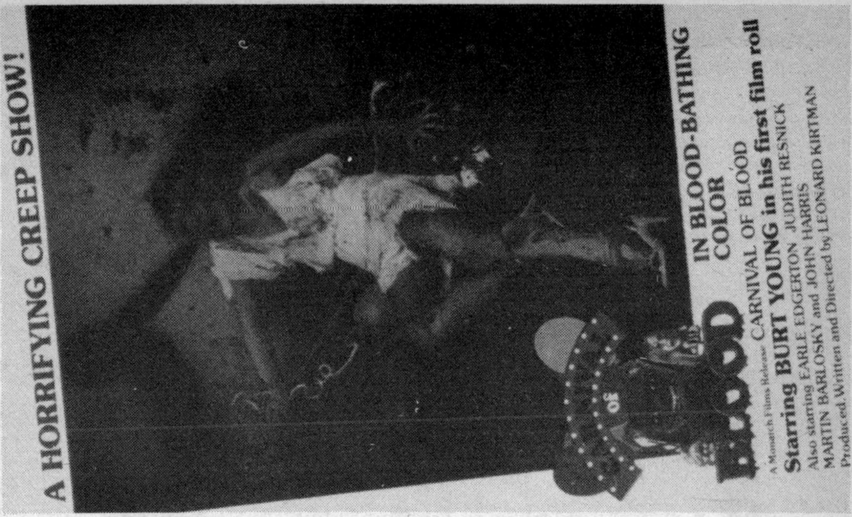

Carnival of Blood (1971)

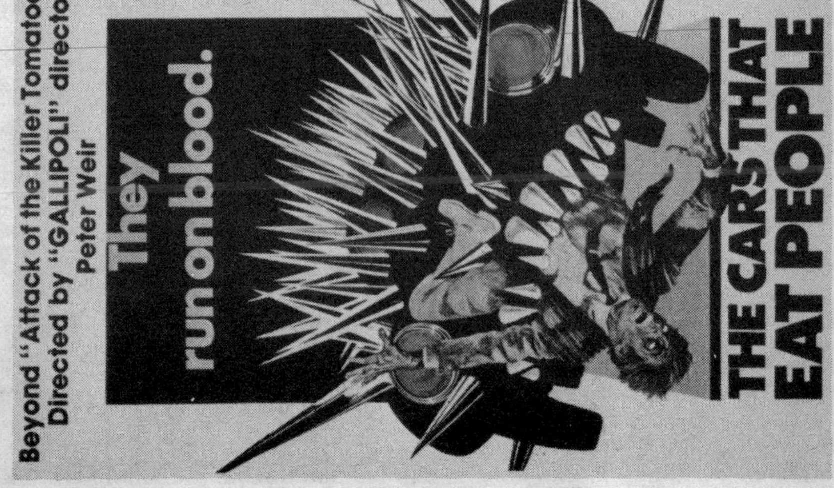

The Cars That Eat People (1977)

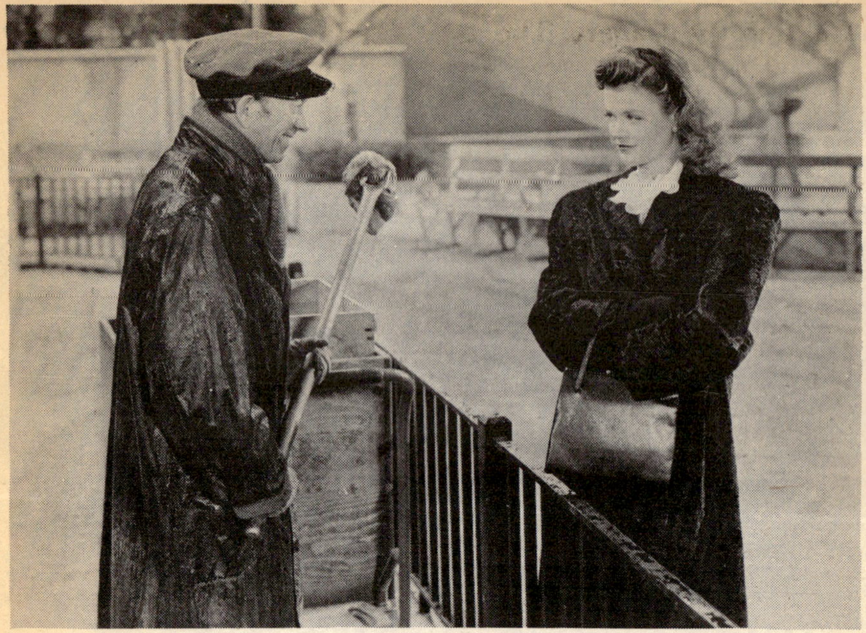

Cat People (1942)

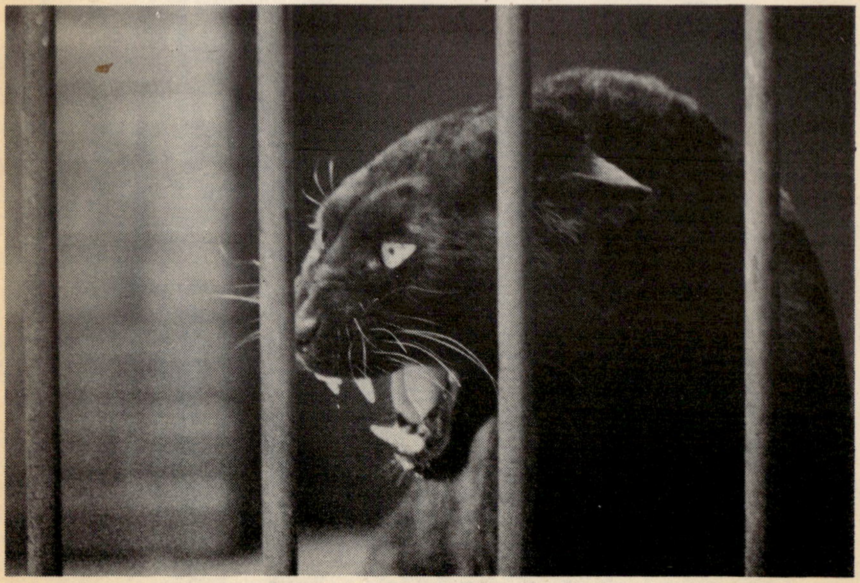

Cat People (1982)

Cat and the Canary, The ★★

(1978) Color, 90 min. Director: Radley Metzger.
Honor Blackman, Michael Callan, Carol Lynley, Olivia Hussey, Edward Fox. Porno filmmaker Metzger made his bid for the mainstream with this updated remake of the silent Paul Leni classic—which had already been remade once before in 1939 as a vehicle for Bob Hope. This time around, Lynley is the beleagured victim of a masked killer who is out to steal her fortune and her sanity. Weak.
(Columbia Pictures Home Entertainment) VC

Cat People ★★★

(1942) B&W, 73 min. Director: Jacques Tourneur.
Simone Simon, Kent Smith, Tom Conway, Jane Randolph. First in the series of now famous Val Lewton-produced horror films of the forties, and one of the best. Simon is convinced that she will turn into a killer cat if she allows her passions to be aroused on her wedding night. Smith is the frustrated bridegroom. Tourneur's now-you-see-it-now-you-don't direction is inspired and succeeds in producing two solid *frissons* that even today have not lost their power to send audiences jumping out of their seats
(Nostalgia Merchant, King of Video) VC

Cat People ★★

(1982) Color, 118 min. Director: Paul Schrader.
Nastassia Kinski, Malcolm McDowell, John Heard, Annette O'Toole. Overlong, overblown remake of Val Lewton's fragile 1942 B-movie classic. The Lewton film moved along at a brisk pace, allowing the viewer little or no time to ponder the essential ridiculousness of the plot. But Schrader shows the cat people bursting out of their human skins, then plods along so that the viewer can't help but ponder such questions as how the cat people metamorphose back into their wrecked human torsos again. Alan Ormsby's script also gets bogged down in trying to create a detailed cat people mythology, something DeWitt Bodeen wisely avoided in the original; he merely sketched in the mythology when needed to propel the plot along. The difference between this *Cat People* and Lewton's is not that the latter is a good film and the former a bad one. It is the difference between skillful cinematic storytelling and ponderousness.
(MCA Videocassette and Disc) VC, LV

Cat Women of the Moon ★

(1953) B&W, 64 min. Director: Arthur Hilton.
Sunny Tufts, Marie Windsor, Victor Jory, Susan Morrow. Astronaut Tufts sets foot on the moon only to discover he is not alone, for below ground there's an empire of telepathic catwomen and above a proliferation of giant spiders. Absolutely horrendous, but boasts one of Elmer Bernstein's earliest film scores.
(Nostalgia Merchant) VC

Cathy's Curse ★ ½

(1980) Color, 91 min. Director: Eddie Matalon.
Alan Scarfe, Randi Allen, Beverly Murray, Roy Witham. Another entry in the let's rip off *The Exorcist* sweepstakes in which a little girl is possessed by the spirit of her long dead aunt, who was burned to death in a car crash. Not very effective Canadian-made chiller.
(Planet Video) VC

Caveman ★★

(1981) Color, 91 min. Director: Carl Gottlieb.
Ringo Starr, Barbara Bach, Dennis Quaid, Jack Gilford, Shelley Long. A prehistoric comedy in the tradition of *Airplane*, but without the latter's zany dialogue—unless you consider lines like "Zug zug!" to be zany. David Allen's stop-motion dinosaurs provide the best, and most amusing, moments.
(CBS/Fox Video) VC

Centerfold Girls

(?) Color, 93 min. Director: John Peyser.
Andrew Prine, Tiffany Bolling. Sexually repressed psycho (Prine) goes on a murder binge with a straight-edged razor, carving up beautiful young women who have posed nude for a girlie magazine called *Bachelor.* Standard mad slasher stuff.
(Media Home Entertainment) VC

Chandu on the Magic Island

(1935) B&W, 67 min. Director: Ray Taylor.
Bela Lugosi, Maria Alba, Clara Kimball Young, Joseph Swickard. Sequel to the serial *Return of Chandu.*
(Video Yesteryear) VC

Changeling, The

(1980) Color, 114 min. Director: Peter Medak.
George C. Scott, Trish Van Devere, Melvyn Douglas, John Colicos. Music teacher Scott, who lost his family in a car accident, moves into an old house which he discovers is haunted by the anguished spirit of a young boy who was murdered there years before. Slick but almost painfully predictable.
(Vestron Video) VC

Chariots of the Gods?

(1974) Color, 97 min. Director: Dr. Harald Reinl.
Documentary based on the internationally best-selling treatise of the same name by Erich Von Daniken, which advances the theory that earth was visited many centuries ago by superior beings from another planet, who left their mark by helping to build the pyramids and other supposedly man-made wonders. A mind-stretching idea dully expressed.
(Video Communications) VC

Charlotte's Web

(1973) Color, 94 min. Directors: Charles Nichols, Iwao Takamoto.
Voices of Debbie Reynolds, Henry Gibson, Paul Lynde, Charles Nelson Reilly, Agnes Moorehead. Delightful animated version of the E.B. White children's classic about a cowardly pig who lives in deathly fear of the slaughterhouse, and the courageous spider who saves his bacon.
(Paramount Home Video, RCA VideoDisc) VC, CED, LV

Charly

(1968) Color, 103 min. Director: Ralph Nelson.
Cliff Robertson, Claire Bloom, Lilia Skala, Leon Janney, Dick Van Patten. Mentally retarded man (Robertson) undergoes advanced scientific experiment which transforms him into a brain. The problem is that the effects of the experiment won't last and so he's doomed to regress. Robertson won an Oscar for his performance though it's hard to see why; he's not really convincing as the retarded Charly. Daniel Keyes' book *Flowers for Algernon,* upon which the film is based, is infinitely more moving.
(CBS/Fox Video) VC, CED)

Child, The ½

(1977) Color, 83 min. Director: Robert Voskanian.
Richard Hanners, Laurel Bennett, Frank Janson, Rosalie Cole. A little girl, who, perhaps, has seen *The Exorcist* one too many times, starts hanging around at the local cemetery where her mother is buried and soon makes friends with a number of flesh-eating ghouls who also happen to be hanging around (in shreds), and uses her supernatural powers to make them do her bidding.
(Family Home Entertainment, AstroVideo) VC

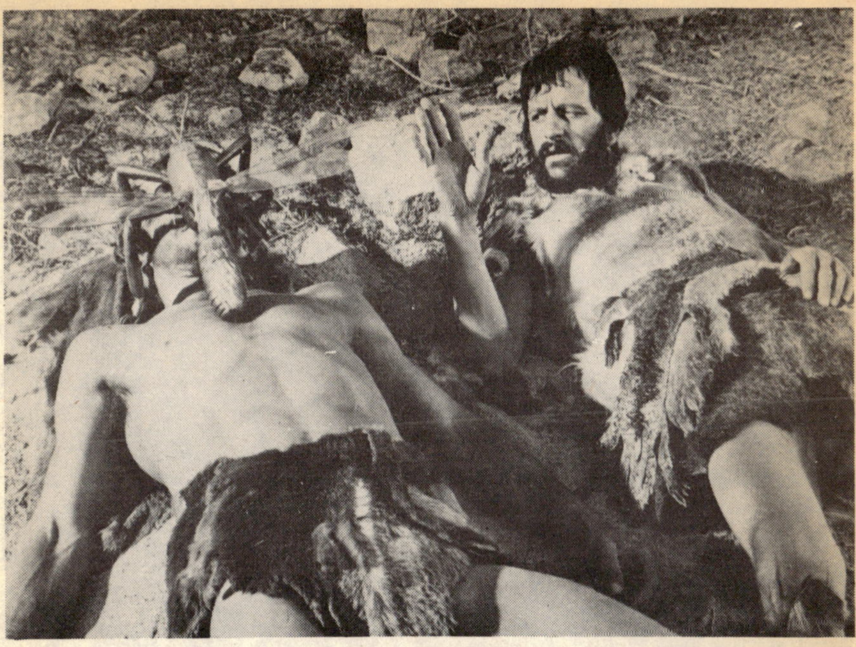

Caveman (1981)

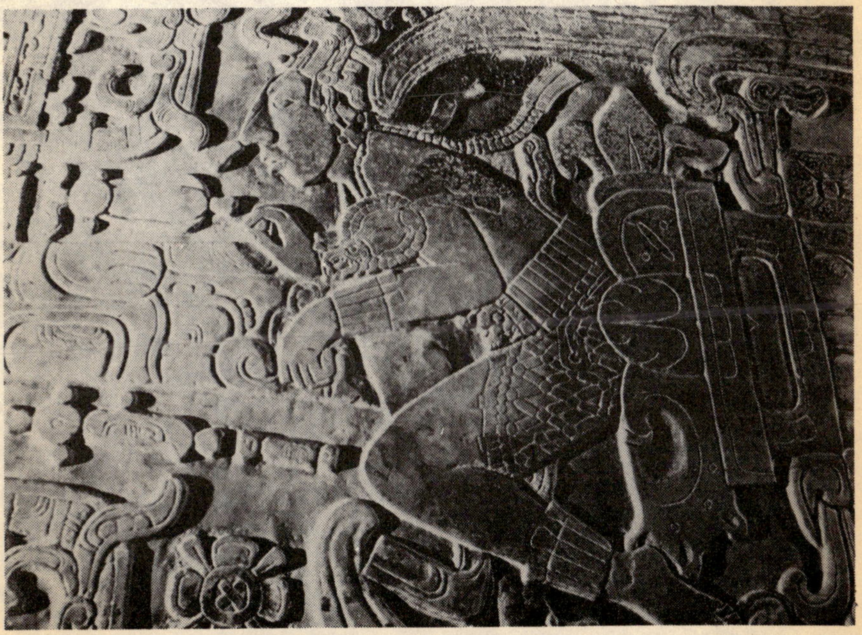

Chariots of the Gods? (1974)

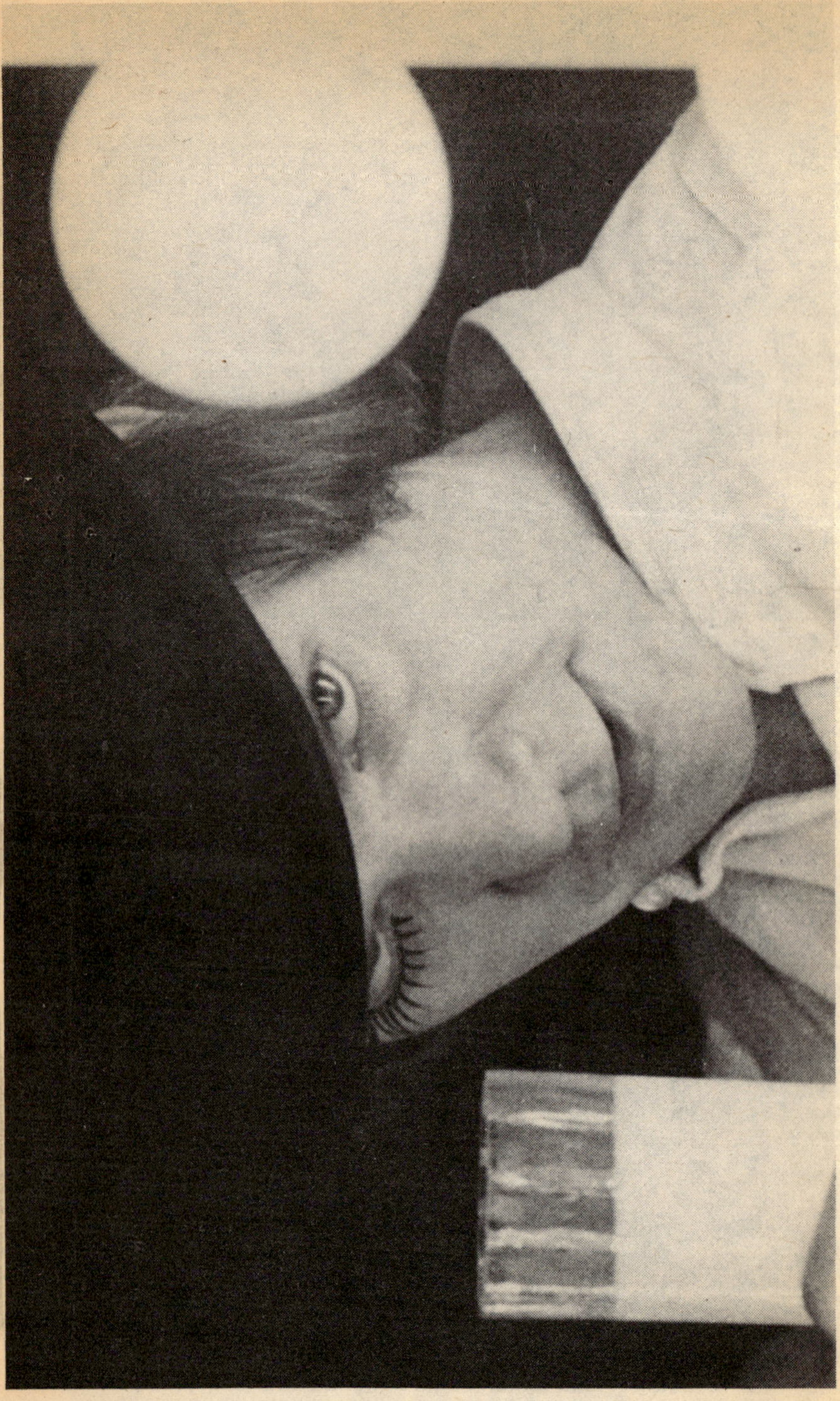

A Clockwork Orange (1971)

Children Shouldn't Play with Dead Things ½

(1972) Color, 85 min. Director: Bob Clark.
Alan Ormsby, Valerie Mauches, Anya Ormsby, Paul Cronin. Low-budgeter filmed in Florida. A group of actors descends upon an abandoned graveyard on a supposedly deserted island to make a horror movie and encounters corpses who rise from their graves to help lend a touch of realism. Half humor, half horror, all amateurish.
(Video Communications) VC

Clash of the Titans

(1981) Color, 127 min. Director: Douglas Hickox.
Harry Hamlin, Burgess Meredith, Judi Bowker, Sir Laurence Olivier, Maggie Smith, Ursula Andress. Popular but under-rated Ray Harryhausen fantasy about the exploits of Perseus (Hamlin) as he attempts to win the hand of the fair Andromeda (Bowker). Great special effects, and a good story too.
(MGM/UA Home Video) VC, CED

Clockwork Orange, A ½

(1971) Color, 137 min. Director: Stanley Kubrick.
Malcolm McDowell, Patrick Magee, Warren Clarke, Michael Bates, Anthony Sharp. Dark, ironic tale of crime and punishment in an ultra-violent future—which has since become the present. McDowell is Alex, a young, conscienceless punk who rapes and kills without remorse until society steps in to re-condition him. First-class filmmaking, chilling, challenging and rough. Based on the book by Anthony Burgess.
(Warner Home Video) VC

Close Encounters of the Third Kind Special Edition

(1977) Color, 134 min. Director: Steven Spielberg.
Richard Dreyfuss, Melinda Dillon, Terri Garr, Cary Guffey, Francois Truffaut. Dreyfuss is a combination Pinocchio and Everyman, who wishes upon a star and actually gets his wish—a visit from benign beings from outer space who spirit him off to a never-never land beyond his wildest middle-class dreams. Technically awesome, marred only by some embarrassing scenes of domestic non-bliss.
(Columbia Pictures Home Entertainment, RCA VideoDisc) VC, CED, LV

Collector, The ½

(1965) Color, 119 min. Director: William Wyler.
Terence Stamp, Samantha Eggar. Psychologically disturbed butterfly collector Stamp kidnaps beauteous Eggar with the object of putting her too under glass. Well acted, but remote chiller based on the novel by John Fowles. Nice score by Maurice Jarre.
(Columbia Pictures Home Entertainment) VC

Color Me Blood Red

(1964) Color, 74 min. Director: Herschell Gordon Lewis.
Don Joseph, Candy Conder, Scott H. Hall, Elyn Warner. A mad artist uses human blood instead of Grumbacher red to spice up his palette. Buckets of gore from one of the pioneers of today's splatter movie trend.
(Video Dimensions) VC

Coma ☐☐

(1978) Color, 112 min. Director: Michael Crichton.
Genevieve Bujold, Michael Douglas, Elizabeth Ashley, Rip Torn, Richard Widmark. Young doctor Bujold discovers an illicit organ bank operating out of her own Boston hospital, where incoming patients are randomly murdered for their precious body parts. Soon her own life is in danger. Interesting idea, but treated too much like *The Perils of Pauline*.
(MGM/UA Home Video) VC, CED

Conan the Barbarian ☐½

(1982) Color, 129 min. Director: John Milius.
Arnold Schwarzenegger, James Earl Jones, Sandahl Bergman, Gerry Lopez. Milius' macho fantasy-adventure about the killer strongman of the Hyborian Age (drawn from the pulp novels and short stories of Robert E. Howard) is spectacular, violent, and tedious. Schwarzenegger certainly looks the part of the muscle-bound hero, and Bergman makes a voluptuous, sword-wielding Valeria, but their characters, like the film itself, never really come alive.
(MCA Videocassette and Disc) VC, LV

Condorman ☐

(1981) Color, 90 min. Director: Charles Jarrott.
Michael Crawford, Oliver Reed, Barbara Carrera. Comic book artist Crawford, a stickler for authenticity, insists that his super hero character, Condorman, not attempt what he himself can't do. So he sets out on a series of James Bond-like misadventures accompanied by a beautiful KGB agent. Dated derring-do.
(Walt Disney Home Video) VC

Cosmic Monsters ☐½

(1958) B&W, 75 min. Director: Gilbert Gunn.
Forrest Tucker, Gaby Andre, Alec Mango, Hugh Latimer. A scientist's bizarre experiment goes awry, ripping a hole in the sky, through which spill aliens and mutant insects bent on conquering earth. Good idea for a Raid commercial.
(Nostalgia Merchant) VC

Crater Lake Monster, The ☐

(1977) Color, 85 min. Director: William Stromberg.
Cardella, Glenn Roberts, Mark Siegel, Kacey Cobb. Mutant, prehistoric monster with flippers hatches from an egg within a mountain lake and crawls—or, rather, flops—up from the depths to terrify absolutely no one, particularly the audience. Model animation effects by David *Caveman* Allen.
(Video Communications, Inc.) VC

Crawling Eye, The ☐☐

(1958) B&W, 85 min. Director: Quentin Lawrence.
Forrest Tucker, Laurence Payne, Janet Munro, Warren Mitchell. The mountainous Swiss town of Trollenberg is suddenly enveloped by a mysterious mist, at the eye of which appears. . .an eye, the biggest peeping tom ever, out not just to stare the residents to death, but to chop off their heads as well. Ludicrous but fun, with a script by Jimmy Sangster.
(Nostalgia Merchant) VC

Crawling Hand, The ☐½

(1963) B&W, 89 min. Director: Herbert L. Strock.
Kent Taylor, Alan Hale, Allison Hayes, Richard Arlen, Peter Breck. An astronaut returns to earth with his own dismembered hand, which has become possessed by an alien life form. The hand decides to go on a murder spree.
(Video Gems) VC

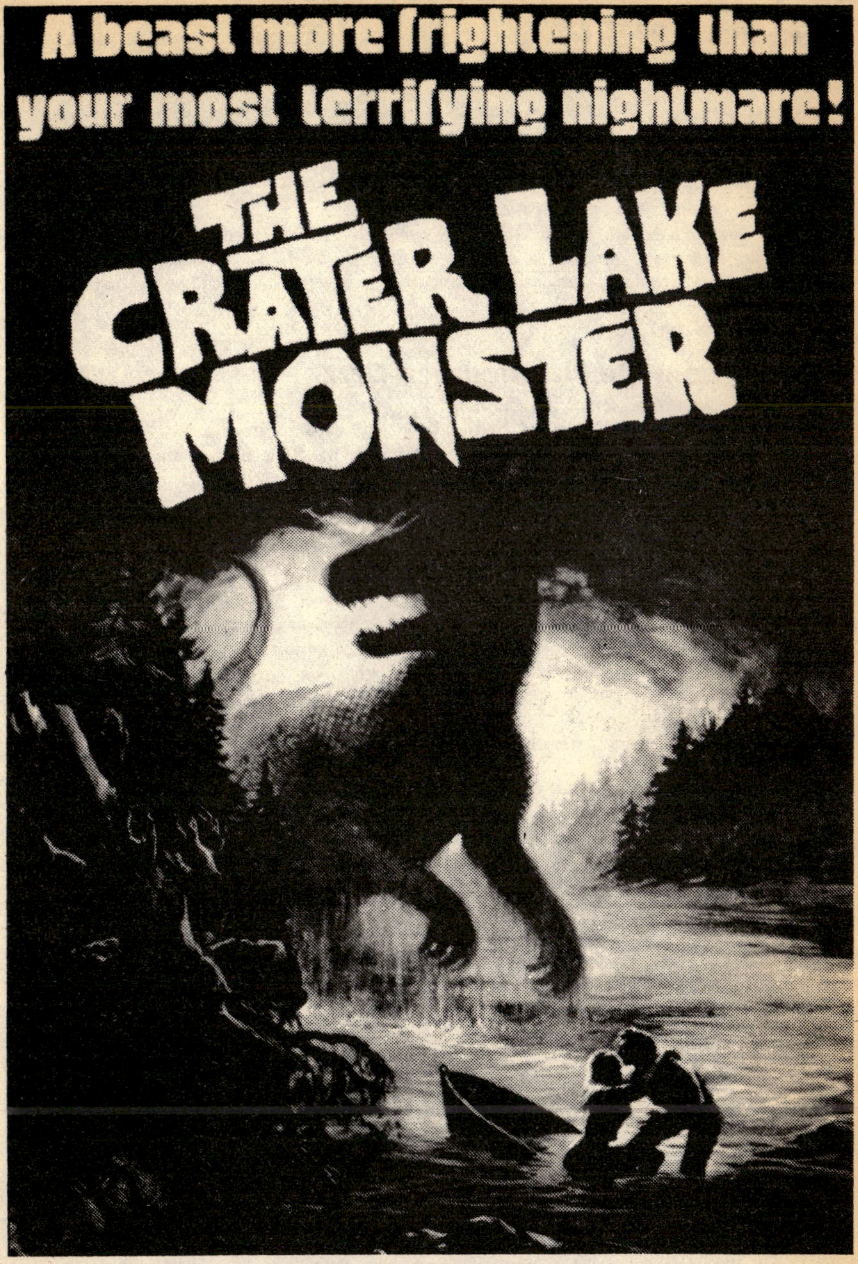
A beast more frightening than
your most terrifying nightmare!
THE
CRATER LAKE
MONSTER

The Crater Lake Monster (1977)

Crazy Ray, The ½

(1923) B&W, 61 min. Director: Rene Clair.
Henri Rollan, Albert Prejean, Madeleine Rodrigue, Marcel Vallee, Charles Martinelli. A ray projected from the top of the Eiffel Tower makes the city of Paris come to a standstill. Inventive.
(Video Archives) VC

Creature from the Black Lagoon, The ½

(1954) B&W, 79 min. Director: Jack Arnold.
Richard Carlson, Julia Adams, Richard Denning, Nestor Paiva, Whit Bissell. An expedition up the Amazon River leads to the discovery of a prehistoric gill man. Cliched sci-fi, but exciting, especially in 3-D, the process in which it was originally filmed and in which it is presently being made available on cassette.
(MCA Videocassette) VC

Creature from the Haunted Sea

(1961) B&W, 63 min. Director: Roger Corman.
Antony Carbone, Betsy Jones-Moreland, Edward Wain. A cheesy undersea monster terrorizes a boat-load of first-class idiots in this low-budget, totally spaced out satire on everything from Bogart to Bond. Hilarious.
(Video Yesteryear) VC

Creeping Flesh, The ½

(1972) Color, 90 min. Director: Freddie Francis.
Peter Cushing, Christopher Lee, George Benson, Lorna Heilbron, Duncan Lamont, Michael Ripper. A Lovecraftian-themed monster movie in which archaeologist Cushing discovers the skeleton of a being belonging to an ancient race of giants. When the creature is doused with rainwater, its flesh reappears and it revives to stalk the countryside. Far-fetched but nicely done. Cushing gives one of his most affecting performances as the sincere scientist who is undone by his discovery.
(Columbia Pictures Home Entertainment) VC

Creeping Terror, The

(1964) B&W, 75 min. Director: A.J. Nelson.
Vic Savage, Shannon O'Neil. Grotesque, macaroni-like creature from outer space lands on earth so that it can wiggle up on people and eat them. Here's a film that's distinguished by its astounding awfulness in every department—bad writing, direction, acting, special effects, music, you name it!
(Video Communications, Inc.) VC

Creepshow

(1982) Color, 122 min. Director: George A. Romero.
Hal Holbrook, Adrienne Barbeau, Fritz Weaver, E.G. Marshall, Stephen King. Romero and best-selling author Stephen King collaborated on this hymn to the popular E.C. horror comics of the early fifties. The film consists of five separate stories each dealing with death, revenge, monsters and such. Marshall's episode in which a man who hates bugs is ultimately done in by thousands of cockroaches is arguably the best. Overlong and not as scary as it might have been, but good tongue-in-cheek fun nonetheless. Tom Savini's special effects are not for the squeamish.
(Warner Home Video) VC

Crucible of Terror

(1971) Color, 91 min. Director: Ted Hooker.
Mike Raven, Mary Maude, James Bolam, Melissa Stribling, Ronald Lacey. British-made cross between Roger Corman's amusing *Bucket of Blood* and Herschell G. Lewis' gorefest *Color Me Blood Red* in which a mad sculptor creates his prize-winning busts by coating his female models in bronze. Assorted sub-plots add to the tedium.
(Video Gems) VC

Crypt of the Living Dead ☐

(1973) Color, 93 min. Director: Ray Danton.
Andrew Prine, Mark Damon, Patty Shepard, Jack La Rue, Jr. The corpse of the vampire bride of a soldier killed during the Crusades is unearthed by a bunch of dummies who have never seen a horror movie and obviously don't know better, and she predictably comes back to life, thirsting for blood. A.k.a. *Young Hannah, Queen of the Vampires.*
(Direct Video) VC

Curse of the Cat People, The ☐☐½

(1944) B&W, 70 min. Directors: Robert Wise, Gunther von Fritsch.
Simone Simon, Kent Smith, Jane Randolph, Elizabeth Russell, Sir Lancelot. Simon's ghost returns not as a cat but as an imaginary playmate for her ex-husband's lonely little daughter. Ethereal Val Lewton film is not really a sequel to *Cat People,* but a totally different kind of film.
(Nostalgia Merchant) VC

Curse of the Crying Woman ☐½

(1961) B&W, 74 min. Director: Raphael Baledon.
Abel Salazar, Rosita Arenas, Rita Macedo, Domingo Soler, Carlos Moctezuma. Mexican horror film star Salazar also produced this tedious recounting of a supposedly well-known Mexican legend about a witch who returns from the grave to curse everybody out.
(Budget Video) VC

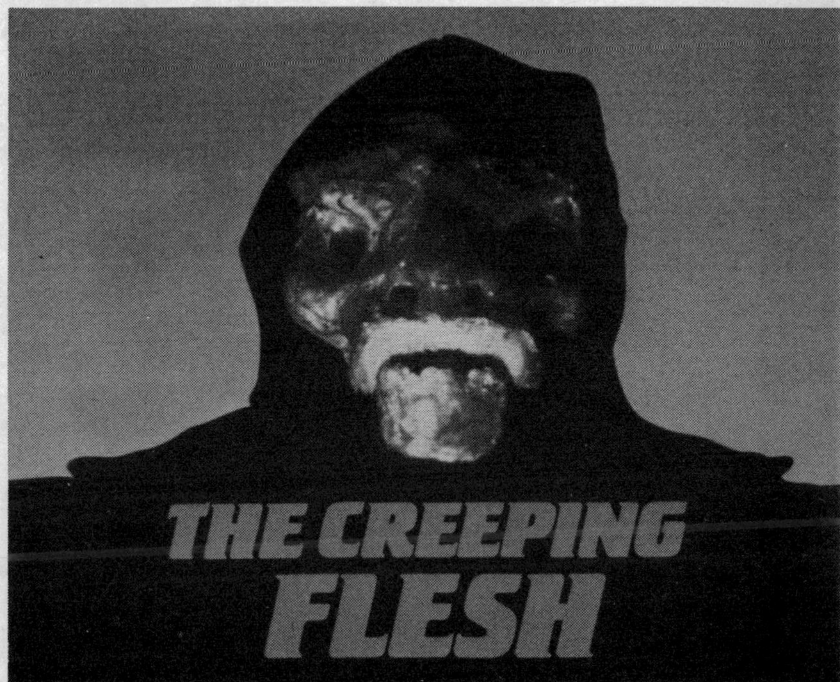

The Creeping Flesh (1972)

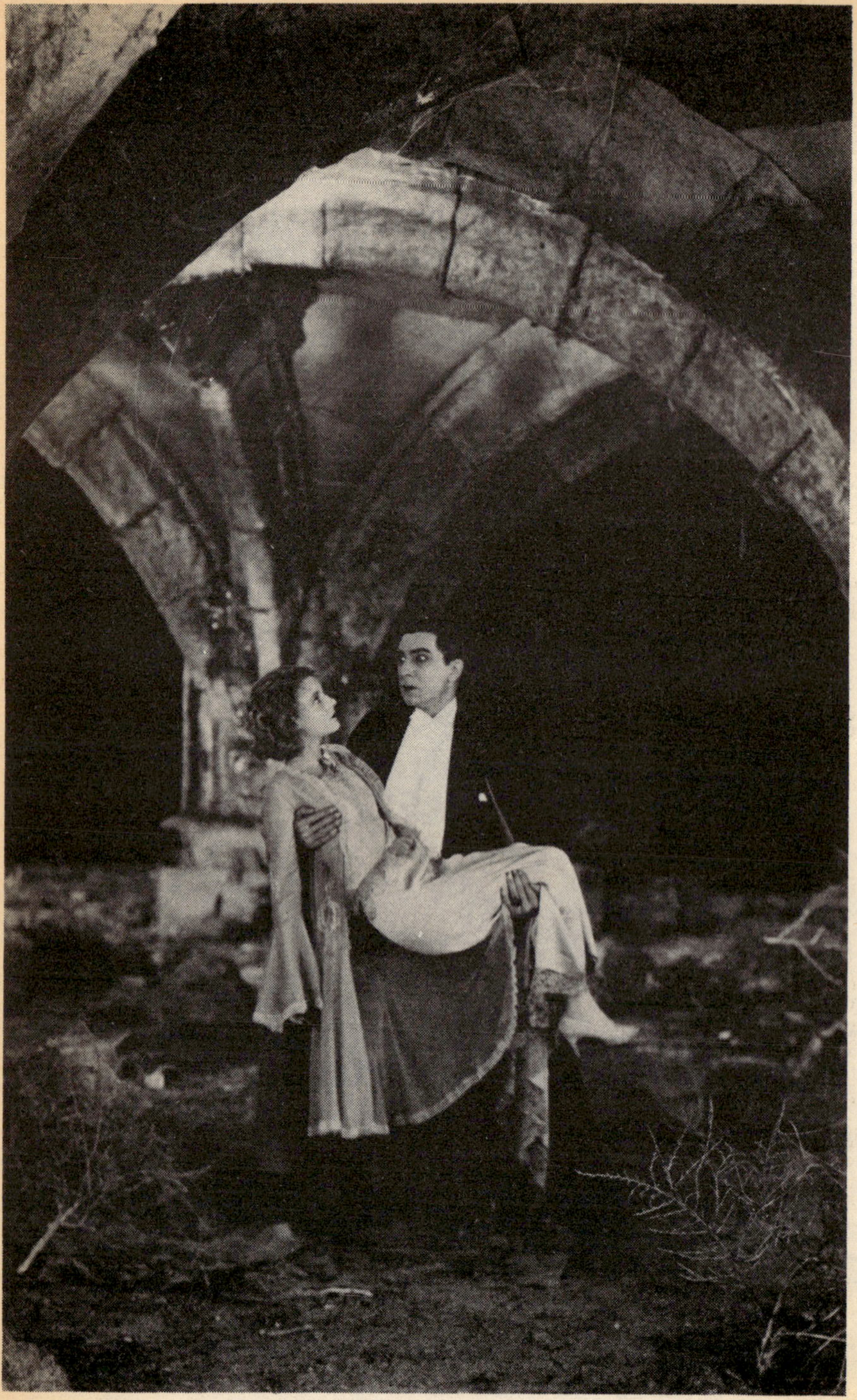

Dracula (1931)

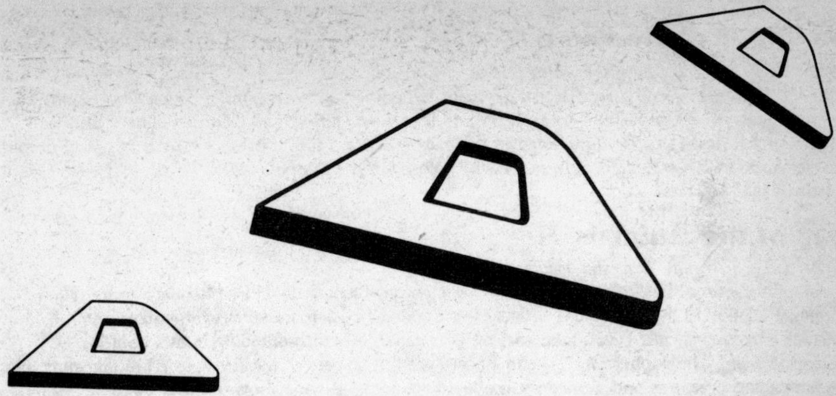

Damien—Omen II ½

(1978) Color, 110 min. Director: Don Taylor.
William Holden, Lee Grant, Lew Ayres, Robert Foxworth, Sylvia Sidney. An interestng idea is thrown away in favor of keeping up the gore score as the devil's child is groomed by villain Foxworth to take over Thorn Industries, a multi-national company capable of hastening Armageddon by throwing the world into political and economic chaos. Sequel to *The Omen.*
(CBS/Fox Video) VC, CED

Darby O'Gill and the Little People

(1959) Color, 93 min. Director: Robert Stevenson.
Albert Sharpe, Janet Munro, Sean Connery, Jimmy O'Dea, Kieron Moore, Estelle Winwood. O'Gill, a caretaker on an old Irish estate, spins so many fanciful stories that no one believes anything he says anymore, especially when it comes to leprechauns, with whom he soon goes into cahoots, matching wits with King Brian of the Leprechauns himself. Colorful Disney fantasy with outstanding special effects. Lots of blarney, but fun all the way.
(Walt Disney Home Video) VC

Dark, The

(1979) Color, 92 min. Director: John "Bud" Cardos.
William Devane, Cathy Lee Crosby, Richard Jaeckel, Keenan Wynn. Los Angeles skid row murders perpetrated by an unknown killer dubbed the "mangler" by the press turn out to be the work of a werewolf-like alien from outer space with glowing red eyes and a really rotten disposition. Absolute junk.
(Media Home Entertainment) VC

Dark Star

(1975) Color, 83 min. Director: John Carpenter.
Dan O'Bannon, Andreijah Pahich, Brian Narelle. Carpenter began this film as an elaborate 16mm short while a student at the University of Southern California, but producer Jack H. Harris smelled commercial potential and helped him expand it into a theatrical feature. An amusing satire of rocket operas, from *Buck Rogers* to *2001.* O'Bannon later went on to write *Alien.*
(Video Communications, Budget Video) VC

Daughter of Horror ✪✪

(1953) B&W, 60 min. Director: John Parker.
Adrienne Barret, Bruno Ve Sota, Ben Roseman. Experimental fantasy full of psychotic illusions like severed hands on the prowl and so forth. Future film music luminaries George Antheil, Shorty Rogers, and Ernest Gold co-contributed to the bizarre score. Marni Nixon, who did the singing for Natalie Wood in *West Side Story*, provides the solos. A.k.a. *Dementia.*
(Thunderbird Films) VC

Day of the Animals ✪

(1977) Color, 95 min. Director: William Girdler.
Christopher George, Leslie Nielsen, Linda Day George, Richard Jaeckel, Michael Ansara, Ruth Roman. Pollution of the earth's ozone layer from overuse of aerosol sprays turns nature's livestock—birds, wildcats, bears, rats, snakes, you name it—into marauding beasts bent on destroying man. Christopher George and Ansara are the leaders of a wilderness party that runs into the rampaging creatures and must do some fast thinking to survive. Lots of gore, but little else.
(Media Home Entertainment) VC

Day of the Triffids ✪✪½

(1963) Color, 94 min. Director: Steve Sekely.
Howard Keel, Nicole Maurey, Janette Scott, Kieron Moore. Disaster strikes on a global scale as a meteorite shower blinds everyone who sees it and causes carnivorous extraterrestrial plants to mutate all over the earth. Okay adaptation of John Wyndham's nifty sci-fi novel of the same name.
(Media Home Entertainment, Budget Video, King of Video) VC

Day of Wrath ✪✪✪

(1943) B&W, 100 min. Director: Carl Dreyer.
Thorkild Roose, Lisbeth Movin, Sigrid Neiiendam, Preben Lerdoff. Ponderous but absorbing—and meticulously detailed—study of religious persecution in 17th century Holland. The atmosphere is overwhelming.
(Cable Films) VC

Day the Earth Caught Fire, The ✪✪✪

(1962) B&W, 90 min. Director: Val Guest.
Edward Judd, Leo McKern, Janet Munro. Simultaneous nuclear tests conducted by the superpowers at the North and South Poles alter the earth's orbit, sending the planet hurtling towards the sun in this cautionary sci-fi chiller that is just as timely today as it was 20 years ago. Much of the film is set in the offices of a large London newspaper and the scenes of the reporters at work on this biggest of all disaster stories are most convincing.
(Thorn/EMI Video) VC

Day the Earth Stood Still, The ✪✪✪

(1951) B&W, 92 min. Director: Robert Wise.
Michael Rennie, Patricia Neal, Sam Jaffe, Hugh Marlowe, Billy Gray. Rennie, a visitor from another planet, arrives on earth accompanied by a strong-armed robot named Gort to warn earthlings that their warlike habits will not be tolerated if they try to extend them to outer space. A topical film when it was made; it remains even more topical now. Great score by Bernard Herrmann.
(CBS/Fox Video) VC

Day Time Ended, The ✪

(1980) Color, 79 min. Director: John "Bud" Cardos.
Jim Davis, Dorothy Malone, Chris Mitchum, Marcy Lafferty. Davis and his family encounter strange, glowing pyramids, gremlins and other phenomena as their remote desert home is beseiged by beings from an alien world. In the end, their house disappears into a time warp. Make sense?
(Media Home Entertainment) VC

Dead of Night ☑☑☑

(1946) B&W, 102 min. Directors: Alberto Cavalcanti, Charles Crichton, Basil Dearden, Robert Hamer.
Michael Redgrave, Googie Withers, Mervyn Johns, Sally Anne Howes. A quartet of ghost stories. Most famous, and finest, is the one in which ventriloquist Redgrave and his dummy lock horns in a deadly game of identity.
(Thorn/EMI Video) VC

Dear Dead Delilah ☑☑

(1972) Color, 95 min. Director: John Farris.
Agnes Moorehead, Will Geer, Patricia Carmichael, Dennis Patrick, Michael Ansara. Moorehead is the wealthy but dying matriarch of a decaying southern clan whose heirs are being systematically butchered by an axe-wielding maniac. In the tradition of *Hush. . .Hush, Sweet Charlotte*, but with gore galore.
(Cinema Concepts) VC

Death Kiss, The ☑☑

(1933) B&W, 75 min. Director: (?)
Bela Lugosi, David Manners, Adrienne Ames. A phantom killer stalks a big time Hollywood movie studio where obviously this film was *not* made.
(Thunderbird Films) VC

Death Machines ☑

(1976) Color, 90 min. Director: Paul Kyriazi.
Ron Marchini, Mari Honjo, Chuck Katzaian, Michael Chong. Dragon Lady mobstress Honjo turns ethnic trio of martial experts into cold-blooded assassins by injecting them with a special serum. You guessed it, she's out to dominate the world. Lots of kung-fu action and other forms of mayhem, but not much else.
(Video Communications) VC

Death Race 2000 ☑☑½

(1975) Color, 85 min. Director: Paul Bartel.
David Carradine, Sylvester Stallone, Simone Griffith, Louisa Moritz. Outrageous satire set in a futuristic America where hit-and-run driving has become the national sport and cross-country racers rack up points for achieving the highest body count. Stallone is particularly funny as a souped-up gangster from Chicago who strives to cheat at every turn. Bloody, but fun.
(Warner Home Videa) VC

Death Smiles on a Murderer ☑

(1974) Color, 79 min. Director: Aristide Massaccesi.
Klaus Kinski, Ewa Aulin, Angelo Bo. Kinski chews up the scenery as a mad doctor bent on reviving the dead in this confusing and gory gothic horror tale.
(Demonique Video) VC

Death Sport ☑☑

(1978) Color, 90 min. Directors: Allan Arkush, Henry Suso.
David Carradine, Claudia Jennings, Richard Lynch. It's the year 3000. Earth is a wasteland roamed by cannibal mutants and gladiators known as Range Guides who do their fighting on motorcycles.
(Warner Home Video) VC

Death Valley ½

(1982) Color, 90 min. Director: Dick Richards.
Paul LeMat, Catherine Hicks, Stephen McHattie. Former TV commercial director Richards has an undeniable flair for the pictorial, but that's about all. This film and his two previous features—*The Culpepper Cattle Company, March or Die*—are striking visually, but except for their taboo scenes of sex and violence, they seem like glorified TV commercials—slick, but empty. This one, about a young couple who are victimized by a deranged young desert rat and who must kill to survive, is no exception. Typical slasher fare, glossy and gory.
(MCA Videocassette) VC

Dementia 13 ½

(1963) B&W, 81 min. Director: Francis Ford Coppola.
William Campbell, Luana Anders, Bart Parton, Patrick Magee. Filmed by newcomer Coppola in Ireland for producer Roger Corman. It's about a weird family, one of whose members died years before in a drowning accident—or was it an axe murder? Some coroner they must have had not to be able to tell the difference. Anyway, now the axeman is back.
(Video Yesteryear, Budget Video) VC

Demon, The

(1981) Color, 94 min. Director: (?)
Cameron Mitchell, Jennifer Holmes. Residents of a small town off the beaten track are being stalked and killed by a bloodthirsty creature who's out to reduce the town's census to zero.
(Video Communications) VC

Demon Lover, The

(1976) Color, 85 min. Directors: Donald G. Jackson, Jerry Younkins.
Gunnar Hansen, Val Mayerik, Christmas Robbins, Tom Hutton. Low budgeter about an occultist who conjures up a hideous demon to do his bidding but then must deal with the beast when it turns on him too. A must-see for those of you who enjoyed Hansen as "Leatherface" in *The Texas Chainsaw Massacre.*
(Unicorn Video) VC

Desperate Living

(1977) Color, 90 min. Director: John Waters.
Liz Renay, Mink Stole, Susan Lowe, Edith Massey, Mary Vivian Pearce, Jean Hill. Released from a mental hospital, socialite Stole later runs off with her 400-pound maid (Hill) when the maid kills Mink's husband by sitting on him and squashing him to death. The pair then holes up in a town called Mortville which is populated by criminals and run by an Idi Amin-worshipping fat lady (Massey).
(Wizard Video) VC

Destination Moon ½

(1950) Color, 91 min. Director: Irving Pichel.
John Archer, Warner Anderson, Tom Powers, Dick Wesson. Pioneer space film about man's first voyage to the moon, acclaimed at the time for its documentary flavor and emphasis on detail rather than action. Dated now, but still interesting. Based on Robert A. Heinlein's novel *Rocket Ship Galileo* and co-scripted by Heinlein himself.
(Nostalgia Merchant) VC

Devil and Max Devlin, The ½

(1979) Color, 96 min. Director: Steven Hilliard Stern.
Elliott Gould, Bill Cosby, Susan Anspach, Adam Rich. Gould is the beleagured manager of a rundown apartment building who is struck and killed one morning by a bus, then makes a deal with the devil that his life be restored to him if he can convince three people to sell their own souls in exchange. Cute story, with Cosby delivering some priceless lines as the devil's fork-tongued assistant, Barney Satin. But not a total success.
(Walt Disney Home Video) VC

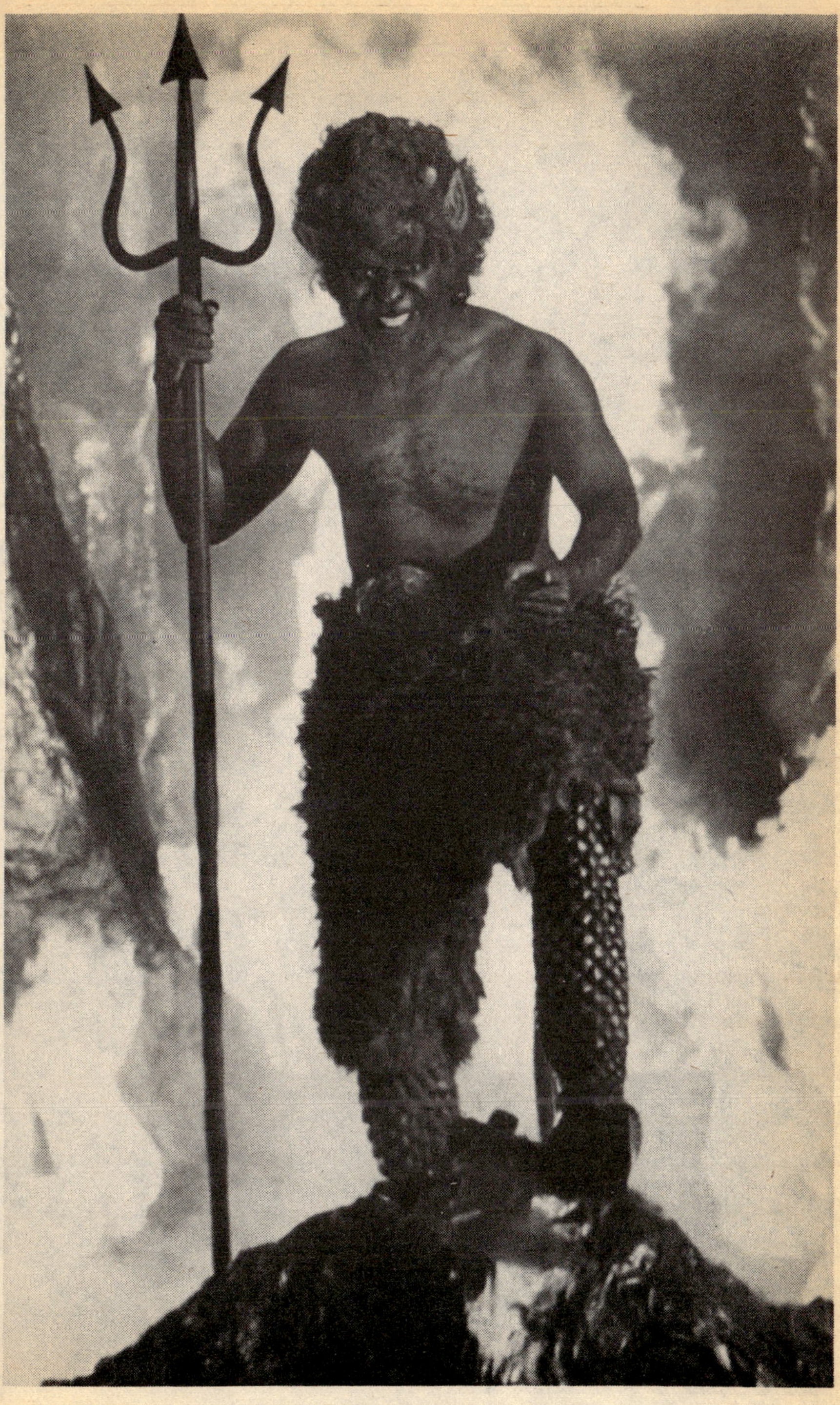

The Devil and Max Devlin (1979)

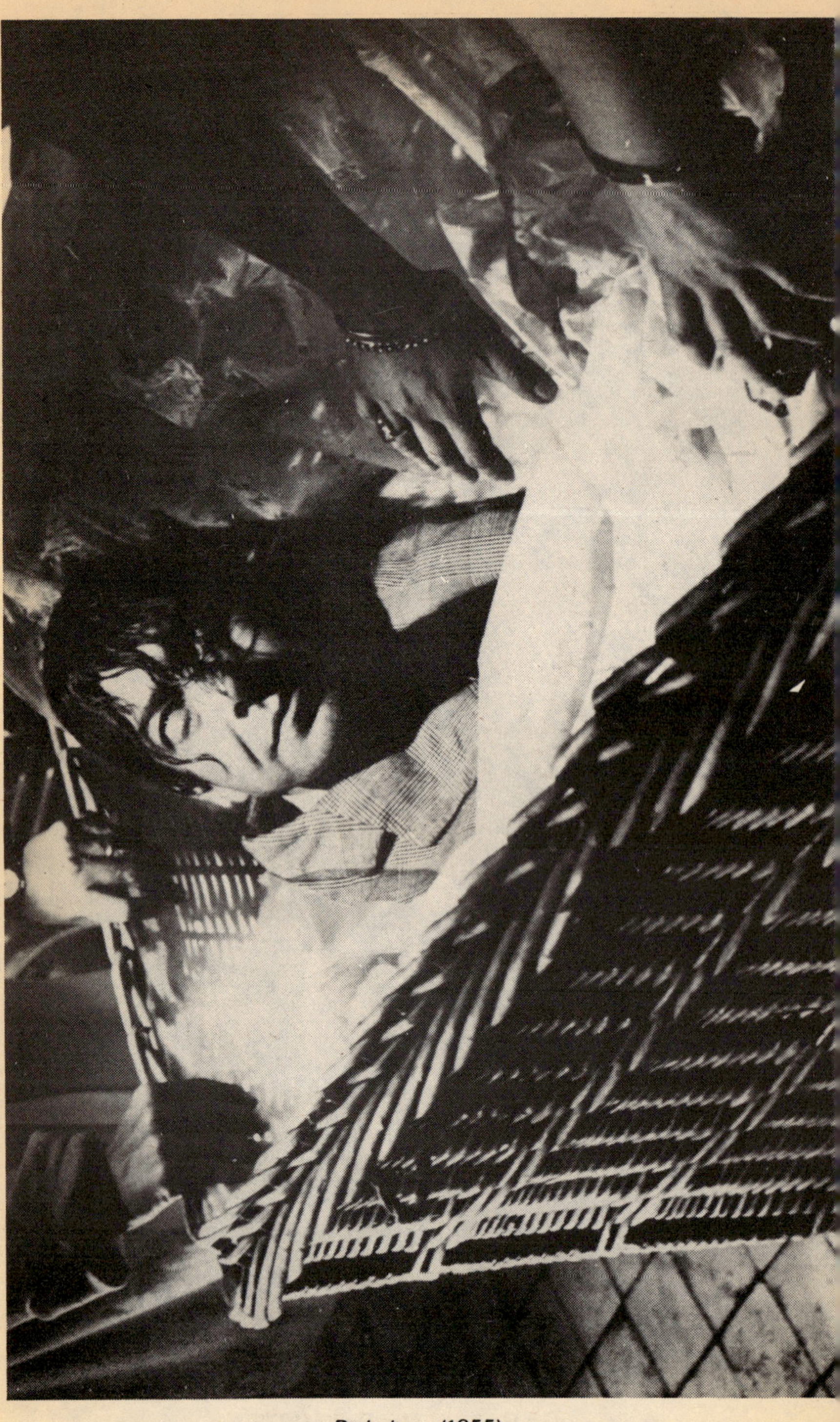

Diabolique (1955)

Devil Girl from Mars ½

(1954) B&W, 76 min. Director: David MacDonald.
Patricia Laffan, Hazel Court, Hugh McDermott, Adrienne Corri, Peter Reynolds. Fifties British sci-fi in which a woman from Mars crash lands in the United Kingdom to begin searching for earthmen with whom she can spawn a breed of space tots.
(Nostalgia Merchant) VC

Devil Times Five

(1979) Color, 90 min. Director: Sean MacGregor.
Gene Evans, Sorrell Booke, Leif Garrett, Carolyn Stellar. Murderous children go on the rampage. Originally released in 1974 as *The Horrible House on the Hill.*
(Media Home Entertainment) VC

Devils, The

(1971) Color, 109 min. Director: Ken Russell.
Oliver Reed, Vanessa Redgrave, Dudley Sutton, Gemma Jones, Michael Gothard. A harrowing, exhausting film drawn from John Whiting's play of the same name and Aldous Huxley's book *The Devils of Loudon.* About a case of religious and sexual hysteria that breaks out in a convent in the self-governing, 17th century city of Loudon, France and the evil men who use the incident to destroy the philandering priest (Reed) who stands in the way of Cardinal Richlieu's plot to hold religious and political dominion over the entire country. Film demands repeated viewings for everything to sink in. But its message of the threat to personal freedom that results from combining church and state is an important one. Especially today.
(Warner Home Video) VC

Devil's Rain, The

(1975) Color, 85 min. Director: Robert Fuest.
Ernest Borgnine, Eddie Albert, Ida Lupino, William Shatner, Keenan Wynn. Satanism and witchcraft flourish in a dusty southwestern town, which is also the gateway to Hell. Hero Shatner tries to abscond with the devil's guest register. In the end, the rain of the title turns all the satanists into pizzas. A real mess. Look for John Travolta in a small role.
(Video Communications) VC

Devil's Wedding Night, The ½

(1973) Color, 85 min. Director: Paul Solvay.
Mark Damon, Sara Bay. An archaeologist discovers a mysterious ring that has the secret power to draw young girls to the mysterious Transylvanian castle near which it was found. The ring, it turns out, once belonged to Count Dracula himself.
(Video Communications) VC

Diabolique ½

(1955) B&W, 107 min. Director: Henri-Georges Clouzot.
Simone Signoret, Vera Clouzot, Paul Meurisse, Charles Vanel. The put-upon wife and mistress of the obnoxious headmaster of a boy's school plot and carry out an intricate scheme to murder him, dumping his crated-up body in the school's swimming pool. Come morning, however, the pool is drained and the crate and body have mysteriously vanished. The victim, apparently, is still alive and lusting for revenge. Scary murder mystery with a neat surprise twist.
(Budget Video, Direct Video) VC

Diamonds Are Forever

(1971) Color, 119 min. Director: Guy Hamilton.

Sean Connery, Jill St. John, Charles Gray, Jimmy Dean. After a hiatus of one film (George Lazenby played 007 in *On Her Majesty's Secret Service*, released the year before), Sean Connery returned to the screen to play Bond for one last time in this seventh entry in the popular series. Too bad he didn't choose *OHMSS* as his swan song; it was a much better film. This time around, Bond is once again on the trail of his arch enemy Ernst Stavro Blofeld (Gray), who, like Dr. No before him, is messing around with the lives of British agents as well as America's space program. The chase leads Bond from London to Las Vegas and climaxes in a battle on an oil rig in the middle of the Gulf of Mexico. Eye-filling, but empty. Bears absolutely no resemblance to the Ian Fleming novel on which it is based and is the worse for it.

(CBS/Fox Video, RCA VideoDisc) VC, CED

Dr. Black, Mr. Hyde

(1976) Color, 87 min. Director: William Crain.

Bernie Casey, Rosalind Cash, Marie O'Henry, Stu Gilliam. Blaxploitation version of the Robert Louis Stevenson story. Casey is the good doctor who experiments with a potion that releases his villainous alter-ego. A.k.a. *The Watts Monster.*

(Video Communications) VC

Dr. Butcher, M.D.

(1981) Color, 80 min. Director: Frank Martin.

Ian McCulloch, Alexandra Cole, Donald O'Brian, Sherry Buchanan. Moreau-style jungle doctor performs backwoods brain surgery on conscious victims, stifling their screams by severing their vocal chords prior to the operation. Charming.

(Paragon Video) VC

Dr. Heckyl and Mr. Hype

(1980) Color, 99 min. Director: Charles B. Griffith.

Oliver Reed, Sunny Johnson, Maia Danziger, Mel Welles, Jackie Coogan, Corinne Calvet. Dr. Heckyl (Reed), a deformed podiatrist, drinks a home-made concoction that turns him into the charming, but loud-mouthed, lady-killer Mr. Hype. Off-beat satire of the familiar Stevenson tale from the writer of Roger Corman's hilarious horror movie spoof *Little Shop of Horrors*, but nowhere near as funny.

(Paragon Video) VC

Dr. Jekyll and Mr. Hyde ½

(1920) B&W, 63 min. Director: John S. Robertson.

John Barrymore, Louis Wolheim, Nita Naldi, Martha Mansfield, Brandon Hurst. Not the first film version of Stevenson's story but the one whose format most subsequent versions have followed. Barrymore eschewed make-up and special effects for his initial transformation scenes in favor of facial contortions and much grimacing and breast-beating. His performance sent shockwaves through audiences of the 1920s, but produces mostly laughter today. Otherwise, the film fairly reeks of atmosphere and is quite well done, if a bit slow moving.

(Blackhawk) VC

Dr. Jekyll's Dungeon of Death

(1979) Color, 91 min. Director: (?)

James Mathers. Low, low, *low*, budget monster-in-the-basement type horror-exploitation film with lots of gore and sadism. Just what the doctor ordered.

(Wizard Video) VC

Dr. Mabuse: The Fatal Passion

(1922) B&W, 90 min. Director: Fritz Lang.
Rudolf Klein-Rogge, Aud Egede Nissen, Alfred Abel, Bernhardt Goetzke, Paul Richter. First of director Lang's series of Expressionistic crime dramas about a Professor Moriarty-like criminal mastermind who is determined to hold all Germany in his icy, Fascist grip. Eerily prescient of Hitler's rise to power. Based on *Dr. Mabuse, Master of Mystery* by Norbert Jacques. A.k.a. *Dr. Mabuse, Der Spieler (The Gambler).*
(Thunderbird Films) VC

Dr. No

(1963) Color, 105 min. Director: Terence Young.
Sean Connery, Joseph Wiseman, Ursula Andress, Jack Lord. First of the James Bond films, the longest running, most successful series in movie history. In his initial outing, 007 (Connery) is sent to Jamaica to investigate the death of a British agent and stumbles upon the island hideaway of the title character, an evil genius with mechanical hands who belongs to a society of sophisticated international terrorists called SPECTRE, and who uses his island as a base from which to sabotage America's missile shots from nearby Cape Canaveral. Still exciting even if it is dated, and Connery remains the definitive Bond.
(CBS/Fox Video, RCA VideoDisc) VC, CED

Don't Answer the Phone!

(1980) Color, 95 min. Director: Robert Hammer.
James Westmoreland, Flo Gerrish, Nicholas Worth, Ben Frank, Pamela Bryant.
Psychotic rapist/strangler prowls the hills of Hollywood in search of victims and finds no shortage. Based on the novel *Nightline* by Michael Curtis. A.k.a. *The Hollywood Strangler.*
(Media Home Entertainment) VC

Don't Go in the House ½

(1980) Color, 82 min. Director: Joseph Ellison.
Dan Grimaldi, Robert Osth, Ruth Dardick. Tormented by his mom, a young boy gets his revenge by murdering her and then cremating her body, an act which drives him psycho but also instills him with a goal; to become an incinerator worker when he grows up. Which he does, then luring unsuspecting young women to his place of business so he can pretend they're mom and burn them up as well. In the end, he gets pretty burned up himself when he imagines all these old flames coming back to life to revenge themselves on him. Not exactly a hot one.
(Media Home Entertainment) VC

Don't Look in the Basement ½

(1972) Color, 95 min. Director: S.F. Brownrigg.
William McGee, Annie MacAdams, Rosie Holotik, Gene Ross, Jessie Lee Fulton. Inmates of a Florida asylum for criminally bad filmmakers plot to take over the studio—er, nut house—in this criminally bad and bloody shocker from the distributors of *Last House on the Left.*
Video Communications) VC

Don't Look Now

(1973) Color, 110 min. Director: Nicolas Roeg.
Donald Sutherland, Julie Christie, Hilary Mason. What could have been a haunting psychological thriller is turned into a stylistic mish-mash by director Roeg who just doesn't seem to know when to put his editing shears away. Christie and Sutherland are a couple whose daughter died in a drowning accident. While in Venice, the pair makes contact with a blind medium who has visions of the child, a tiny figure in a red raincoat, still alive. Based on a short story by Daphne DeMaurier.
(Paramount Home Video, RCA VideoDisc) VC, CED

Dracula ★★

(1931) B&W, 75 min. Director: Tod Browning.

Bela Lugosi, Helen Chandler, Dwight Frye, David Manners, Edward Van Sloan. Undeniably a classic, but dull nevertheless. The first half hour, detailing Frye's trip to Castle Dracula, provides the film's eeriest and most atmospheric moments, but the film declines precipitously thereafter, becoming little more than a photographed stage play. Lugosi lays on a thick slice of ham as the Count. Based on the stage play by Hamilton Deane and John L. Balderston.

(MCA Videocassette) VC

Dracula ★★

(1979) Color, 109 min. Director: John Badham.

Frank Langella, Sir Laurence Olivier, Kate Nelligan. Langella's tour-de-force performance in the Broadway revival of the thirties play by Deane and Balderston prompted producer Walter Mirisch to bankroll yet another screen version of the classic tale. Langella plays the king of vampires as sort of a Byronic hero, an interpretation which worked on Broadway due to his strong charisma, but fails to work here because that charisma doesn't always come across on screen. Elegant, but undistinguished.

(MCA Videocassette and Disc) VC, LV

Dracula and Son ★★

(1976) Color, 105 min. Director: Eduardo Molinaro.

Christopher Lee, Benard Menez, Marie-Helene Breillat, Raymond Bussieres. Dracula (Lee) and son (Menez) are forced into exile by the communist party leaders of present day Transylvania. So they take up residence in England where they secure jobs as movie vampires. Comedy/satire from the director of *Le Cage Aux Folles.*

(Columbia Pictures Home Entertainment) VC

Dracula's Dog ★★½

(1977) Color, 88 min. Director: Albert Band.

Michael Pataki, Jan Shutan, Libbie Chase, Reggie Nalder, Jose Ferrer. An explosion uncovers the tomb of one of Dracula's vampire servants along with the servant's dog, also a vampire. Together, they embark on a plan to draw new human and canine victims into their cult. A.k.a. *Zoltan. . .Hound of Dracula.*

(Video Communications) VC

Dracula's Last Rites ★★

(1980) Color, 88 min. Director: Dominic Paris.

Patricia Lee Hammond, Gerald Fielding, Victor Jorge, Mimi Weddell. Story of a village of vampires lorded over by a mortician named Lucard—which is guess what spelled backwards? A.k.a. *Last Rites.*

(Paragon Video) VC

Dracula Sucks ★

(1978) Color, 91 min. Director: Philip Marshak.

Jamie Gillis, Annette Haven, John Holmes, Serena, John Leslie. X-rated combination of Warholian camp fun and standard porno action, featuring some of porndom's most durable "performers." In this outing, the Count doesn't just go for the throat. Amusing in spots, but the acting, as is usual in porno flicks, is abysmal.

(Media Home Entertainment) VC

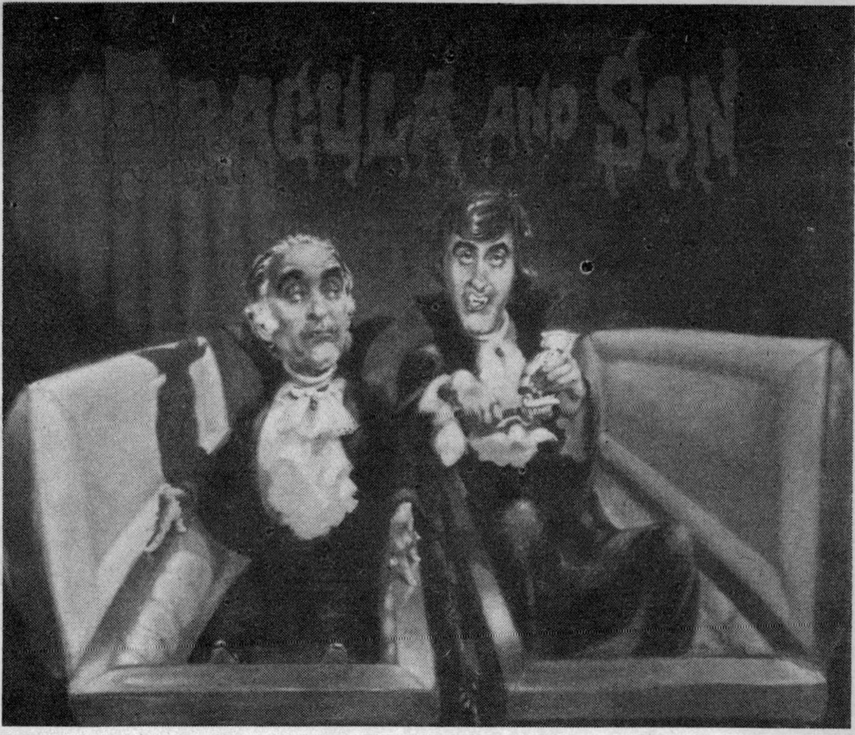

Dracula and Son (1976)

". . .from the director of *Le Cage Aux Folles*. ."

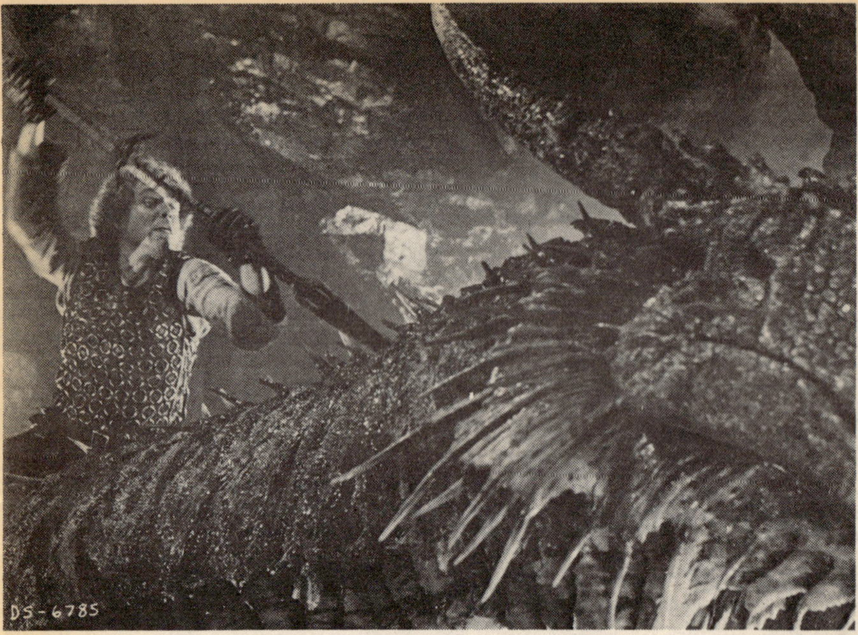

Dragonslayer (1981)

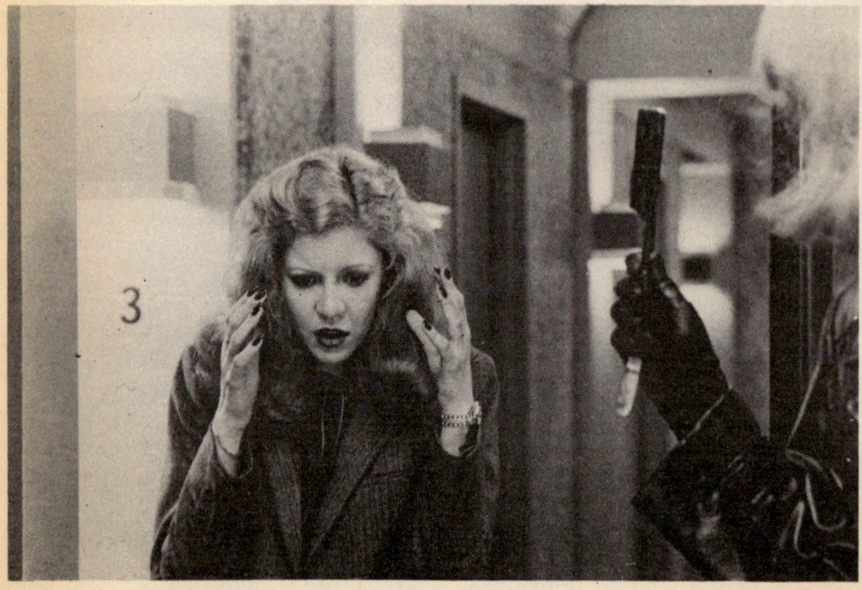

Dressed to Kill (1980)

Dragonslayer ½

(1981) Color, 110 min. Director: Matthew Robbins.

Peter MacNicol, Caitlin Clarke, Ralph Richardson. A fire-breathing monster dragon is terrorizing the 6th century British countryside. The citizens' only hope is an aging sorcerer (Richardson), but when he is killed before he can save them, the task falls on his young apprentice (MacNicol), whose mission is complicated by resistance from the king and by his falling in love. Occasionally ponderous sword and sorcery epic, but the scenes with the dragon are magnificent.

(Paramount Home Video, RCA VideoDisc) VC, CED

Dressed to Kill ½

(1946) B&W, 72 min. Director: Roy William Neill.

Basil Rathbone, Nigel Bruce, Patricia Morrison, Edmond Breon, Frederick Worlock. The final entry in the long-running Universal Sherlock Holmes series with Rathbone and Bruce. This time Holmes is on the trail of a gang of thieves out to claim a set of engraving plates stolen from the Bank of England years before by a master criminal who is now serving time in jail. Holmes' chief clue: encoded notes played by a set of music boxes that were made by the criminal as a way of letting his colleagues know where the plates are located. Good fun.

(Electric Video) VC

Dressed to Kill

(1980) Color, 105 min. Director: Brian De Palma.

Michael Caine, Angie Dickinson, Nancy Allen. Caine is a New York City psychiatrist whose chief clients include a housewife (Dickinson) with sexual problems and a transsexual named Bobbi, who is about to take the big step, but then panics with murder on his/her mind. Film is so derivative that it cannibalizes its entire structure from *Psycho* and lifts whole scenes not only from that film but from other Hitchcock films like *Vertigo* and *Rear Window* and even from some of De Palma's own past films as well. Effective, but it leaves you with the feeling that you've been ripped off by a real pro.

(Warner Home Video, RCA VideoDisc) VC, CED

Driller Killer

(1979) Color, 90 min. Director: Abel Ferrara.

Jimmy Laine, Carolyn Marz, Baybi Day, Tony Coca-Cola and the Roosters. A frustrated artist goes bonkers and starts killing people with a carpentry drill. Nice guy. Gore galore.

(Wizard Video) VC

Drive-In Massacre

(1976) Color, 78 min. Director: Stuart Segall.

Jake Barnes, Adam Lawrence, Douglas Gudbye. A restless crowd and a bad double feature lead to two brutal killings at a drive-in where a dollar a carload turns out to be no bargain. A real brain splatterer!

(Cult Video) VC

Duel ½

(1971) Color, 73 min. Director: Steven Spielberg.

Dennis Weaver. It's man vs. machine as a traveling businessman named Mann (Weaver) is pitted against a monster truck piloted by a malevolent but faceless driver bent on destroying him in a road race to the death. This taut, very skillfully made-for-TV movie earned director Spielberg his spurs and the rest, as they say, is movie history. Based on a short story by Richard Matheson.

(MCA VideoDisc) LV

Dumbo

(1941) Color, 65 min. Director: Ben Sharpsteen.
Animated Disney musical about a little circus elephant who learns to fly by flapping his abnormally large ears. The kids will love it and adults will too.
(Walt Disney Home Video, RCA VideoDisc) VC, LV, CED

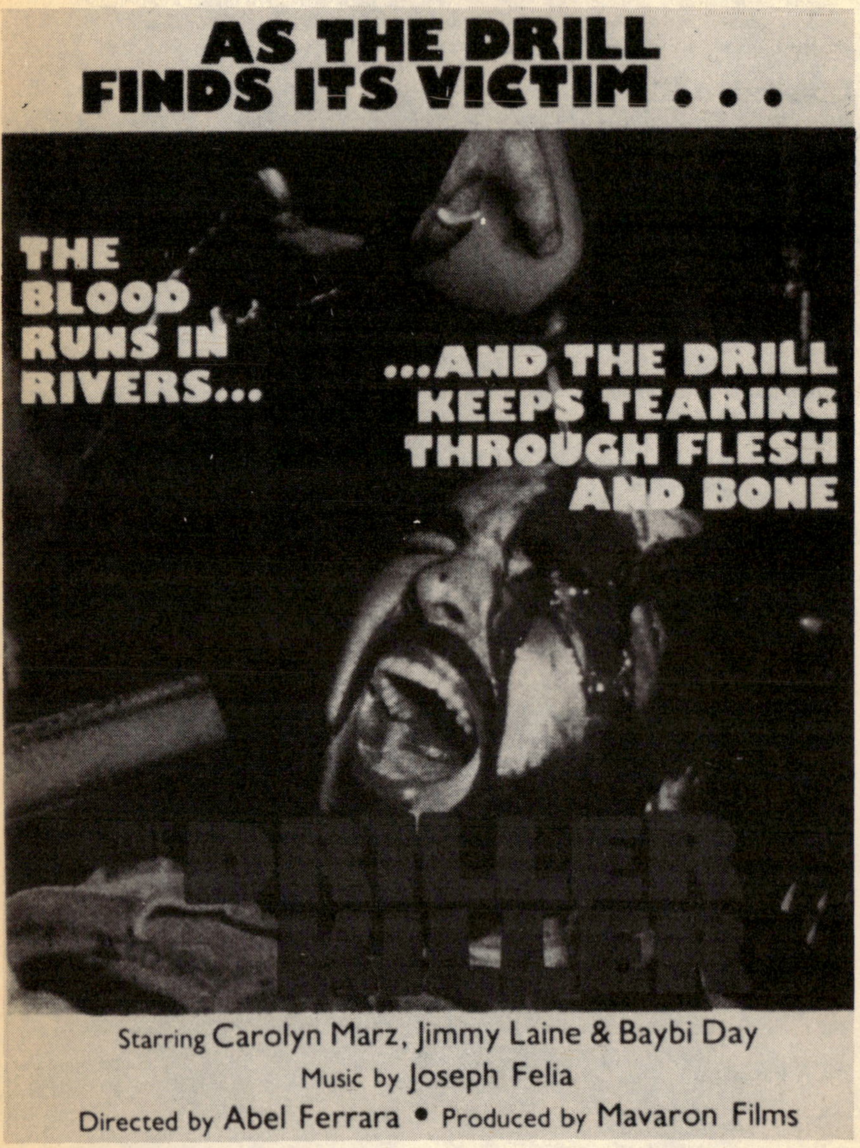

The Driller Killer (1979)

Earthquake

(1974) Color, 129 min. Director: Mark Robson.

Charlton Heston, Genevieve Bujold, Ava Gardner, Lorne Greene. Los Angeles is at last devastated in lovingly graphic detail by the monster quake seismologists and soothsayers have been warning Angelenos about ever since the San Andreas fault first started to grumble. The special effects are truly marvelous, but the stock characters are either so banal or so unlikeable that one doesn't really care what happens to them.

(MCA Videocassette) VC, LV

Eerie Midnight Horror Show, The

(1974) Color, 87 min. Director: Mario Gariazzo.

Stella Carnacina, Chris Avram, Lucretia Love, Luigi Pistilli, Gabriele Tinti. Post-*Exorcist* conglomeration of obsession/possession themes coupled with religious metaphors about Satan, Barabbas and other bad and good guys from the Bible, plus a weak story about a statue that comes to life. Made in Italy as *The Tormented.*

(Planet Video) VC

Elephant Man, The

(1980) B&W, 123 min. Director: David Lynch.

Anthony Hopkins, John Hurt, Anne Bancroft, Sir John Gielgud, Wendy Hiller. In a bid for instant *auteur* status, director Lynch transformed the painful but uplifting true story of deformed Victorian John Merrick into a stylistic re-hash of his only other film, *Eraserhead.* This is directorial conceit at its most damaging, for *The Elephant Man* could have been a great movie. Instead, like its predecessor, it is bleak, boring, and pretentious.

(Paramount Home Video, RCA VideoDisc) VC, CED, LV

Encounter with Disaster

(1979) Color/B&W, 101 min.

Documentary consisting of old news clips of famous disasters like the crash of the Hindenburg and the eruption of Mt. Etna in Italy, combined with new footage of the disaster sites today. The old clips are quite dramatic. A.k.a. *13 Great Disasters that Shook the World.*

(Video Communications) VC

Encounter with the Unknown

(1972) Color, 87 min. Director: Harry Thomason.
Rosie Holotick, Gene Ross, Annabelle Weenick. Narrated by Rod Serling. Docudrama recounting three supposedly authenticated cases of contact with spirits and other ghostly phenomena.
(Video Communications) VC

End of the World

(1977) Color, 92 min. Director: John Hayes.
Christopher Lee, Lew Ayres, Dean Jagger, MacDonald Carey, Sue Lyon. A priest (Lee) is killed by an alien organism which then proceeds to take over his identity and turn his church into a nesting place for other aliens bent on taking over the world. Standard fare.
(Media Home Entertainment) VC

Equinox

(1971) Color, 82 min. Director: Jack Woods.
Edward Connell, Barbara Hewitt, Fritz Leiber. While looking for a missing archaeologist, four teenagers stumble upon an old book about devil worship and are thereafter pursued by a giant winged creature that wants the book for itself. Jim Danforth's low-budget model animation effects are the only plus in this bomb.
(Wizard Video) VC

Eraserhead

(1977) B&W, 90 min. Director: David Lynch.
Jack Nance, Charlotte Steward, Jeanne Bates, Laurel Near. Disgusting, downbeat, dream-like (or nightmare-like) tale of a fish-like monster baby whose birth turns its parents' lives upside down (not that their lives were all that rightside up in the first place). The film itself spins wildly out of control with allegorical/symbolic/nonsensical fantasy images of grotesque doings. Made by the cheerless David Lynch before he went on to ruin *The Elephant Man.* A cult favorite—but then, isn't everything these days?
(Columbia Pictures Home Entertainment) VC

Escape from New York ½

(1981) Color, 99 min. Director: John Carpenter.
Kurt Russell, Lee Van Cleef, Donald Pleasence, Isaac Hayes, Harry Dean Stanton, Ernest Borgnine, Adrienne Barbeau. A comic-strip satire of the future—specifically the year 1997, in which Manhattan has been turned into a maximum security prison in order to accommodate the three-million-plus criminals who have helped to push America's growing crime rate over the 400% mark. Enroute to a summit meeting, the president (Pleasence) is forced to crash land in this hell hole and becomes a hostage. Newly convicted Snake Plissken (Russell) is then offered his freedom if he'll go in and get the pres back. Not as excitng as it could be, nor as much fun, given the wild plot ingredients, but the film has its moments, and Russell's impersonation of Clint Eastwood at his grittiest is quite amusing.
(Embassy Home Entertainment, RCA VideoDisc) VC, CED

Escape to Witch Mountain ½

(1975) Color, 97 min. Director: John Hough.
Eddie Albert, Ray Milland, Kim Richards, Ike Eisenmann, Donald Pleasance. Two orphans with supernatural powers are pursued by millionaire Milland who wants to use those powers for his own ends. Amusing, imaginative fantasy marred by some occasional lapses into typical Disney cuteness.
(Walt Disney Home Video, RCA VideoDisc) VC, CED, LV

Everything You Always Wanted to Know About Sex... But Were Afraid to Ask ½

(1972) Color, 87 min. Director: Woody Allen.
Lynn Redgrave, Burt Reynolds, Gene Wilder, Louise Lasser, John Carradine. Episodic comedy/fantasy based (very loosely) on Dr. David Reuben's popular guidebook. Funniest episodes include a segment about a marauding breast that spoofs a typical Hollywood monster movie of the fifties and the final segment in which Woody plays a sperm that is about to face the "moment of truth." Uneven, but funny.
(CBS/Fox Video, RCA VideoDisc) VC, CED

Evil Mind, The ½

(1935) B&W, 72 min. Director: Maurice Elvey.
Claude Rains, Fay Wray, Jane Baxter, Mary Clare, Donald Calthrop. A fake medium discovers that his powers are for real when he predicts a disaster that actually comes true. The rub comes when he then envisions his own death. Can he prevent it? Script by Edgar Wallace. A.k.a. *The Clairvoyant.*
(Thunderbird Films, Direct Video) VC

Evilspeak

(1981) Color, 91 min. Director: Eric Weston.
Clint Howard, Charles Tyner, R.G. Armstrong. Howard turns in a grotesque performance as a crazy student at a military school who uses the school's sophisticated (that's for sure!) computer system to call forth the forces of evil, which include a wild pack of demonic pigs. As you can see, Howard isn't the only thing that's grotesque about this mess.
(CBS/Fox Video) VC

Excalibur

(1981) Color, 140 min. Director: John Boorman.
Nicol Williamson, Nigel Terry, Helen Mirren, Nicholas Clay, Paul Geoffrey. A haunting and moving hymn to the legend of King Arthur and his Knights of the Round Table, which trumpets the rise of Christian civilization out of the magic, murder and chaos of the Dark Ages while at the same time expressing some discouragement over the cost of that rise—man's loss of his sense of wonder. While some of the lesser roles are acted with too much hysteria, Terry is quite perfect as the once and future king and Williamson is wonderfully droll as the wizard Merlin. The film is quite bloody, but it is also spectacularly beautiful, almost magical. Destined to become a once and future classic.
(Warner Home Video) VC

Exorcist, The ½

(1973) Color, 120 min. Director: William Friedkin.
Ellen Burstyn, Jason Miller, Linda Blair, Max von Sydow, Lee J. Cobb. A pyrotechnical wonder designed to pulverize audiences into a single gagging mass. Virginal Blair is possessed by the devil and becomes a foul-minded, foul-mouthed, vomit-spewing little monster. Miller and von Sydow are the exorcists who are called in to drive the demon out. Dick Smith's astonishing make-up and prosthetic effects are the real stars. But the film itself does not wear well because once one becomes inured to the shocks, the plot and characters reveal themselves as being both contrived and empty.
(Warner Home Video, RCA VideoDisc) VC, CED

Exorcist II—The Heretic

(1977) Color, 118 min. Director: John Boorman.
Richard Burton, Louise Fletcher, Linda Blair, Max von Sydow, James Earl Jones. In an effort to overcome comparison with the original, Boorman elected to make a very different kind of movie—a farce. Fletcher delivers her lines as if suffering from tired blood. Burton constantly looks pained, as if suffering from a severe case of gastritis. And the script is completely unmotivated, untied-together, and ultimately uninvolving. One of the worst sequels in movie history.
(Warner Home Video) VC

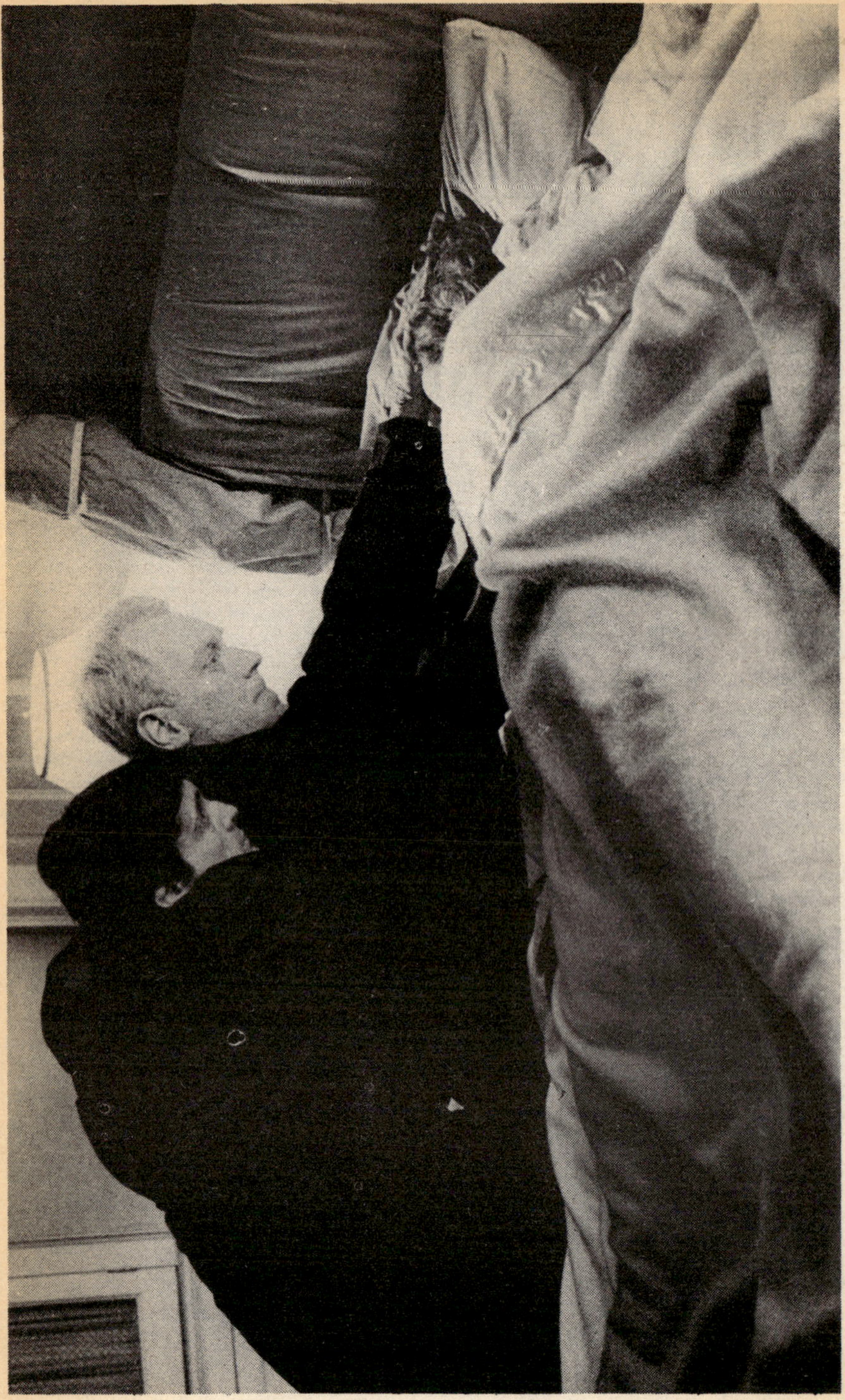

The Exorcist (1973)

Eyes of a Stranger 🎞🎞

(1980) Color, 85 min. Director: Ken Wiederhorn.
Lauren Tewes, John Disanti, Peter Dupre, Jennifer Jason Leigh. TV reporter Tewes discovers that the psychotic killer of young women whose escapades she has been headlining each night lives in the apartment across the way from her. The question is how to prove it so that the police will be convinced? On her own, she decides to smoke him out. Occasionally tense tale laced with graphic violence that is weakened by some wild implausibilities toward the end. Special effects by Tom *Friday the 13th* Savini.
(Warner Home Video) VC

Eyes of Laura Mars, The 🎞

(1978) Color, 103 min. Director: Irvin Kershner.
Faye Dunaway, Tommy Lee Jones, Brad Dourif, Raul Julia, Rene Aburjonois. Fashion photographer Dunaway, who combines scenes of eroticism with violence in her picture spreads for *Vogue* and other such magazines, gets a taste of the real thing when she starts "seeing" the violent mutilation murders of various women through her mind's eye. Able to predict the murders but unable to stop them, she seeks solace in the arms of the detective (Jones) assigned to the case, but gets a big surprise instead. Designed as a high class thriller, this is really a low-class exploitation film full of sleazy non-characters and contrived situations, including an ending that's downright unbelievable. John *Halloween* Carpenter wrote the original story (though he disavows what was done to it) and Jack *The Blob* Harris executive produced. Dunaway should have shot her cameraman; she looks positively anemic throughout.
(Columbia Pictures Home Entertainment, RCA VideoDisc) VC, CED

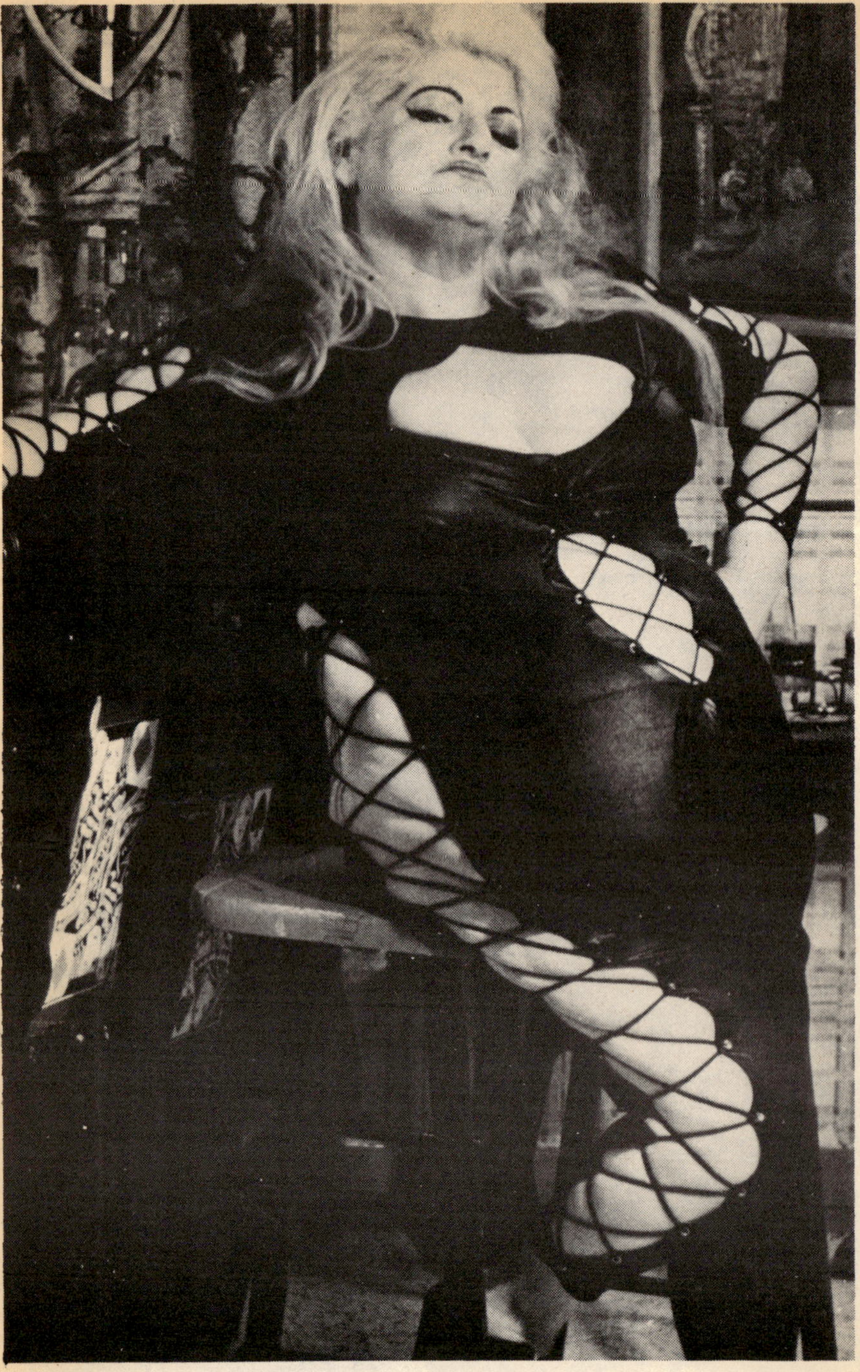

Female Trouble (1974)

Fabulous World of Jules Verne ½

(1961) B&W, 83 min. Director: Karel Zeman.
Louis Tock. Ernest Navara, Milo Hall, Francis Sherr. Czechoslovakian film which combines live-action with animation to bring elements from some of Verne's most fabulous novels and stories to life.
(Video Communications) VC

Fade to Black

(1980) Color, 100 min. Director: Vernon Zimmerman.
Dennis Christopher, Linda Kerridge, Tim Thomerson, Morgan Paull, Marya Small. Deranged film fan Christopher goes over the edge and starts killing those who have victimized him, modeling his murders after scenes from his favorite movies. A promising idea insufficiently realized. Kerridge is probably the definitive Marilyn Monroe lookalike. Christopher scored big in *Breaking Away.* Maybe this film should have been called *Breaking Apart.*
(Media Home Entertainment) VC

Fail-Safe

(1964) B&W, 111 min. Director: Sidney Lumet.
Henry Fonda, Walter Matthau, Fritz Weaver, Dan O'Herlihy. Computer malfunction prompts an accidental nuclear strike on Russia. U.S. President Fonda races against time to convince the Soviet Premier that it was all a mistake so that an all-out nuclear war can be avoided. Tense drama based on the cautionary novel by Eugene Burdick and Harvey Wheeler.
(Columbia Pictures Home Entertainment) VC

Fall of the House of Usher, The ½

(1960) Color, 85 min. Director: Roger Corman.
Vincent Price, Mark Damon, Myrna Fahey, Harry Ellerbe. The first of Corman's popular series of broad-stroked adaptations of the works of Edgar Allen Poe—designed to introduce gothic horror American-style to a film-going public convinced that only the British could bring off such tales. Price is obsessed by the death of his wife and the imminent collapse of his home.
(Warner Home Video) VC

Fall of the House of Usher, The ★

(1979) Color, 100 min. Director: James L. Conway.
Martin Landau, Charlene Tilton, Ray Walston. Undistinguished, over-inflated adaptation of the familiar Poe tale about the doomed Usher family. Landau is even hammier than Vincent Price.
(Video Communications) VC

Fan, The ★

(1981) Color, 95 min. Director: Edward Bianchi.
Lauren Bacall, James Garner, Maureen Stapleton, Hector Elizondo, Michael Biehn. Bacall is a glamorous Broadway star who becomes stalked by a spurned, psychotic fan. Pointless, gory thriller that wastes a lot of high-priced talent.
(Paramount Home Video) VC

Fantastic Planet ★★½

(1973) Color, 72 min. Director: Rene Laloux.
Voices of Barry Bostwick, Nora Heflin, Cynthia Alder (American version). Animated fantasy satire about a futuristic planet which holds the survivors (Ohms) of a devastated Earth as captive pets.
(Video Yesteryear) VC

Fantastic Voyage ★★½

(1966) Color, 100 min. Director: Richard Fleischer.
Stephen Boyd, Raquel Welch, Edmond O'Brien, Donald Pleasence, Arthur O'Connell. A medical team is reduced to microscopic size and injected into the bloodstream of the dying U.S. president so that it can journey to his brain and perform a complex surgical operation from the inside, the only way to save his life. Complications arise when one member of the team starts sabotaging the equipment and endangering the others' lives—for this baddie's a foreign agent in more ways than one. Unique plot is supported by some unusual and imaginative special effects, but the characters and situations are fairly predictable.
(CBS/Fox Video) VC, CED

Faust ★★★

(1926) B&W, 90 min. Director: F.W. Murnau.
Emil Jannings, William Dieterle, Eric Barclay, Gosta Ekman, Camilla Horn. The classic story by Goethe of the perils of dealing with the devil. Jannings chews up the scenery as Mephisto, but the film is intensely atmospheric, full of ingenious camera trickery, and on the whole one of Murnau's best.
(Thunderbird Films) VC

Fear in the Night ★★★

(1972) Color, 85 min. Director: Jimmy Sangster.
Judy Geeson, Ralph Bates, Peter Cushing, Joan Collins. Young bride Geeson, recovering from a nervous breakdown, moves onto the campus of the boys' school where husband Bates teaches, starts hearing voices and encountering other fearsome phenomena and begins to think she's suffering a relapse. In fact, she's being terrorized quite on purpose. Serviceable Hammer Films thriller that offers few surprises but is nicely done. A throwback to the series of films (*Paranoiac, The Maniac)* which the company turned out in the wake of *Psycho.*
(Thorn/EMI Video) VC

Female Trouble ★★

(1974) Color, 92 min. Director: John Waters.
Divine, David Lochary, Mary Vivian Pearce, Mink Stole, Edith Massey. Dawn Davenport (Divine) pursues her life of crime as if it were a form of show business, determined to win a cherished Oscar for best performance by a mass murderer in an electric chair. A film in amusing bad taste from the unhinged director of *Pink Flamingos* and *Polyester.*
(Wizard Video) VC

Fiend Without a Face ★★

(1958) B&W, 74 min. Director: Arthur Crabtree.
Marshall Thompson, Terence Kilburn. Dumb but entertaining sci-fi thriller about American and Canadian Air Force officers and scientists who discover that the earth is being invaded by invisible creatures that suck out people's spines. When finally revealed, the creatures look like brains with tails.
(Blackhawk) VC

Fiendish Plot of Dr. Fu Manchu, The ★

(1980) Color, 100 min. Director: Piers Haggard.
Peter Sellers, Helen Mirren, Sid Caesar, Simon Williams, Steve Franken, David Tomlinson. A depressingly witless footnote to the career of Peter Sellers, who died shortly before the film was released (escaped?). In it, Sellers plays both masterfiend Fu and his lifelong adversary, Nayland Smith of Scotland Yard. The plot has something to do with Fu's theft of the crown jewels and other assorted fabulous riches in order to create an elixir that will restore youth to his 168-year-old body. Overall, the film seems to have been made by no one even remotely adept at comedy.
(Warner Home Video) VC

Final Conflict, The ★½

(1981) Color, 108 min. Director: Graham Baker.
Sam Neill, Rossano Brazzi, Don Gordon, Lisa Harrow. After murdering what seems like hundreds of innocent people in his two previous escapades, *The Omen* and *Damien-Omen II,* the son of Satan is at last given his comeuppance. One expects at least armageddon, but Damien goes out with a whimper instead.
(CBS/Fox Video) VC

Final Programme, The ★½

(1973) Color, 89 min. Director: Robert Fuest.
Jon Finch, Jenny Runacre, Patrick Magee, Hugh Griffith, Sterling Hayden. End of the world sci-fi/fantasy/comedy with Finch as superagent Jerry Cornelius who eventually saves the human race by undergoing an offbeat experiment in unisex mutation. Dumb. Based on a novel by Michael Moorcock. A.k.a. *The Last Days of Man on Earth.*
(Thorn/EMI Video) VC

Firefox ★½

(1982) Color, 137 min. Director: Clint Eastwood.
Clint Eastwood, David Huffman, Freddie Jones, Warren Clarke, Ronald Lacey. U.S. fighter pilot Eastwood infiltrates Soviet security in order to steal an ultra sophisticated Russian fighter plane (the Firefox) for the West. Ponderous action yarn that suffers from extreme length as well as Eastwood's shortcomings as an action director. He should have let Don Siegel direct this one for him. The last 20 minutes are exciting, though, due to effects master John Dykstra's fabulous orchestration of Eastwood's high speed getaway aboard the Firefox with the Russians in hot pursuit.
(Warner Home Video) VC

First Spaceship on Venus

(1959) Color, 80 min. Director: Kurt Mätzig.
Yoko Tani, Oldrich Lukes, Ignacy Machowski. Scientists land on Venus and discover remnants of a civilization similar to that of earth, but which has long since vanished as the result of an atomic explosion. Based on a novel by Stanislaw Lem.
(Video Communications) VC

Flash Gordon

(1980) Color, 111 min. Director: Mike Hodges.
Sam J. Jones, Melody Anderson, Topol, Max von Sydow, Timothy Dalton. Multi-million dollar comic strip produced by Dino DeLaurentiis in the hopes of climbing aboard the *Star Wars* bandwagon. Flash is a football player who becomes involved with Dale Arden and Dr. Zarkoff on a mission to the planet Mongo, where Ming the Merciless still reigns supreme. Flashy, but only for kids. Music by Queen.
(MCA Videocassette and Disc) VC, LV

Flash Gordon: Mars Attacks the World

(1938) B&W, 82 min. Directors: Ford Beebe, Robert Hill.
Buster Crabbe, Jean Rogers, Charles Middleton, Frank Shannon. Emperor Ming the Merciless threatens Earth's existence with a device that removes all nitrogen from the planet's atmosphere. Flash goes to the rescue. Lackluster feature culled from the 15-part serial *Flash Gordon's Trip to Mars* released the same year.
(Media Home Entertainment) VC

Flash Gordon: Rocketship

(1936) B&W, 82 min. Director: Frederick Stephani.
Buster Crabbe, Jean Rogers, Charles Middleton, Frank Shannon. The planet Mongo is on a collision course with Earth. Flash, Dale, and Dr. Zarkoff blast off to divert it. Feature drawn from the original 13-part serial released the same year. A.k.a. *Spaceship to the Unknown.*
(Media Home Entertainment) VC

Flesh and Blood Show, The ½

(1973) Color, 97 min. Director: Pete Walker.
Jenny Hanley, Ray Brooks, Luan Peters, Patrick Barr, Robin Askwith, Judy Matheson. A group of actors is called to audition for a Grand Guignol-type stage production, but it's all a ruse perpetrated by a madman who plans to kill the troupe in a supreme act of revenge against all actors. Appropriately titled splatter movie full of wall-to-wall sex and violence.
(Wizard Video) VC

Flesh Gordon

(1972) Color, 70 min. Directors: Howard Ziehm, Michael Benveniste.
Jason Williams, Suzanne Fields, Joseph Hudgins, William Hunt, John Hoyt. X-rated satire in which Flesh, Dale Ardor, and Dr. Jerkoff do battle in space with the evil Emperor Wang and his libidinous minions. Uneven, but the animated effects by Jim Danforth and Dave Allen provide some definite high spots.
(Media Home Entertainment) VC

Flight to Mars

(1951) Color, 72 min. Director: Lesley Selander.
Cameron Mitchell, Marguerite Chapman, Arthur Franz. An expedition to Mars reveals the existence of an underground civilization with plans to take over the earth. More Red Menace.
(Nostalgia Merchant) VC

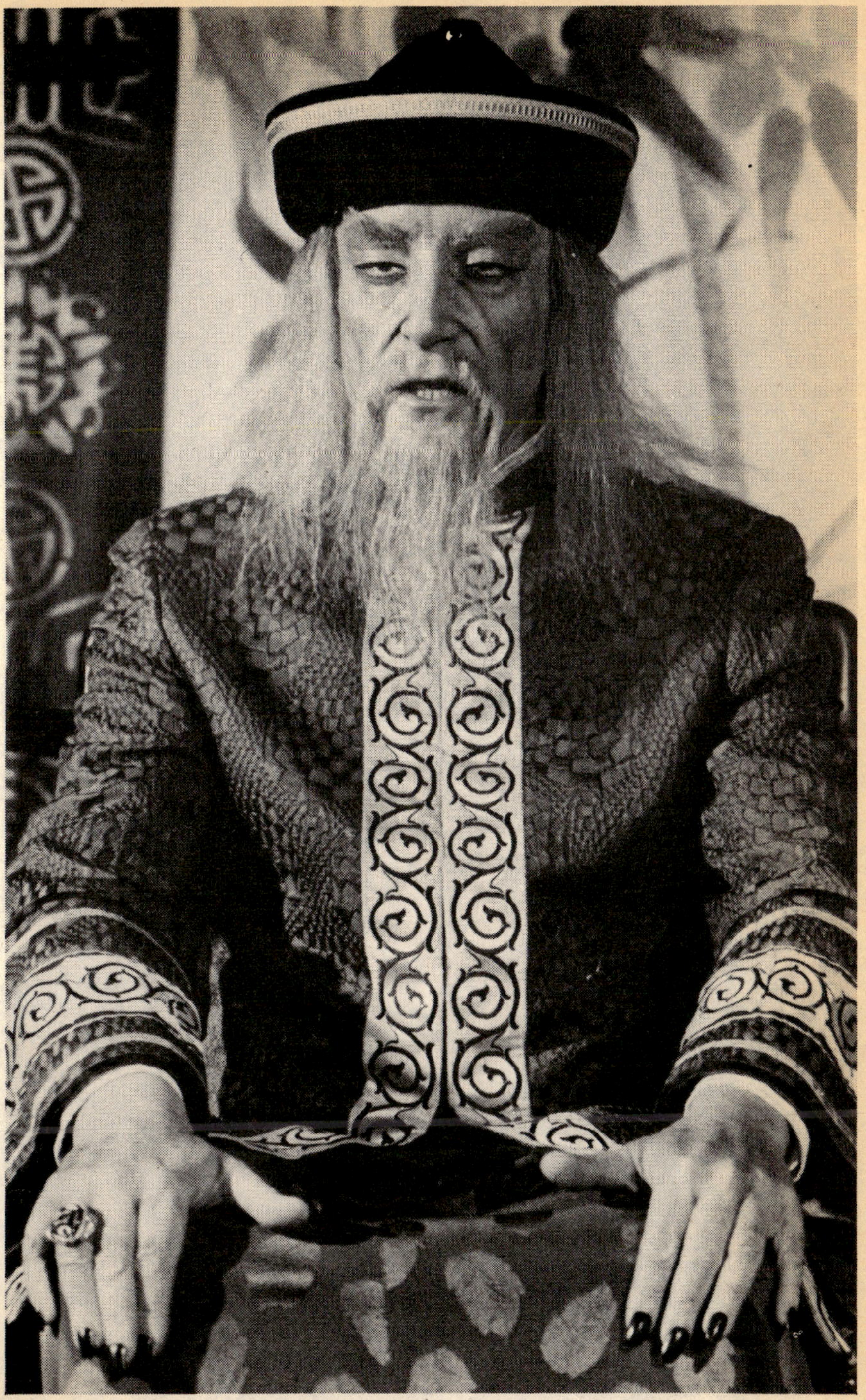

The Fiendish Plot of Dr. Fu Manchu (1980)

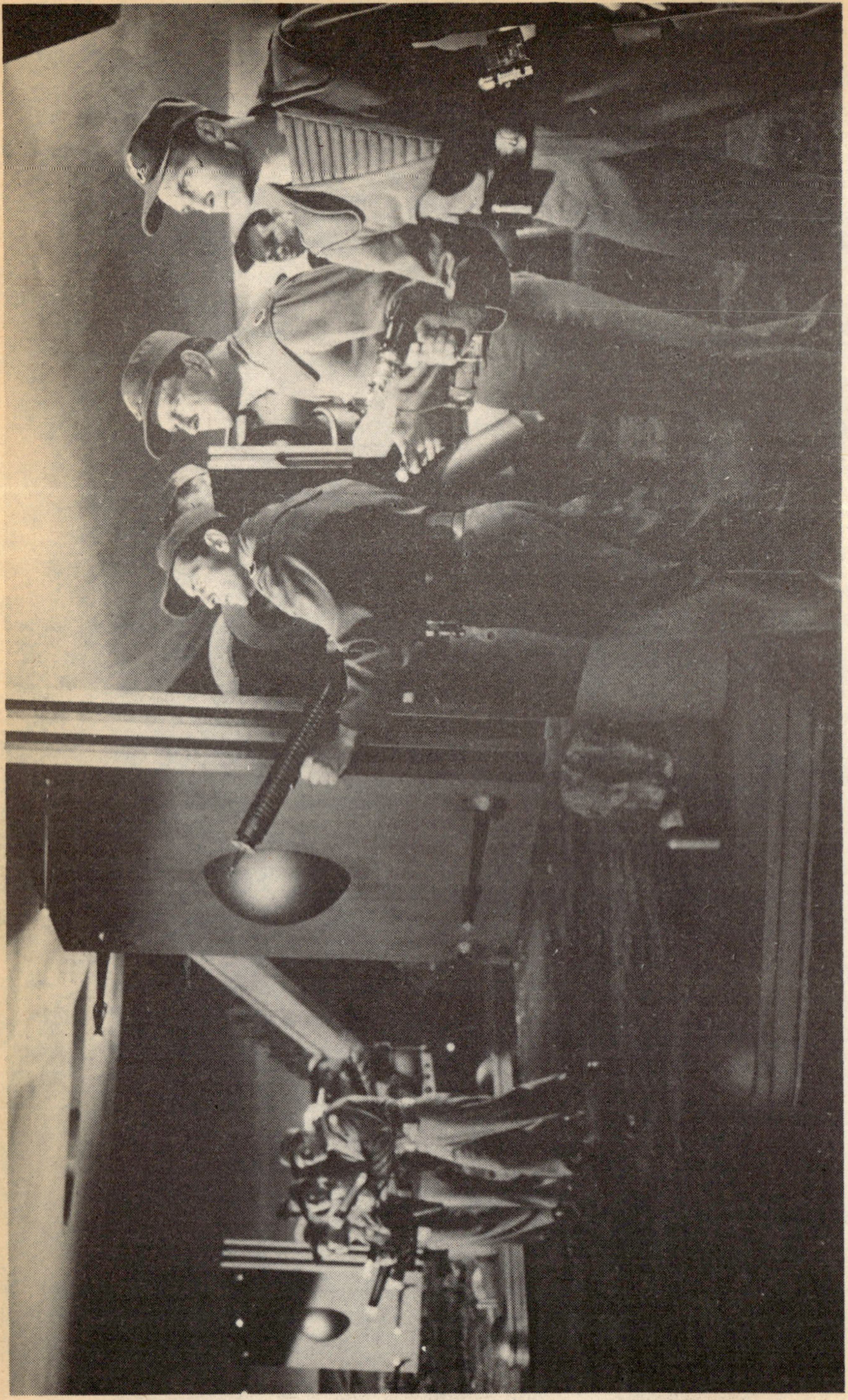

Forbidden Planet (1956)

Flying Saucer ½

(1950) B&W, 69 min. Director: Mikel Conrad.

Mikel Conrad, Pat Garrison, Denver Pyle. A pre-*Thing* sci-fi tale about an American agent sent to the North Pole to investigate rumors that Soviet agents have uncovered a spaceship from another planet. Trite.

(Nostalgia Merchant) VC

Fog, The

(1980) Color, 91 min. Director: John Carpenter.

Hal Holbrook, Janet Leigh, Adrienne Barbeau, Jamie Lee Curtis, John Houseman. A ghost ship whose crew was murdered for the gold on board returns in the fog to seek vengeance on the descendants of those who perpetrated the deed. Transparent characters and telegraphed scares, not to mention an ending that seems tacked on for its shock value alone, sink this contemporary ghost story from the director of the popular *Halloween.*

(CBS/Fox Video, RCA VideoDisc) VC, CED, LV

Fog Island ½

(1945) B&W, 72 min. Director: Terry Morse.

George Zucco, Lionel Atwill, Veda Ann Borg, Jerome Cowan. A diverse group of people is brought together by a man recently released from prison who wishes to determine who in the group sent him there. Despite the teaming of the always accomplished Atwill and Zucco, a bore.

(Thunderbird Films) VC

For Your Eyes Only ½

(1981) Color, 127 min. Director: John Glen.

Roger Moore, Carol Bouquet, Topol, Lynn-Holly Johnson, Julian Glover. Bond's assignment this time is to uncover a stolen missile guidance system. In doing so, he becomes involved with dope smugglers as well as the KGB. Gimmicks are forsaken for non-stop action, but the result is the same: tedium on a spectacular scale.

(CBS/Fox Video) VC, CED

Forbidden Planet

(1956) Color, 98 min. Director: Fred McLeod Wilcox.

Walter Pidgeon, Anne Francis, Leslie Neilsen, Jack Kelly, Earl Holliman, Robbie the Robot. A team of American astronauts lands on Altair Four to rescue a group of colonists, but discovers only a planet paradise whose sole inhabitants (Pidgeon and daughter Francis) have no desire to be rescued—even though there's a serpent in this paradise, a marauding, invisible monster. Imaginative sci-fi loosely based on Shakespeare's *The Tempest.*

(MGM/UA Home Video) VC, CED

Force Beyond, The ½

(1978) Color, 85 min. Director: William Sachs.

Don Elkins, Peter Byrne, Renee Dahinden, Frances Farrelly. Teens sight flying saucers, then spot aliens, conclude that something is definitely "up" and determine to convince their elders of the truth behind UFOs. For the kids.

(Media Home Entertainment) VC

Frankenstein ★★★

(1931) B&W, 71 min. Director: James Whale.
Colin Clive, Mae Clarke, John Boles, Boris Karloff, Dwight Frye. First feature version of the oft-filmed Mary Shelley tale is shot through with Expressionist touches drawn from the silent German cinema. Clive overacts as Frankenstein, but Karloff's portrayal of the pathetic creature who was spurned by his creator remains definitive. A classic.
(MCA Videocassette and Disc) VC, LV

Frankenstein's Castle of Freaks ★

(1975) Color, 89 min. Director: Robert H. Oliver.
Rossano Brazzi, Michael Dunn, Edmund Purdom, Christine Royce, Gordon Michael. A potpourri of creatures run riot over the countryside thanks to more handiwork from the mad Dr. F and his latest life-giving device, the Electric Accumulator—a good name for a rock group, don't you think?
(AstroVideo) VC

Frankenstein's Daughter ★

(1958) B&W, 85 min. Director: Dick Cunha.
John Ashley, Sandra Knight, Donald Murphy, Sally Todd, Harold Lloyd Jr. A descendent of you-know-who sets loose another reign of terror by creating a woman who's a real chip off the old block. Grade-Z.
(Nostalgia Merchant) VC

Freaky Friday ★★½

(1976) Color, 95 min. Director: Gary Nelson.
Barbara Harris, Jodie Foster, John Astin, Patsy Kelly, Dick Van Patten, Sorrel Booke. Mother Harris and daughter Foster magically switch personalities for a day, resulting in a lot of screwball mis-adventures for each of them. Harris pulls off her reversion to teenager quite nicely, but Foster is a bit stiff trying to play an adult. An overabundance of slapstick also tends to mar this otherwise entertaining Disney outing.
(Walt Disney Home Video) VC

Frenzy ★★★½

(1972) Color, 116 min. Director: Alfred Hitchcock.
Jon Finch, Barry Foster, Barbara Leigh-Hunt, Anna Massey. Innocent Finch is suspected of being a psychopathic killer of young women whom Scotland Yard has dubbed The Necktie Murderer on account of the method he uses to strangle his victims. The real culprit is Foster, a garrulous British grocer, who, all smiles and deceit, pretends to be Finch's friend. Hitchcock's first British film in quite some time is a cold, disturbing affair, but top-notch.
(MCA Videocassette) VC

Friday the 13th ★½

(1980) Color, 95 min. Director: Sean S. Cunningham.
Adrienne King, Betsy Palmer, Harry Crosby. A summer camp that was closed down after two counselors were brutally murdered prepares to re-open for business. One by one, the new counselors are stalked and slaughtered by a faceless killer. This is the controversial box-office smash that propelled the gore film into the big time and spawned a host of gruesome imitations. Effects by Tom Savini.
(Paramount Home Video, RCA VideoDisc) VC, CED, LV

Friday the 13th—Part Two ★

(1981) Color, 87 min. Director: Steve Miner.
Amy Steel, John Furey, Adrienne King, The body count continues.
(Paramount Home Video) VC, LV

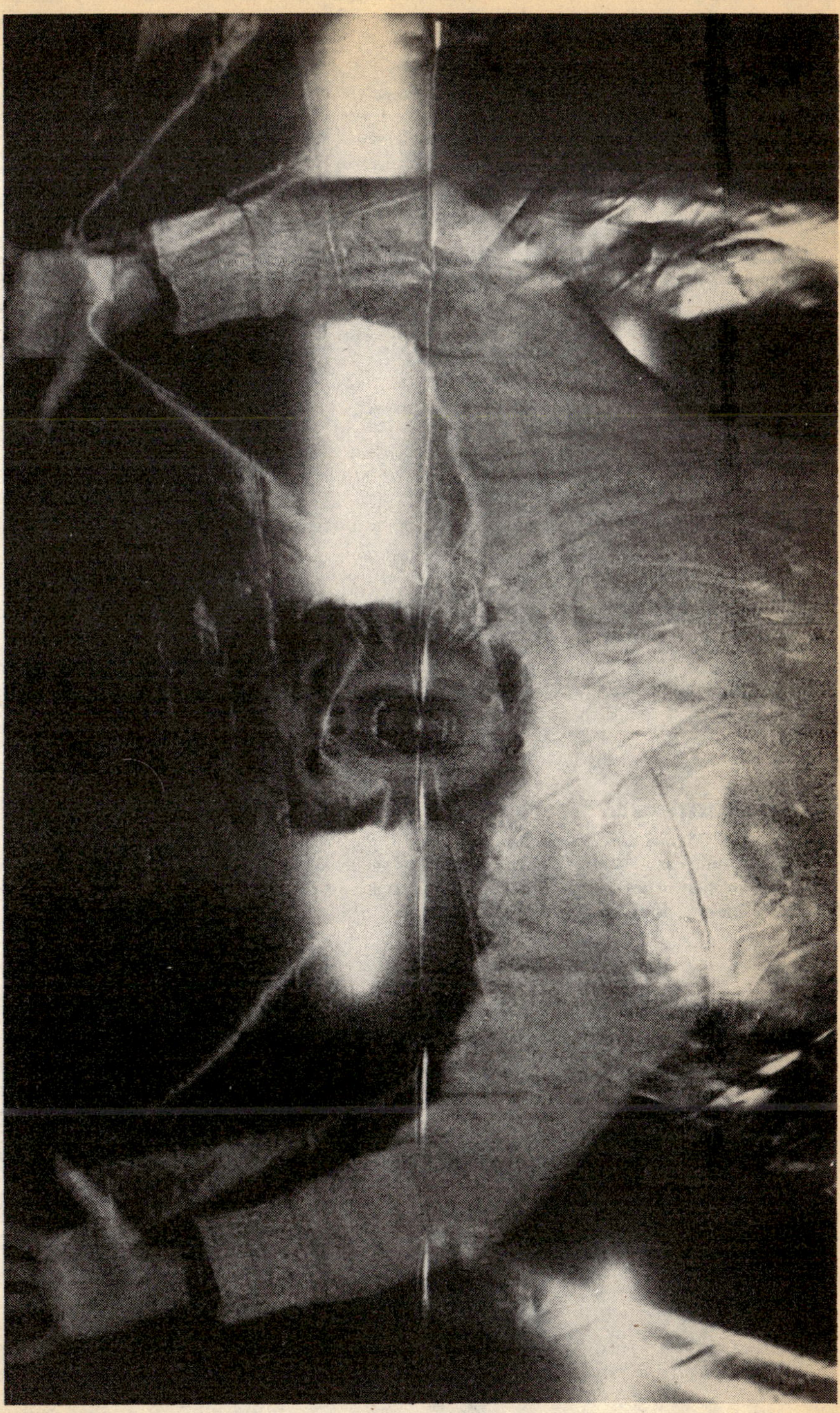

Friday the 13th (1980)

From Russia, With Love

(1964) Color, 118 min. Director: Terence Young.
Sean Connery, Daniela Bianchi, Lotte Lenya, Pedro Armendariz, Robert Shaw. This second of James Bond's screen adventures is also one of the best. Agent 007 is sent to Istanbul to steal a secret decoder device from the Russians and gets involved with a beautiful Russian spy who is being used as a dupe by SPECTRE to trap the unsuspecting Bond. Colorful, exciting, and faithful adaptation of the Ian Fleming novel that doesn't rely on gimmicks to keep the audience's attention.
(CBS/Fox Video, RCA VideoDisc) VC, CED

From the Earth to the Moon ½

(1958) Color, 100 min. Director: Byron Haskin.
George Sanders, Joseph Cotten, Debra Paget, Don Dubbins. Three men and a woman rocket to the moon during the closing days of the American Civil War. Based on Jules Verne's novel of the same name.
(Video Communications) VC

Funhouse, The ½

(1981) Color, 94 min. Director: Tobe Hooper.
Elizabeth Berridge, Cooper Huckabee, Largo Woodruff, Miles Chapin, Kevin Conway, Sylvia Miles, William Finley. Four teenagers decide to spend the night in a carnival funhouse and encounter all manner of horrors, including a deformed monster with two faces. Short on sense, but effective nonetheless.
(MCA Videocassette) VC

Fury, The ½

(1978) Color, 117 min. Director: Brian De Palma.
Kirk Douglas, John Cassavetes, Carrie Snodgress, Andrew Stevens, Amy Irving. Two young psychics are pursued by government agents and international terrorists who want to put their powers to use as the ultimate weapon. After this one, De Palma should have gone back to making underground films. Based on the novel by John Farris.
(CBS/Fox Video) VC

Futureworld

(1976) Color, 104 min. Director: Richard Heffron.
Peter Fonda, Arthur Hill, Blythe Danner. Ostentatious sequel to the low-keyed and enjoyable *Westworld* which stretches credulity more than the imagination.
(Warner Home Video) VC

Galactica III: Conquest of the Earth ½

(1980) Color, 99 min. Directors: Sidney Hayers, Sigmund Neufeld, Jr., Barry Crane.
Kent McCord, Robert Reed, Lorne Greene, Wolfman Jack. More outer space nonsense spliced together into feature film form from various episodes of the *Battlestar Galactica* TV series. Producer Glen Larson sure manages to get a lot of mileage out of the same footage.
(MCA Videocassette) VC

Galaxina

(1981) Color, 96 min. Director: William Sachs.
Dorothy Stratten, Avery Schreiber, Stephen Macht, James David Hinton. Lame satire of space operas in general and *Alien* in particular. Stratten is a gorgeous robot who comes to develop human feelings and by movie's end falls in love with an intergalactic policeman. Film's funniest moments involve Schreiber's efforts to elude the space creature he has given birth to *Alien*-style and which now pursues him relentlessly because it thinks he's its mother.
(MCA Videocassette and Disc) VC, LV

Ghidrah, the Three-Headed Monster ½

(1965) Color, 85 min. Director: Inoshiro Honda.
Yosuke Niozumi, Emi Ito. One time Japanese monster movie villains Mothra, Rodan, and Godzilla don the white hats this time to combat another post-nuclear fiend, Ghidrah. Once again, the city of Tokyo is their stomping ground.
(Budget Video, Direct Video) VC

Ghost Story ½

(1981) Color, 108 min. Director: John Irvin.
Fred Astaire, Melvyn Douglas, Douglas Fairbanks Jr., John Houseman, Alice Krige, Craig Wasson. Four old-timers who committed an act of manslaughter in their youth are haunted in their waking and non-waking moments by the vengeful ghost of the victim whose body they tried to conceal. Jack Cardiff's stunning, atmospheric photography of northern New York and Vermont's wintry landscapes and Alice Krige's other-worldly performance as the spiteful spirit are the only two elements that work in this otherwise disjointed and not very frightening adaptation of the popular Peter Straub novel.
(MCA Videocassette and Disc) VC, LV

Ghosts on the Loose

(1943) B&W, 65 min. Director: William Beaudine.

Leo Gorcey, Huntz Hall, Bobby Jordan, Stanley Clements, Bela Lugosi, Ava Gardner. The Bowery Boys become involved with foreign agents who are using a haunted house as a blind for their counterfeiting ring. Zany, but not necessarily funny.

(Thunderbird Films, Budget Video) VC

Ghosts That Still Walk ½

(1978) Color, 96 min. Director: James T. Flocker.

Matt Boston, Ann Nelson, Jerry Jensen, Caroline Howe, Phil Catalli. Spirit of an Indian mummy possesses a young boy, who then proceeds to kill numerous members of his family. Meanwhile, boulders come to life in the surrounding mountains, begin rolling down hills and terrorizing passing motorists. It's all part of an Indian curse against the white man for stealing Indian land.

(Video Communications) VC

Ghoul, The ½

(1974) Color, 90 min. Director: Freddie Francis.

Peter Cushing, Veronica Carlson, John Hurt. A doctor's son, victim of a curse, requires flesh and blood to survive. Nicely handled period thriller set in the 1920s, which has the look of a Hammer Film, but isn't one. Structured a bit like *Psycho* with an unexpected murder occurring halfway through.

(Electric Video) VC

Giant from the Unknown ½

(1958) B&W, 77 min. Director: Richard E. Cunha.

Buddy Baer, Sally Fraser, Ed Kemmer, Morris Ankrum, Bob Steele. A giant Spanish Conquistador returns from the dead to reclaim a small California village as his own. Make-up is by veteran Jack *(Frankenstein)* Pierce.

(Nostalgia Merchant) VC

Gladiators, The ½

(1969) Color, 90 min. Director: Peter Watkins.

Arthur Pentelow, Frederick Danner. Documentary-like forerunner of *Rollerball* which takes place in the year 1994. Teams from the East and West meet on TV every Saturday night to duel to the death as part of a series of international peace games held in an effort to avert broader war. Grim, but challenging drama filmed in Sweden. Grand Prize Winner at the 1970 International Science-Fiction Festival in Trieste.

(Wizard Video) VC

Glen or Glenda?

(1953) B&W, 67 min. Director: Edward D. Wood, Jr.

Bela Lugosi, Dolores Fuller, Daniel Davis (Ed Wood), Lyle Talbot. Transvestite director Wood's plea for tolerance of his "condition" mixes bizarre fantasy sequences with straightforward dramatic (though unintentionally hilarious) scenes of him explaining to his girlfriend how much he'd like to wear her sweater. Lugosi is the on-camera narrator, a doctor who steps in now and then to explain what's going on. A perfectly dreadful movie.

(Video Dimensions) VC

Godsend, The

(1977) Color, 93 min. Director: Gabrielle Beaumont.

Cyd Hayman, Malcolm Stoddard, Angela Pleasence, Patrick Barr. Another post-*Exorcist* terror tale about a really rotten kid. This one's a blonde, but she doesn't necessarily have more fun. And neither does the audience.

(Vestron Video) VC

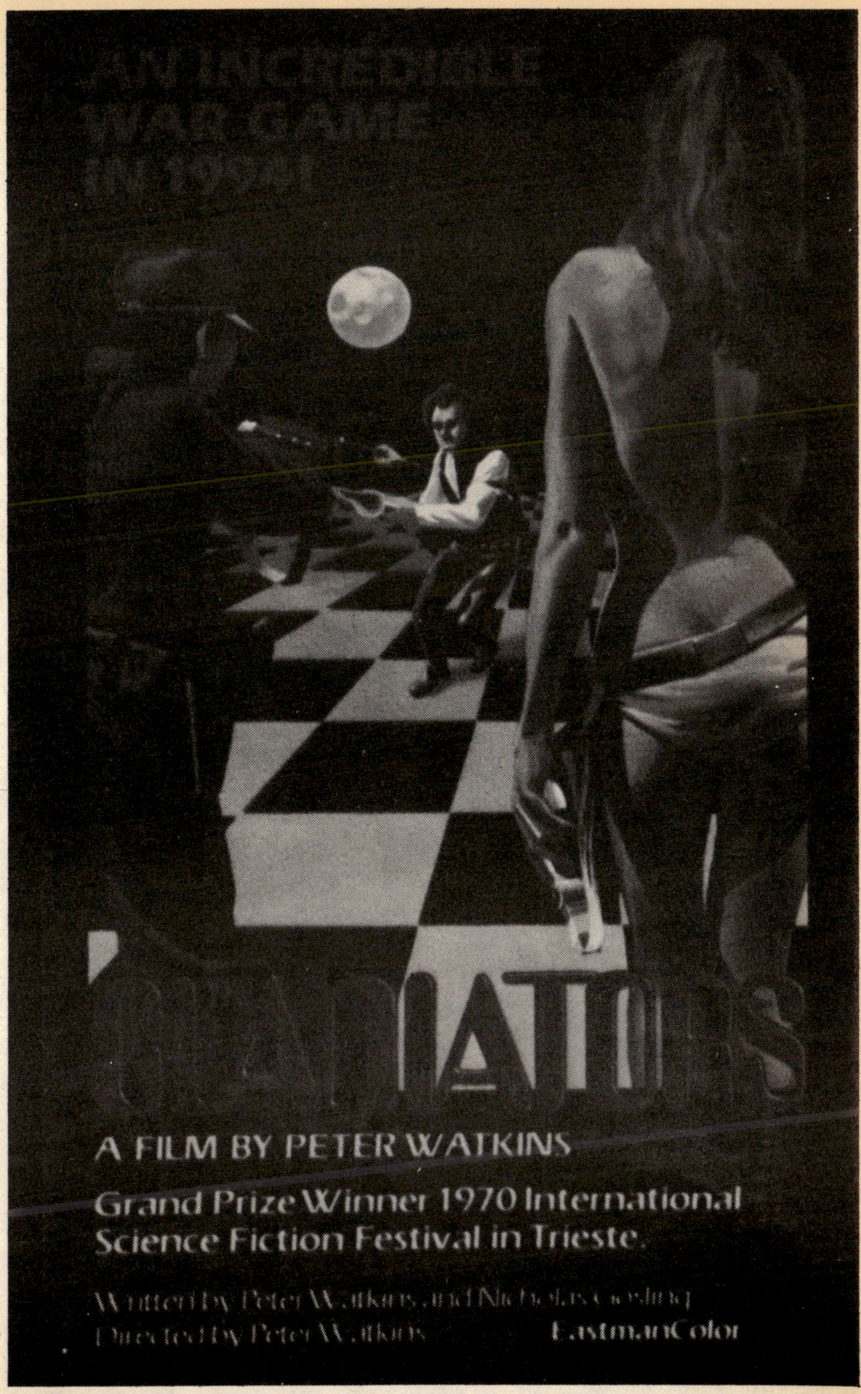

The Gladiators (1969)

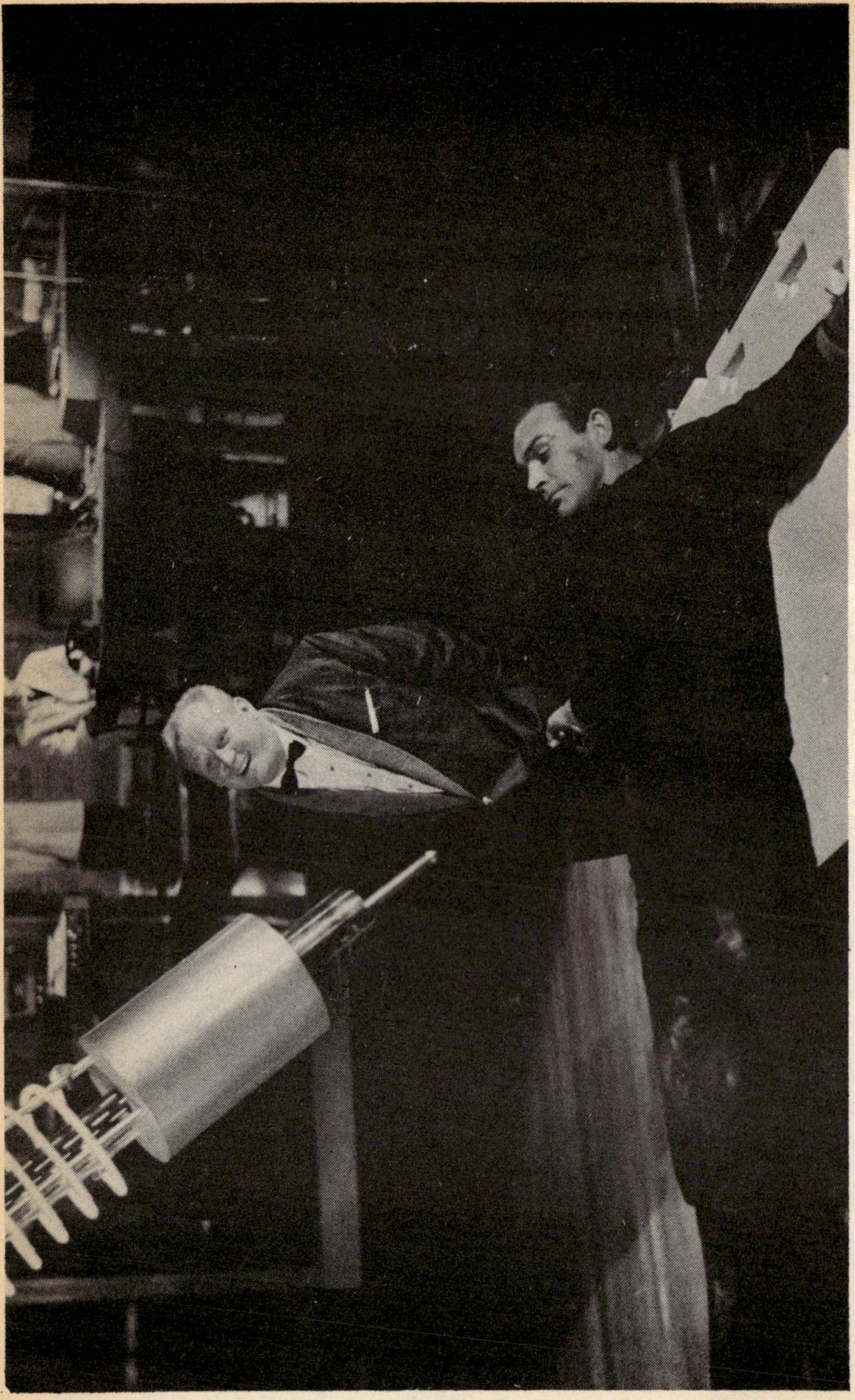

Goldfinger (1964)

Goldengirl ☐☐

(1979) Color, 117 min. Director: Joseph Sargeant.
Susan Anton, Curt Jurgens, Harry Guardino, James Coburn, Robert Culp, Leslie Caron. Neo-Nazi doctor and physical fitness nut Jurgens uses his daughter as a guinea pig in an experiment designed to produce a superwoman. He conditions her with drugs until she is mentally and physically ready to become the world's greatest Olympic track star. Dumb.
(CBS/Fox Video) VC

Golden Voyage of Sinbad, The ☐☐½

(1974) Color, 105 min. Director: Gordon Hessler.
John Phillip Law, Tom Baker, Caroline Munro, Douglas Wilmer. Sinbad (Law) and a helpful homunculus embark on a strange voyage in search of a mythical golden crown and encounter the beautiful Munro plus many wonderful Ray Harryhausen special effects along the way. The acting overall is weak—Law makes a completely colorless hero, the music score by Miklos Rosza works against the film rather than with it, and the story by Brian Clemens is just so-so. But despite these shortcomings, the film remains an exciting entry in the Harryhausen Sinbad series.
(Columbia Pictures Home Entertainment) VC

Goldfinger ☐☐☐

(1964) Color, 112 min. Director: Guy Hamilton.
Sean Connery, Honor Blackman, Gert Frobe, Shirley Eaton, Bernard Lee, Harold Sakata. Third entry in the James Bond series has agent 007 hot on the trail of international gold smuggler Frobe, whose latest nefarious scheme is to explode a nuclear bomb inside Fort Knox, thereby rendering its gold reserves radioactive for the next hundred years. Sakata is Frobe's silent but deadly bodyguard who's not only an expert at karate, but wields a mean iron hat as well. Lavish adventure with the emphasis on suspense rather than gimmicks.
(CBS/Fox Video, RCA VideoDisc) VC, CED

Gorath ☐

(1962) Color, 89 min. Director: Inoshiro Honda.
Ryo Ikebe, Jun Tazaki, Yumi Skirakawa. A runaway planet is on a collision course with earth, but misses due to some quick thinking by scientists, who use rockets to divert it. But hold on, folks, that's not all. The gravitational pull of the passing planet causes a major earthquake which releases a prehistoric monster in the shape of a giant walrus! No, I'm not kidding.
(Discount Video) VC

Gore, Gore Girls, The ☐

(1972) Color, 90 min. Director: Herschell Gordon Lewis.
Frank Kress, Amy Farrell, Henny Youngman. Gory whodunit from splatter-master Lewis about a psychopathic slayer-mutilator of beautiful go-go dancers who work for nightclub owner Youngman. A.k.a. *Blood Orgy.*
(Midnight Video) VC

Gorgo ☐☐½

(1961) Color, 76 min. Director: Eugene Lourie.
Bill Travers, William Sylvester, Vincent Winter, Bruce Seton, Christopher Rhodes. An undersea explosion off the Irish coast releases a baby monster which is then captured and put on exhibit in a London circus. But then, Mama comes to call. Good special effects.
(Nostalgia Merchant) VC

Gorilla, The ✪✪

(1939) B&W, 67 min. Director: Allan Dwan.
The Ritz Brothers, Patsy Kelly, Anita Louise, Bela Lugosi, Lionel Atwill. Comedy/mystery in the tradition of *The Cat and the Canary*—and based on a play by Ralph Spence that's just about as old—but a lot zanier due to the participation of the madcap brothers Ritz. A man commits a series of murders in a gorilla suit to make his crimes look like the work of a killer ape. Silly, but fun.
(Budget Video) VC

Graduation Day ✪✪

(1981) Color, 85 min. Director: Herb Reed.
Christopher George, Patch MacKenzie, E. Danny Murphy, Michael Pataki, E.J. Peaker. Death on campus as track stars are stalked and killed by standard horror movie psycho whose face is concealed until the not too surprising finish.
(Columbia Pictures Home Entertainment) VC

Great Gabbo, The ✪✪½

(1929) Color/B&W, 70 min. Director: James Cruze.
Erich von Stroheim, Betty Compson, Don Douglas, Marjorie Kane. Early talkie offers von Stroheim as an insane ventriloquist who comes to believe that his dummy is alive and victimizing him. Based on Ben Hecht's short story *The Rival Dummy.*
(Thunderbird Films) VC

Great Movie Stunts & The Making of Raiders of the Lost Ark ✪✪✪

(1981) Color, 100 min.
Originally aired separately on network TV, these two behind-the-scenes looks at the phenomenonally successful George Lucas/Steven Spielberg collaboration about the adventures of Indiana Jones (Harrison Ford) and his search for the lost Ark of the Covenant have been combined onto one cassette. Together, the two documentaries contain just about every exciting scene from *Raiders.* The "Stunts" episode demonstrates how major action sequences were designed and carried out while the "Making" film captures the cast and crew in the studio and on location. A real collector's item.
(Paramount Home Video, RCA VideoDisc) VC, CED

Great Muppet Caper, The ✪✪½

(1981) Color, 95 min. Director: Jim Hensen.
The Muppets, Charles Grodin, Diana Rigg, John Cleese, Robert Morley, Peter Falk, Jack Warden. Theft of fabulous jewel, the "Baseball Diamond," sparks the caper of the title and a host of take-offs on various famous scenes from familiar movies. Most successful is Miss Piggy's nautical ballet a la Esther Williams.
(CBS/Fox Video, RCA VideoDisc) VC, CED

Green Room, The ✪✪½

(1978) Color, 90 min. Director: Francois Truffaut.
Francois Truffaut, Nathalie Baye, Jean Daste, Jean-Pierre Moulin. A journalist erects a secret shrine to the dead, including his young bride, who was killed shortly after their marriage. A love story with ghostly overtones, based on Henry James' *Altar of the Dead.*
(Warner Home Video) VC

Gruesome Twosome, The ☐½

(1967) Color, 72 min. Director: Herschell Gordon Lewis.
Elizabeth Davis, Chris Martel, Gretchen Welles, Rodney Bedell. Wigged out son (Martel) of equally wigged out wig shop owner Davis scalps young women with a battery-operated electric knife and other handy tools in order to collect hair for mom's business. Ultra-realistic gore effects mixed with absurdism make for a passably funny ghoulish "comedy."
(Midnight Video) VC

Gulliver's Travels ☐☐

(1939) Color, 77 min. Director: Dave Fleischer.
Early animated feature with music based on the Jonathan Swift satire about an English traveler who finds himself captive in a land of little people. For the kids.
(Nostalgia Merchant, Media Home Entertainment, Direct Video) VC

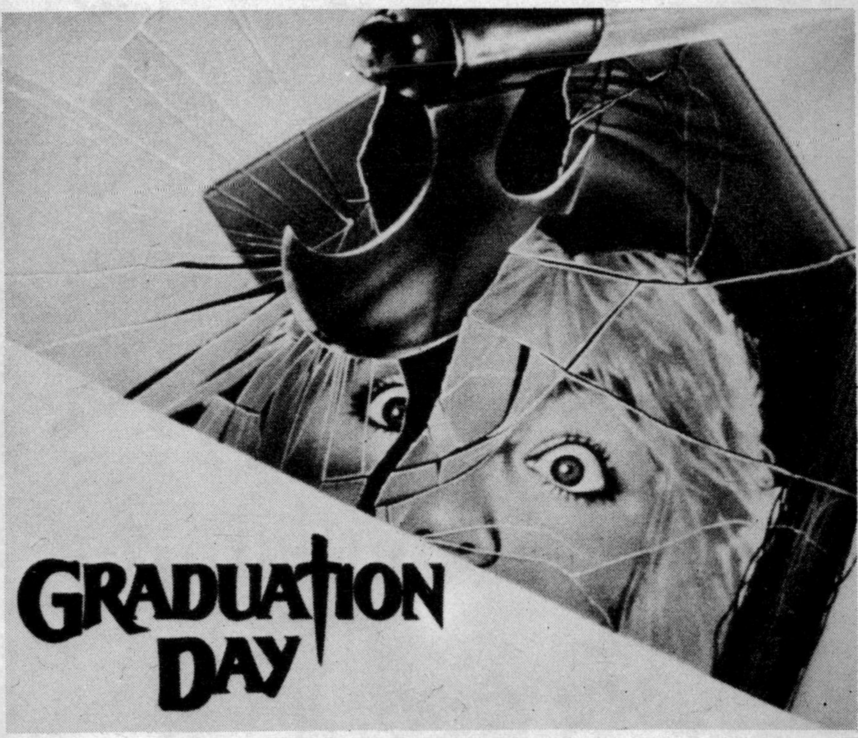

Graduation Day (1981)

"Death on campus. . ."

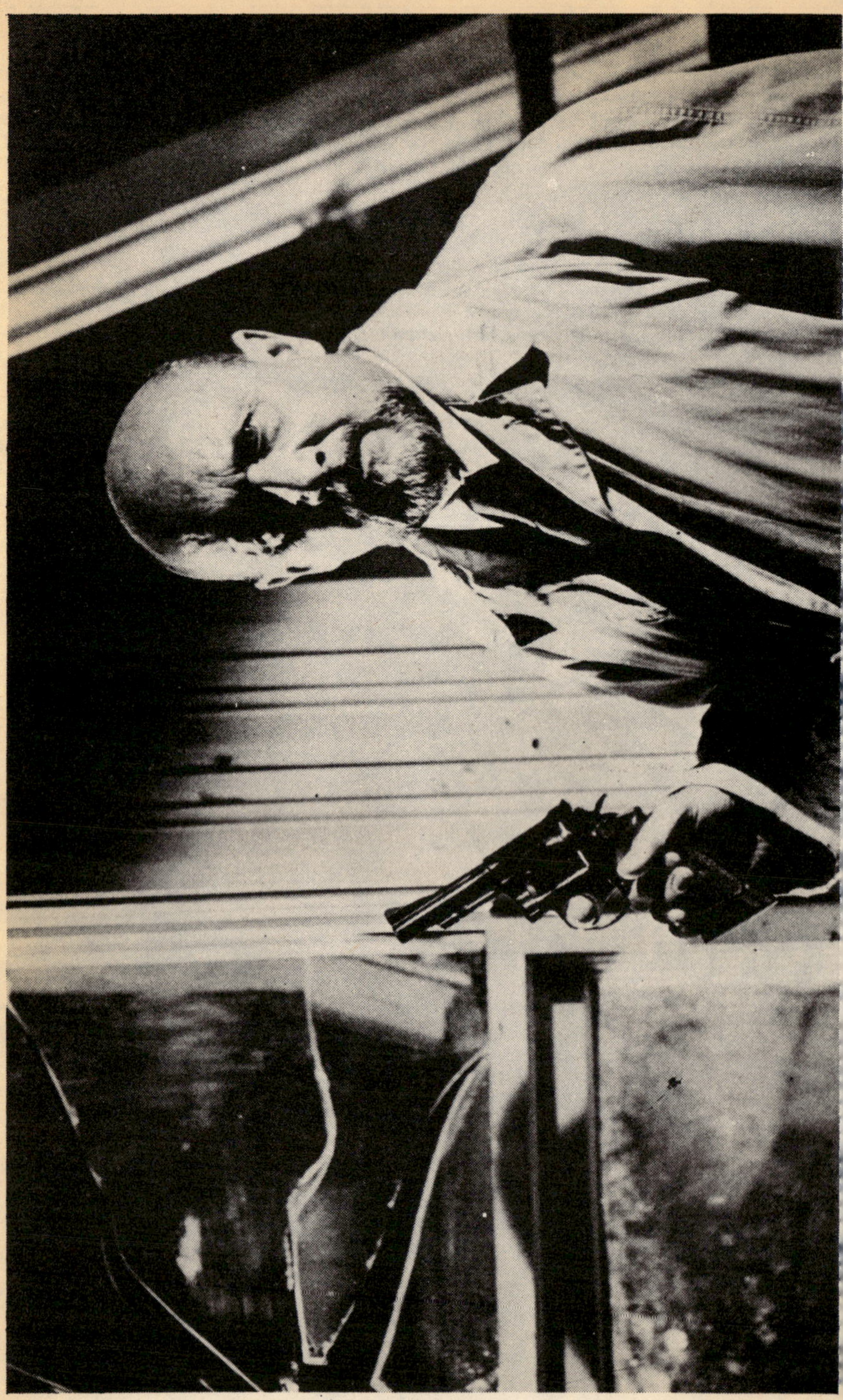

Halloween (1978)

H

Halloween

(1978) Color, 90 min. Director: John Carpenter.
Jamie Lee Curtis, Donald Pleasence, Nancy Loomis, P.J. Soles. A psychotic masked killer—and stand-in for the boogey man—busts out of the asylum where he was sent after murdering his sister some years back and returns to the scene of the crime, his old home town. His target this time: a trio of delectable baby-sitters. This low-budget nod to Hitchcock's *Psycho* (the Pleasence character, for example, is named Sam Loomis after the part played by John Gavin in the Hitchcock classic) went on to become one of the most successful independent films ever made and boosted Carpenter's career considerably. But the film itself is so simple-minded, so full of inconsistencies and wild improbabilities that it leaves one with the feeling of having been tricked rather than treated.
(Media Home Entertainment) VC

Halloween II ½

(1981) Color, 92 min. Director: Rick Rosenthal.
Jamie Lee Curtis, Donald Pleasence, Charles Cyphers, Jeffrey Kramer. The Shape returns to stalk lone survivor Curtis one last time. One hopes, at any rate.
(MCA Videocassette) VC

Hand, The

(1981) Color, 105 min. Director: Oliver Stone.
Michael Caine, Andrea Marcovicci, Annie McEnroe. Caine is a mild-mannered cartoonist who loses his drawing hand and his cool in a freak accident. Thereafter he uses the symbol of the missing hand as a way to unleash all his long suppressed hostilities, including a desire to commit murder. Occasionally convoluted terror tale which lapses all too frequently into undiluted hokum. Caine is good, though. Would make a great double bill with David Cronenberg's *The Brood.* Based on the novel *The Lizard's Tail* by Marc Brandel.
(Warner Home Video) VC

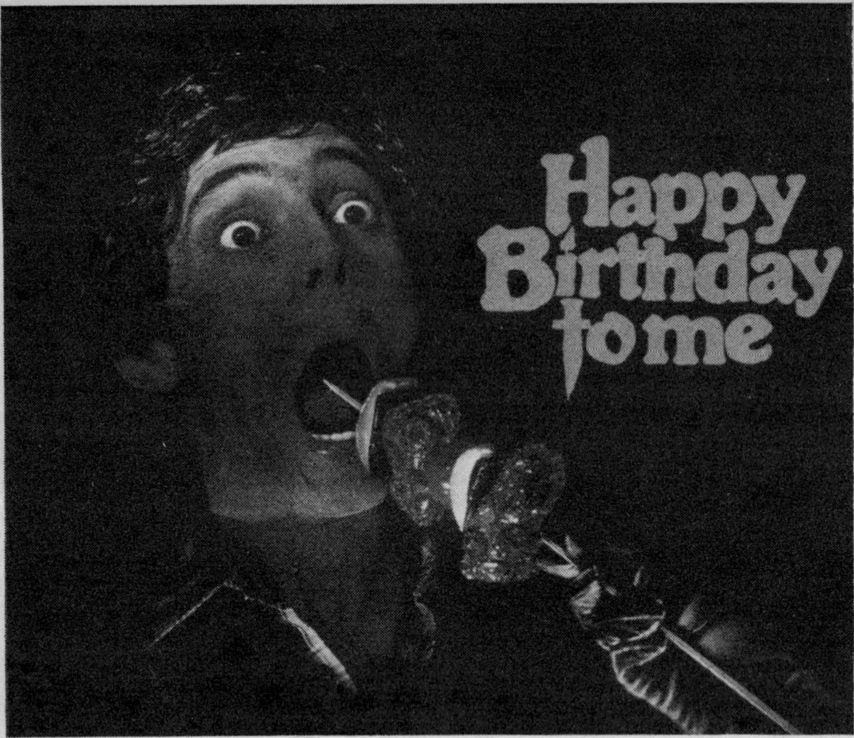

Happy Birthday to Me (1981)

". . .makes no sense at all. . ."

Hansel and Gretel

(1970) Color, 82 min. Director: F.J. Gottlieb.
Barbara Klingered, Francy Fair, Dagobert Walter, Herbert Fux, Karl Dall. A not entirely kiddie-oriented re-telling of the familiar Grimm fairy tale about the woodcutter's children who venture into a forest to pick strawberries and are caught by a witch who turns children into gingerbread. A.k.a. *Hands Off Gretel.*
(Media Home Entertainment) VC

Happy Birthday to Me

(1981) Color, 108 min. Director: J. Lee Thompson.
Melissa Sue Anderson, Glenn Ford, Tracy Bregman, Jack Blum. Returning to college after recuperating from a car crash that killed her mother and put her out of commission for months, Anderson discovers herself experiencing blackouts—after which some of her friends start turning up dead. Is she the guilty party? Well, it takes a party to find out—a birthday party, that is—at which the killer is finally revealed in an ending that is so poorly established that it virtually makes no sense at all. With his longstanding screen reputation, Ford should be ashamed for having appeared in a piece of junk like this, but then his part is so insignificant and his appearances so infrequent that he probably thought it didn't matter. It does.
(Columbia Pictures Home Entertainment) VC

Hardware Wars and Other Film Farces

(1981) Color, 48 min. Directors: Ernie Fosselius, Marv Newland, Rick Harper.
A quartet of spoofs on some of Hollywood's most famous blockbusters, including *Hardware Wars,* a send-up of you-know-what; *Porklips Now,* a deflating of Coppola's Vietnam epic; *Closet Encounters of the Nerd Kind;* and the immortal *Bambi Meets Godzilla.* Inventive and very funny.
(Warner Home Video) VC

Hatchet Murders, The ½

(1975) Color, 98 min. Director: Dario Argento.
David Hemmings, Daria Nicolodi, Gabriele Lavia, Macha Meril. Mind reader tunes into the deranged thoughts of a homicidal maniac, actually sees grisly murders through the killer's eyes, but cannot identify the killer's face until the last reel. A.k.a. *Deep Red.*
(HomeVision) VC

Haunted, The

(1977) Color, 85 min. Director: Michael de Gaetano.
Aldo Ray, Virginia Mayo, Ann Michelle, Jim Nigele. The ancient curse of an Indian woman haunts a present day family, and the body of a young girl is possessed by a vengeful spirit to fulfill the curse. You see, it all started the day they installed a phone booth on the Indians' burial grounds.
(Direct Video) VC

Haunted Strangler, The

(1958) B&W, 81 min. Director: Robert Day.
Boris Karloff, Anthony Dawson, Jean Kent, Elizabeth Allen, Vera Day. Writer Karloff probes the death of a murderer executed at Newgate prison years before and gets so immersed in the details of the man's case that he starts taking on his bad habits as well. Turns out that there's a good reason for this sudden transformation—as revealed in a not-so-surprise ending. Nice Victorian atmosphere, though.
(Media Home Entertainment) VC

Haunting of Julia, The ★★½

(1981) Color, 98 min. Director: Richard Loncraine.
Mia Farrow, Kier Dullea, Tom Conti, Jill Bennett, Cathleen Nesbitt. Farrow's daughter dies in a freak choking accident and her marriage to Dullea dissolves thereafter. Later, when she moves into a home of her own, she finds it to be haunted by the spirit of a lost, lonely, and, as it turns out, very evil little girl. Despite the fact that many important plot threads are left hanging and that some of the plotting makes no sense at all, this film does manage to generate a certain amount of unease. By no means a success, but interesting nonetheless. Dullea is terrible by the way. Based on the novel *Julia* by Peter Straub. A.k.a. *Full Circle.*
(Media Home Entertainment) VC

Hearse, The ★★

(1980) Color, 95 min. Director: George Bowers.
Trish Van Devere, Joseph Cotten, David Gautreaux, Donald Hotton. Heroine Van Devere seeks rest and quiet by moving into an old house that's located well off the beaten track and is also haunted. The ghost, however, is not dead, but a neighbor who has made a pact with the devil to achieve immortality and wants Trish for his eternal bride. Come nightfall, he sends a phantom hearse to fetch her, but she proves to be no pushover. Nicely mounted but totally predictable, standard horror movie fare.
(Media Home Entertainment) VC

Heartbeeps ★½

(1981) Color, 79 min. Director: Allan Arkush.
Andy Kaufman, Bernadette Peters, Randy Quaid, Kenneth McMillan, Melanie Mayron. Futuristic comedy about two robots that fall in love. Not too funny. Stan Winston's make-up effects are brilliant, though.
(MCA Videocassette) VC

Heaven Can Wait ★★

(1978) Color, 100 min. Directors: Warren Beatty, Buck Henry.
Warren Beatty, Julie Christie, James Mason, Jack Warden, Dyan Cannon, Charles Grodin. Lightweight romantic fantasy about footballer Beatty who is mistakenly recalled to the great beyond before his time and bargains with angel Mason to be allowed to return to earth in another man's body to live out his justly remaining years. Film has few comic high spots—nor romantic high spots either, and Beatty is miscast as a light, romantic lead. Re-make of *Here Comes Mr. Jordan.*
(Paramount Home Video, RCA VideoDisc) VC, CED, LV

Hell Night ★½

(1981) Color, 100 min. Director: Tony DeSimone.
Linda Blair, Vincent Van Patten, Peter Barton, Kevin Brody, Jenny Neuman. Just when you thought it was safe to go back to the frat house. . .it turns out to be the very place where a fellow frat brother witnessed his father slay the rest of his family several years back. Needless to say, the concept of hell night (hazing) triggers the prankster in him, and he starts killing off his brothers as well as some of his sisters from an associate sorority. For those of you who thought *Terror Train* was a classic.
(Media Home Entertainment) VC

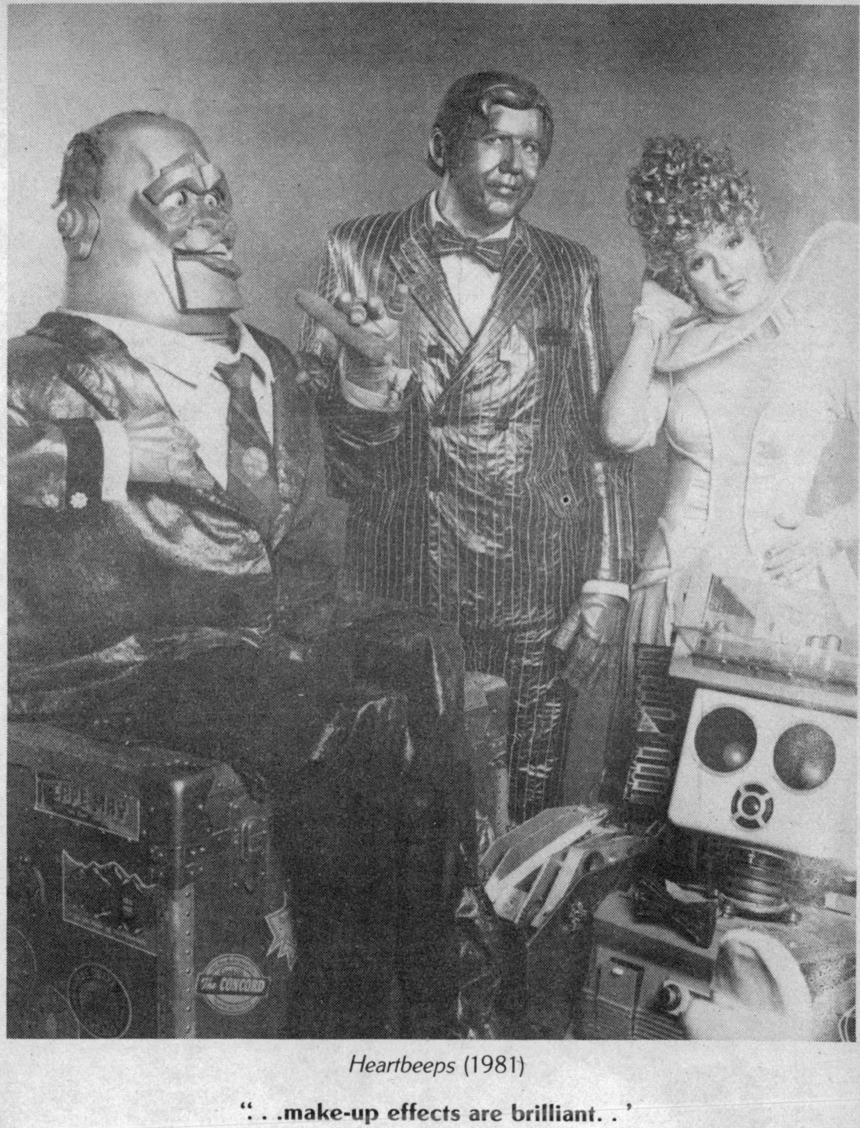

Heartbeeps (1981)

". . .make-up effects are brilliant. . '

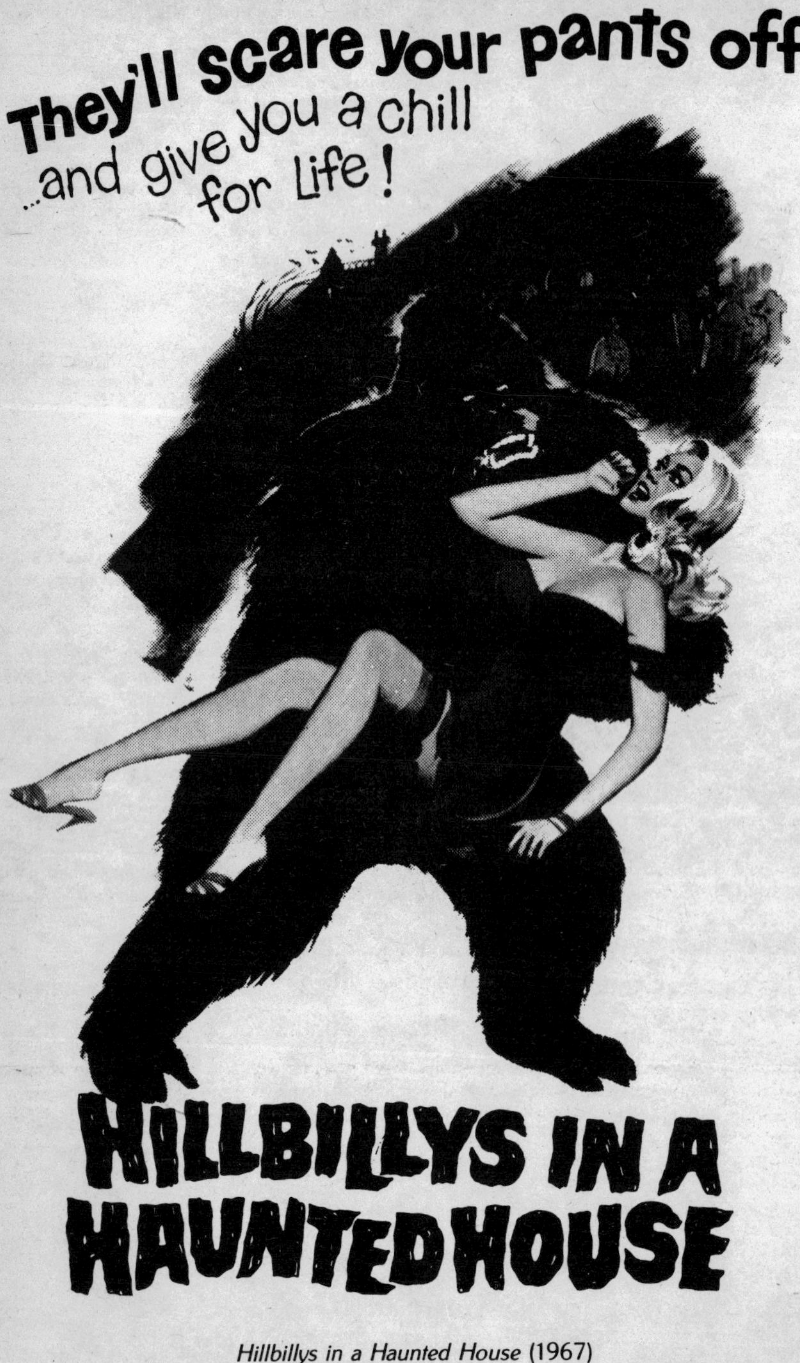
They'll scare your pants off
...and give you a chill
for Life!
HILLBILLYS IN A
HAUNTED HOUSE

Hillbillys in a Haunted House (1967)

Herbie Rides Again ½

(1974) Color, 88 min. Director: Robert Stevenson.
Helen Hayes, Stefanie Powers, Ken Berry, Keenan Wynn, John McIntire, Huntz Hall. Villain Wynn, a greedy land developer, has to combat Hayes, whose land he wants to develop, as well as her superpowered volkswagen in this popular sequel to the even more popular *The Love Bug.*
(Walt Disney Home Video, RCA VideoDisc) VC, CED

Here Comes Mr. Jordan ½

(1941) B&W, 93 min. Director: Alexander Hall.
Robert Montgomery, Claude Rains, Evelyn Keyes. See *Heaven Can Wait* for plot summary. Montgomery fares much better than Beatty in the lead role because of his surer comic touch. And in this film he's a boxer rather than a football star.
(Columbia Pictures Home Entertainment) VC

Hideous Sun Demon

(1959) B&W, 74 min. Directors: Robert Clarke, Thomas Cassarino.
Robert Clarke, Patricia Manning, Alan Peterson, Patrick Whyte, Fred La Porta. An accident in a radiation lab turns a scientist into a scaly monster whenever he gets an overdose of sunlight. As the film is set in California, you can bet this guy's in for trouble. A.k.a. *Terror from the Sun* and *Blood on His Lips.*
(Nostalgia Merchant) VC

High Plains Drifter ½

(1973) Color, 105 min. Director: Clint Eastwood.
Clint Eastwood, Verna Bloom, Marianna Hill, Jack Ging. Eastwood reprises his celebrated spaghetti western character "the-man-with-no-name" but in a very different context, for the film more closely resembles Poe's ghostly *The Masque of the Red Death* than it does a western. In it, Clint takes over as sheriff of a town whose previous sheriff was murdered—or was he?—by a gang of cutthroats while the townsfolk stood by and watched. A la *High Noon,* the gang is set to return and the townsfolk decide they need protection. Eastwood agrees, but not before he makes some very unusual demands. First, he has them literally paint the town red and then he himself gives the town a new name—Hell. Not a total success, but offbeat enough to be worth watching.
(MCA Videocassette and Disc) VC, LV

Hillbillys in a Haunted House

(1967) B&W, 88 min. Director: Jean Yarbrough.
John Carradine, Lon Chaney, Jr., Basil Rathbone, Ferlin Husky, Joi Lansing, Mamie Van Doren. Antiquated old, dark house thriller complete with masked killer and sliding wall panels. Film's only concession to modernity are its busty heroines and abysmal country and western score. Not exactly a classic.
(Video Communications) VC

Hills Have Eyes, The

(1977) Color, 90 min. Director: Wes Craven.
James Whitworth, John Steadman, Janus Blythe, Dee Wallace, Michael Berryman. Suburban middle class vacationers on a drive through the desert meet up with a murderous clan of deranged desert rats (when their car breaks down) and must fight for survival. A gore film with a ghoulishly comic edge that generates quite a fair amount of tension. From the director of the execrable *Last House on the Left.*
(Harmony Vision) VC

Hobbit, The ✪✪½

(1977) Color, 78 min. Director: Arthur Rankin, Jr.

Voices of Orson Bean, John Huston, Otto Preminger, Richard Boone. Animated film with music based on the first of J.R.R. Tolkien's vastly popular series of books about the land of Middle Earth and its population of elves and goblins. Occasionally enchanting, but, as usual with such things, the tunes are very forgettable.

(RCA VideoDisc) CED

Horror Express ✪✪

(1972) Color, 95 min. Director: Eugenio Martin.

Peter Cushing, Christopher Lee, Telly Savalas, Alberto de Mendoza. The body of a recently discovered prehistoric creature that is being shipped aboard the Trans-Siberian Express from China to Moscow is soon discovered by the passengers to be exerting strange power over them, forcing them to commit murder. An Italian-English-Spanish co-production with lots of close-ups of blazing red eyes, if you like that sort of thing.

(Media Home Entertainment, King of Video, Budget Video) VC

Horror Hospital ✪✪½

(1973) Color, 91 min. Director: Antony Balch.

Michael Gough, Robin Askwith, Vanessa Shaw, Dennis Price. Modestly amusing satire of horror films about a doctor who turns his patients into zombies *without* the use of an anesthetic. A dwarf with a Marxist (Groucho, that is) wit provides some of the brighter lines of dialogue.

(Video Communications) VC

Horror Hotel ✪✪½

(1960) B&W, 76 min. Director: John Moxey.

Christopher Lee, Betta St. John, Venetia Stevenson, Patricia Jessel, Valentine Dyall. A student involved in the study of witchcraft (101, perhaps?) stumbles upon a Salem-like Massachusetts town where the craft is still being practiced. Unassuming, but atmospheric and occasionally quite effective minor shocker.

(Thunderbird Films) VC

Horror of Frankenstein ✪✪✪

(1970) Color, 95 min. Director: Jimmy Sangster.

Ralph Bates, Kate O'Mara, Graham Jones, Veronica Carlson, Dennis Price. Sangster satirizes his own script for Hammer's earlier *Curse of Frankenstein* in this tongue in cheek remake. A lot of people dislike this movie because they take it seriously. It's not supposed to be. If you have any doubts about that, just check out Dennis Price's delightful cameo as a droll gravedigger. It's, well. . .priceless.

(Thorn/EMI Video) VC

Horror Rises from the Tomb ✪

(1973) Color, 80 min. Director: Carlos Aured Alonso.

Paul Naschy, Emma Cohen, Vic Winner, Helga Line, Christina Suriana, Luis Ciges. Spirit of villainous knight, who was beheaded for his crimes, returns to plague his ancestors, possessing them and forcing them to re-enact his gruesome crimes. Spanish horror film.

(Demonique Video) VC

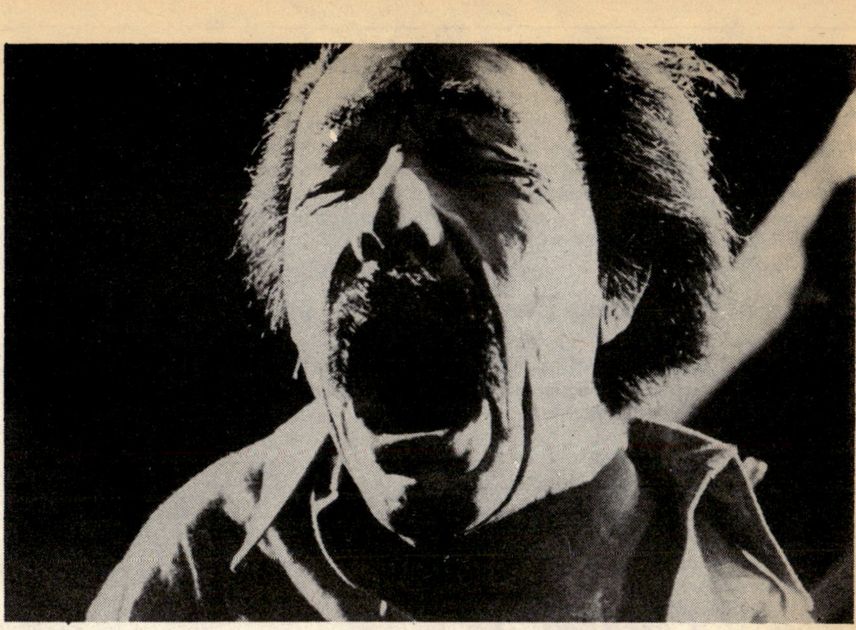

Humanoids from the Deep (1980)

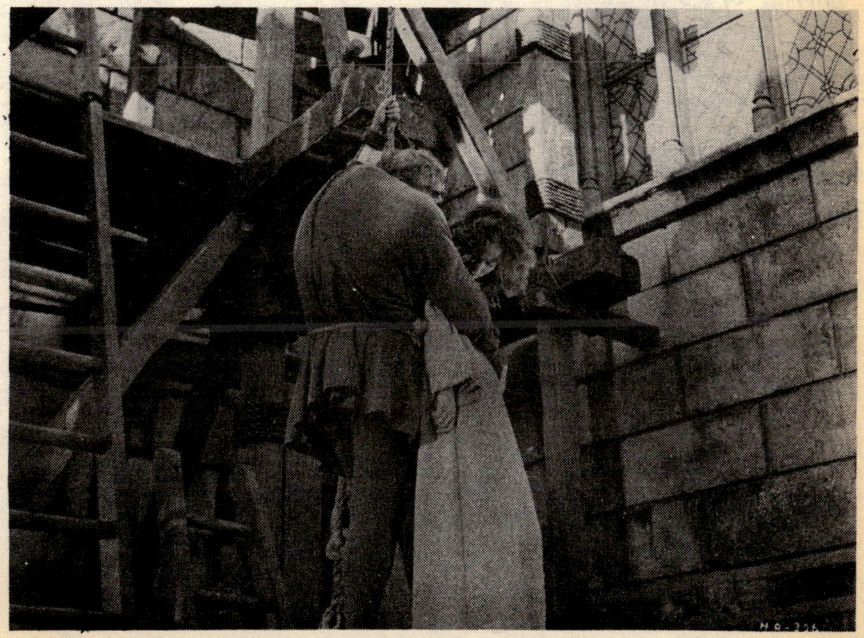

The Hunchback of Notre Dame (1939)

Hound of the Baskervilles, The

(1959) Color, 84 min. Director: Terence Fisher.
Peter Cushing, Christopher Lee, Andre Morell. Conan Doyle's well known Sherlock Holmes mystery about the phantom hound which has cursed and killed the Baskerville line for centuries is given lush, but not very frightening treatment in this low-budget period thriller from England's Hammer Films. Cushing is the embodiment of the effete, neurotic super sleuth, and Morell's stalwart and intelligent Watson remains the closest to Doyle's original conception that the screen has yet given us. An example of Hammer Horror at its best.
(CBS/Fox Video) VC, LV

House of the Living Dead

(1973) Color, 87 min. Director: Ray Austin.
Mark Burns, Shirley Anne Field, David Oxley. A curse on a South African family starts coming true when family members start getting knocked off by a caped killer. A.k.a. *Doctor Maniac.*
(Video Communications) VC

House of the Seven Corpses, The

(1972) Color, 90 min. Director: Paul Harrison.
John Ireland, Faith Domergue, John Carradine. The title explains all in this turkey that is so bad that it was never even released to theatres, but was sold straight to television—which, naturally, accepted it with open arms.
(Video Gems) VC

House That Vanished, The ½

(1973) Color, 84 min. Director: Joseph Larraz.
Andrea Allan, Karl Lanchbury. A young girl is held captive for a night in a house of horror, but when she escapes and returns with the police, the house seems to have disappeared. Was she imagining it all? Not quite. Entertaining mystery/thriller with some erotic soft core sequences.
(Video Communications) VC

Howling, The ½

(1981) Color, 91 min. Director: Joe Dante.
Dee Wallace, Patrick MacNee, Dennis Dugan, Christopher Stone. Sexy werewolf tale which mixes comedy and horror much more successfully than *An American Werewolf* but to just as little purpose. Rob Bottin's werewolf transformation effects are the film's high point, arguably even better than those in *Werewolf.* One of Dante's many in-jokes is to provide most of the film's characters with names of well known horror filmmakers—George Waggner, R. William Neill, Terry Fisher, Fred Francis, Erle Kenton and so on.
(CBS/Fox Video, RCA VideoDisc) VC, CED

Human Experiments

(1980) Color, 82 min. Director: J. Gregory Goodell.
Linda Haynes, Geoffrey Lewis, Ellen Travolta, Aldo Ray, Jackie Coogan, Lurene Tuttel. A prison psychiatrist rids inmates of their criminal impulses through brainwashing techniques which erase their memories completely, after which they are given new identities.
(VidAmerica) VC

Human Monster, The ½

(1939) B&W, 76 min. Director: Walter Summers.
Bela Lugosi, Hugh Williams, Greta Gynt. If you swallow this plot-line whole then I have some swamp property in Florida that I'd like to talk over with you. Con man and insurance swindler Lugosi uses *blind* vagrants to carry out his complex schemes. Based on the novel *The Dark Eyes of London* by Edgar Wallace.
(Thunderbird Films) VC

Humanoids from the Deep ½

(1980) Color, 82 min. Director: Barbara Peeters.
Doug McClure, Ann Turkel, Vic Morrow. A California fishing village is terrorized by a modern ecological horror that is half-man, half-fish, and all horny: sea beasts that are compelled to mate with village women in order to preserve their species. Absurd splattery thriller with some good effects by Rob Bottin.
(Warner Home Video) VC

Hunchback of Notre Dame, The ½

(1923) B&W, 95 min. Director: Wallace Worsley.
Lon Chaney, Patsy Ruth Miller, Norman Kerry. Ponderous, but spectacular first filming of the familiar Victor Hugo novel about the deformed Parisian bellringer and his unrequited love for a beautiful gypsy girl. The pains Chaney went through to create his make-up for the role and the pain he then went through to perform it are the stuff of Hollywood legend. His performance, a sublime example of silent screen pantomime, remains the best thing about the film.
(Blackhawk) VC

Hunchback of Notre Dame, The ½

(1939) B&W, 117 min. Director: William Dieterle.
Charles Laughton, Maureen O'Hara, Edmond O'Brien, Thomas Mitchell, Cedric Hardwicke. This elaborate and expensive remake of the Chaney silent eclipes the original in almost every way. Script, direction and performances are all first rate with Laughton a standout as the pathetic Quasimodo.
(Nostalgia Merchant, RCA VideoDisc) VC, CED

Hunted, The

(1974) Color, 84 min. Director: Douglas Fithian.
Lee Remick, Michael Hinz, Ivan Desny, Jose Caffarel, Jan White, Ingrid Garbo. Variation on the classic tale *The Most Dangerous Game* in which a crazed sportsman hunts down humans and kills them to get his macho kicks.
(Direct Video) VC

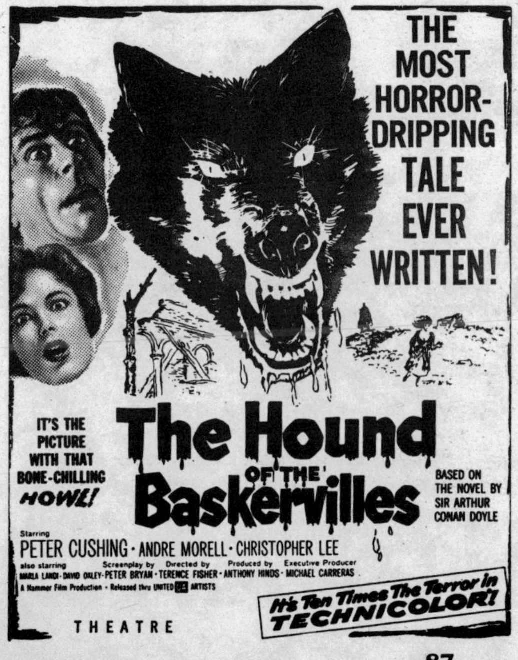

The Hound of the Baskervilles (1959)

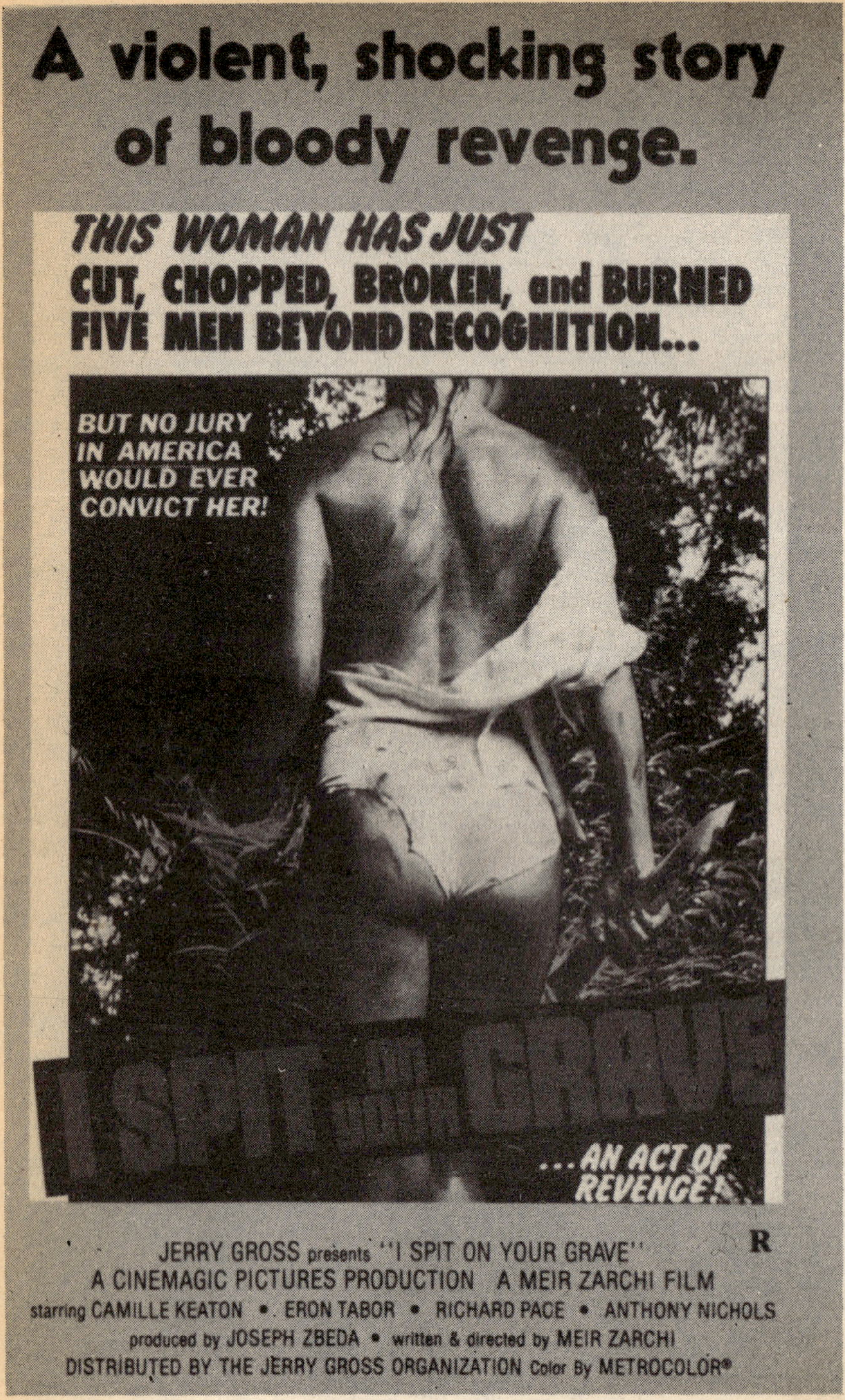

I Spit on Your Grave (1980)

I Bury the Living ½

(1958) B&W, 76 min. Director: Albert Band.
Richard Boone, Theodore Bikel, Peggy Maurer, Herb Anderson. A cemetery owner sticks white pins in the chart on his office wall to indicate those graves which are owned but unoccupied. The black pins indicate those which are both. One day, however, he gets confused and sticks a black pin where a white one should go, and, presto, the living owner suddenly keels over dead. Is it that old black magic, or just part of an ingenious murder scheme? Effective chiller, but the ending doesn't hold up.
(Wizard Video) VC

I Dismember Mama ½

(1974) Color, 81 min. Director: Paul Leder.
Zooey Hall, Joanne Moore Jordan, Greg Mullavey, Marlene Tracy. With this one, the title really does tell all. A deranged young man, sick and tired of his domineering mother, decides to chop her up into little bitty pieces.
(AstroVideo) VC

I Eat Your Skin

(1971) B&W, 82 min. Director: Del Tenney.
William Joyce, Heather Hewitt, Betty Hyatt Linton, Dan Stapleton, Walter Coy. An adventurer and his fair maiden battle a mad scientist and a voodoo priest who have created a race of cannibal-zombies to protect their island hideaway. A.k.a. *Voodoo Blood Bath.* Which title do you think provides the subtler touch?
(Wizard Video) VC

I Married a Monster From Outer Space

(1958) B&W, 78 min. Director: Gene Fowler, Jr.
Tom Tryon, Gloria Talbot. Bridegroom Tryon goes outside to investigate a noise, discovers an alien spaceship instead, then has his body taken over by one of the ugly beings because it wants to roam around the neighborhood undetected. It picked the right actor. Tryon is as stiff as they come. Only blushing bride Talbot knows the truth of the matter, so she tries to blow the whistle on him/it before the bodies of any more earthlings are possessed. This film is not exactly a high-water mark among fifties science-fiction films, but it's good camp fun and is especially recommended for viewing by married couples on their anniversary, a time when each partner will find something in the film to identify with.
(Paramount Home Video) VC

I Spit On Your Grave ✪

(1980) Color, 98 min. Director: Meir Zarchi.
Camille Keaton, Aaron Tabor, Richard Pace, Anthony Nichols. Keaton (Buster's niece, by the way) is raped by a quartet of thugs, after which she exacts her revenge in an orgy of violence that makes what they did to her look positively pleasant by comparison. A film in the tradition of *Last House on the Left,* which is so horrendous that even John Waters admits he was grossed out by it.
(Wizard Video) VC

I Walked with a Zombie ✪✪✪✪

(1943) B&W, 69 min. Director: Jacques Tourneur.
Tom Conway, Frances Dee, James Ellison, Christine Gordon. Intensely atmospheric Val Lewton film set in Haiti which borrows plot elements from *Jane Eyre,* but gives them a voodoo twist. Planter Conway's wife (Gordon) suffers from a strange, catatonic malaise, which the natives believe to be zombie-ism. Dee is the nurse he hires to take care of her. Director Tourneur, whose best film this is, provides some stunning set pieces, including a hair-raising journey by Dee and Gordon through the haunted, Haitian marshes during a wind storm to get to a voodoo ceremony which Dee hopes will result in Gordon's cure. A great one.
(Nostalgia Merchant) VC

If ✪✪ ½

(1969) Color/B&W, 111 min. Director: Lindsay Anderson.
Malcolm McDowell, David Wood, Richard Warwick, Peter Jeffrey, Christine Noonan. Drama of life in a repressive English boarding school for boys leading to a finale (possibly fantasized?) in which the boys rebel against their authoritarian masters with machine guns. Vastly overpraised when it first came out.
(Paramount Home Video) VC

In Search of Ancient Astronauts ✪✪✪

(1973) Color, 52 min. Director: Alan Landsburg.
Narrated by Rod Serling. Erich van Daniken's best-selling *Chariots of the Gods?,* which suggested that earth was visited by extra-terrestrials many millions of years ago and that they left much evidence of their visit behind, spawned this mind-stretching documentary which was originally aired nationally by NBC during prime time. The evidence the film presents may not be conclusive, but the questions it raises certainly are challenging. Serling's presence on the soundtrack makes the whole affair seem like the ultimate adventure in *The Twilight Zone.*
(Thunderbird Films) VC

In Search of Noah's Ark ✪

(1976) Color, 95 min. Director: James L. Conway.
Narrated by Brad Crandall. A pseudo documentary which, in its advertising, claims to have found and photographed the original lost ark of Biblical legend, but then shows nothing except a bunch of boards in the shape of what might have been a boat located somewhere near Mount Ararat in Turkey. A real rip-off. It was sold to and appeared on network TV just two months after its saturation debut in theatres nationwide, which gives you some idea of the philosophy that guided its producers: take the money and run.
(Video Communications) VC

Incredible Hulk, The ✪✪

(1978) Color, 104 min. Director: Kenneth Johnson.
Bill Bixby, Lou Ferrigno, Jack Colvin. Feature length pilot for the TV series that made "green is beautiful" a household phrase. Bixby gets an overdose of gamma rays and turns into green-skinned, muscle-bound Ferrigno whenever his ire is aroused. Fun, but some of the individual series episodes were a lot more so.
(MCA Videocassette) VC

Incredible Shrinking Man, The ☒☒☒½

(1957) B&W, 81 min. Director: Jack Arnold.

Grant Williams, Randy Stuart, April Kent, William Schallert. While boating, Williams is subjected to a strange, radioactive mist which later causes him to start shrinking in size. Attacked by the family cat, he flees into the cellar where, continuing to shrink, he must do battle with a common spider to survive. One of the best science-fiction films of the fifties full of terrific special effects, suspenseful direction by Arnold, and a thought-provoking script by Richard Matheson based on his own novel *The Shrinking Man*. Tops.

(MCA VideoDisc) LV

Incredible Shrinking Woman, The ☒½

(1981) Color, 88 min. Director: Joel Schumacher.

Lily Tomlin, Charles Grodin, Ned Beatty, Rick Baker. Tomlin is a suburban housewife whose overexposure to aerosol sprays and other housekeeping ingredients results in her dwindling in size. She is then set upon by spies and counterspies who wish to discover the cause of her shrinkage in order to develop a secret weapon. Excellent special effects and an amusing performance by Baker disguised in gorilla suit as an ape named Sidney are the only redeeming elements in this otherwise silly variation on Richard Matheson's novel *The Shrinking Man* and the classic 1957 film made from it.

(MCA Videocassette and Disc) VC, LV

Invaders from Mars ☒½

(1953) Color, 78 min. Director: William Cameron Menzies.

Leif Erickson, Jimmy Hunt, Arthur Franz, Helena Carter, Morris Ankrum. A little boy with an overactive imagination spots a red glow emanating from behind the hill which overlooks his bedroom window, goes to investigate, and discovers evidence of an alien landing. But when he tells his parents in the morning, they won't believe him. Then his father (Erickson) is taken over by the aliens and returns home as a zombie in their control. Like many genre fans my age, this film scared me half to death when I first saw it. Now, however, it seems not only quite tame, but quite awful—badly acted, obvious and trite. Must be that it was made for kids. Nice color camerawork, though.

(Nostalgia Merchant) VC

Invasion from Inner Earth ☒

(1977) Color, 100 min. Director: Bill Rebane.

Paul Bentzer, Debbie Pick. A strange, earth-spawned disease wipes out a whole town—a result, no doubt, of massive exposure to this movie.

(Video Communications) VC

Invasion of the Blood Farmers ☒

(1972) Color, 80 min. Director: Ed Adlum.

Norman Kelley, Tanna Hunter. How ya' gonna' keep 'em down on the farm after they've been pureed? A half-baked religious sect, the Druids, cooks up a wild scheme to keep its catatonic, anemic, dying Queen—boy, is *she* a wreck!—alive by using ritual sacrifices involving gallons of human blood. Yummy.

(Thunderbird Films) VC

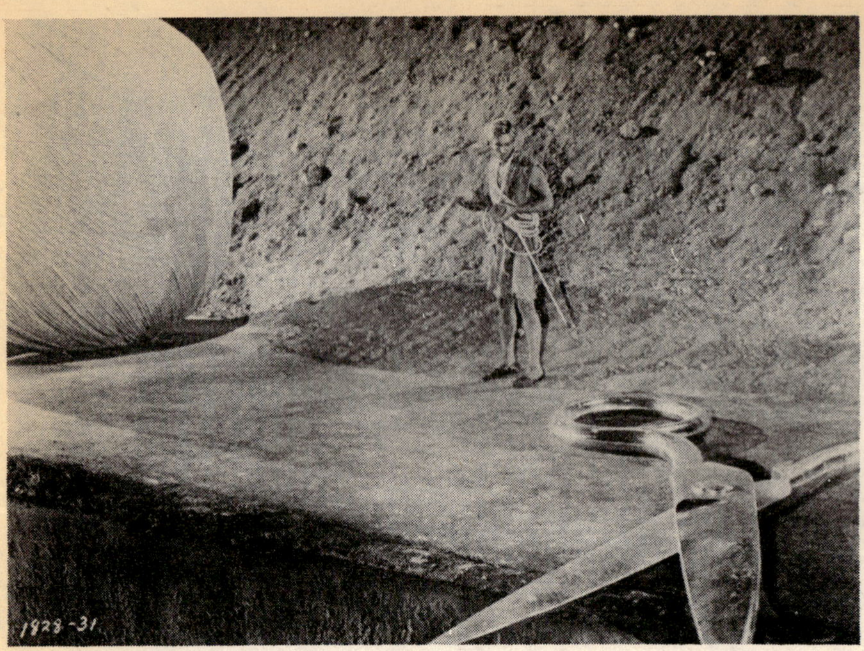

The Incredible Shrinking Man (1957)

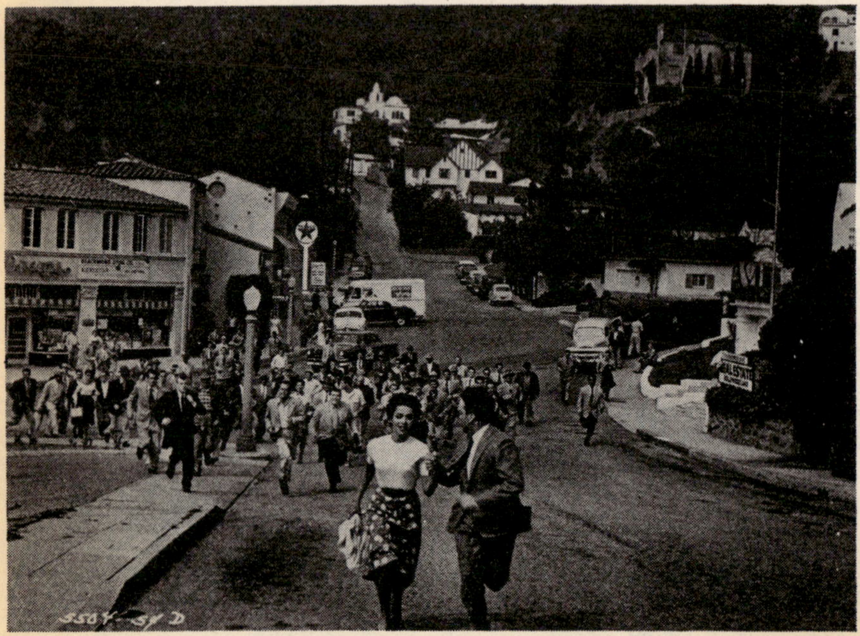

Invasion of the Body Snatchers (1956)

Invasion of the Body Snatchers ★★★½

(1956) B&W, 80 min. Director: Don Siegel.
Kevin McCarthy, Dana Wynter, Larry Gates, King Donovan, Carolyn Jones, Sam Peckinpah. The sleepy little town of Santa Mira, California, is suddenly invaded by body snatching spores from outer space, which overnight turn many of the townspeople into cold, unfeeling "pods." Fast-paced and effective sci-fi chiller that is also deeply reflective of the time it was made—the rabidly anti-communist, witchhunting fifties, a time when friends, relatives, and lovers literally did turn overnight into unfeeling enemies—government informers, Red baiters, and so on. One of the best.
(Nostalgia Merchant, RCA VideoDisc, NTA Home Entertainment) VC, CED

Invisible Ghost, The ★

(1941) B&W, 64 min. Director: Joseph H. Lewis.
Bela Lugosi, Polly Ann Young, John McGuire, Betty Compson, Jack Mulhall. The ghost of Lugosi's wife—actually she's not dead at all—comes back from the great beyond to hypnotize the poor dolt into committing murder for her. One of the endless series of low-grade thrillers that helped to seal the coffin on poor Lugosi's foundering screen career. A.k.a. *The Phantom Killer.*
(Video Ten) VC

Island, The ★

(1980) Color, 113 min. Director: Michael Ritchie.
Michael Caine, David Warner, Angela Punch-McGregor. Newsmagazine reporter Caine and his incredibly snotty son fly to the Bahamas to investigate a series of unsolved missing persons cases and stumble upon a cult of pirate cutthroats, descendants of the infamous buccaneers, who are still living in the old style, plundering and killing unsuspecting tourists for booty. A piece of far-fetched drivel in which Caine literally sleepwalks through his role, and the pirates, who speak a patois of gibberish, are about as fearsome as The Three Stooges. Based on a novel by Peter Benchley.
(MCA Videocassette) VC

Island of Dr. Moreau, The ★

(1977) Color, 98 min. Director: Don Taylor.
Burt Lancaster, Michael York, Barbara Carrera, Richard Basehart. Transparent adaptation of H.G. Wells' novel about vivisectionist Moreau (Lancaster) and his evil experiments to turn animals into humans through surgery. *Humanimals,* he calls them. Lancaster is miscast, Carrera is gorgeous, but wasted, and the humanimal make-ups on the whole are not very terrifying or convincing. *Isle of Lost Souls* (1933), also based on the Wells' book, is far superior.
(Warner Home Video) VC

Isle of the Dead ★★★

(1945) B&W, 72 min. Director: Mark Robson.
Boris Karloff, Ellen Drew, Marc Cramer, Katherine Emery, Jason Robards, Sr. Karloff is a Greek general who takes time off from his war duties to visit the grave of his wife on a remote island. The island is subsequently quarantined due to an outbreak of plague, and he and some of the other travelers are left stranded. One by one they die. But is it from the plague, or from some more sinister disease—like vampirism? Spooky Val Lewton chiller.
(Nostalgia Merchant) VC

It Came from Outer Space ★★½

(1953) B&W, 81 min. Director: Jack Arnold.
Richard Carlson, Barbara Rush, Charles Drake. An alien space ship crash lands in the desert, and its crew immediately starts assuming the identities of various humans in the area in order to move about unobserved, collecting needed parts to repair the ship. Astronomer Carlson makes contact with the ugly but benign beings, then must prevent the police and angry townsfolk from closing in for the kill until the aliens can fix their ship and head back for home. Originally filmed in 3-D and available on videocassette in that format. Based on a short story by Ray Bradbury.
(MCA Videocassette) VC

It's a Wonderful Life ♆♆♆

(1946) B&W, 129 min. Director: Frank Capra.
James Stewart, Donna Reed, Henry Travers, Lionel Barrymore. Good guy Stewart struggles hard to help his friends and his town flourish during hard times, but fails, and decides to commit suicide. Angel Travers intervenes to show Jimmy just how bad things would have been had he never lived. Corny but heartfelt Capra comedy/fantasy that endures because of the sincere performances of everyone involved.
(Nostalgia Merchant) VC

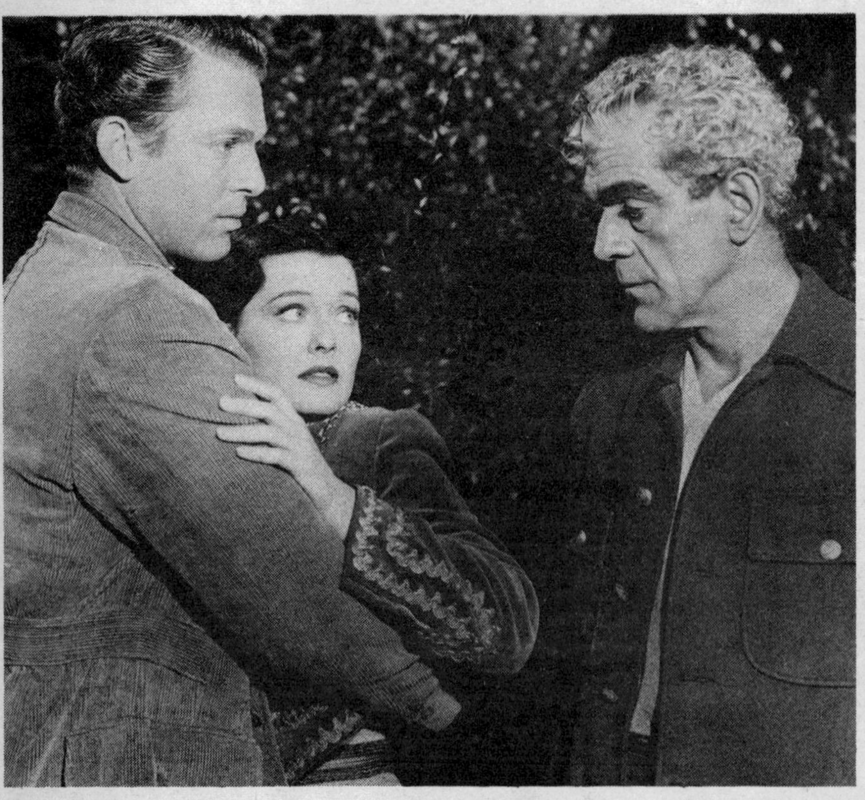

Isle of the Dead (1945)

"Spooky Val Lewton chiller."

Jack and the Beanstalk ★★

(1952) B&W/Color, 87 min. Director: Jean Yarbrough.
Bud Abbott, Lou Costello, Dorothy Ford, Buddy Baer, Barbara Brown. Frequently funny Abbott & Costello farce based on the well-known fairy tale. Very good for kids, but not as amusing to adults as some of A&C's other comedies are.
(Video Communications) VC

Jack the Ripper ★½

(1979) Color, 105 min. Director: Jesus Franco.
Klaus Kinski, Josephine Chaplin. The phantom killer of the London fog strikes again. Klaus is quite convincing as Jack—but then, isn't he *always* convincing as a psycho, even if he's not playing one?—but the film is just standard, gory stuff.
(Demonique Video) VC

Jaws ★★★½

(1975) Color, 124 min. Director: Steven Spielberg.
Roy Scheider, Robert Shaw, Richard Dreyfuss, Lorraine Gary, Murray Hamilton. A 25-foot Great White Shark invades the waters off Amity Island at the outset of the summer tourist season and starts gobbling up visiting swimmers. Police chief Scheider wants to close the beaches, but mayor Hamilton won't let him. As a result, the team of Scheider, Dreyfuss and Shaw must venture out in a boat and try to kill the shark at sea. An expertly directed, nail-biting thriller based on the novel by Peter Benchley.
(MCA Videocassette and Disc) VC, LV

Jaws II ★★

(1978) Color, 116 min. Director: Jeannot Szwarc.
Roy Scheider, Lorraine Gary, Murray Hamilton. Another Great White Shark descends upon Amity Island again, arguably to avenge the death of its mate three years ago. Scheider is very good, but otherwise the film is a total rehash of the original, only not anywhere near as suspenseful. For one thing, director Szwarc (which rhymes with shark) shows us so many close-ups of the beast that eventually it loses its fearsomeness altogether and looks just like the mechanical creature it is.
(MCA Videocassette and Disc) VC, LV

Jesus Christ Superstar ★★★

(1973) Color, 103 min. Director: Norman Jewison.
Ted Neeley, Carl Anderson, Yvonne Elliman, Barry Dennen, Joshua Mostel. Moving film adaptation of the best-selling rock album and successful Broadway rock opera which recounts the life of Christ in a lively format that younger people—theoretically, anyway—would be more inclined to identify with. Anderson's Judas is a dynamo.
(MCA Videocassette and Disc) VC, LV

Journey into the Beyond ★★

(1973) Color, 83 min. Director: Rolf Olsen.
Narrated by John Carradine. Documentary which takes viewers on an expedition to lands where supernatural rituals, exorcism, spiritualism, and sacrificial offerings, not to mention other bizarre and gruesome activities, are still being practiced.
(Family Home Entertainment) VC

Judex ★★½

(1963) B&W, 95 min. Director: Georges Franju.
Channing Pollock, Francine Berge, Edith Scob, Sylva Koscina. Updated remake of the comic book-style 1916 French serial by Louis Feuillade, which was also remade in 1933 by Maurice Champreux, about Judex (Pollock), a masked magician, and his efforts to save the City of Light from the clutches of an evil, but beautiful master criminal. Stylish nonsense.
(Budget Video) VC

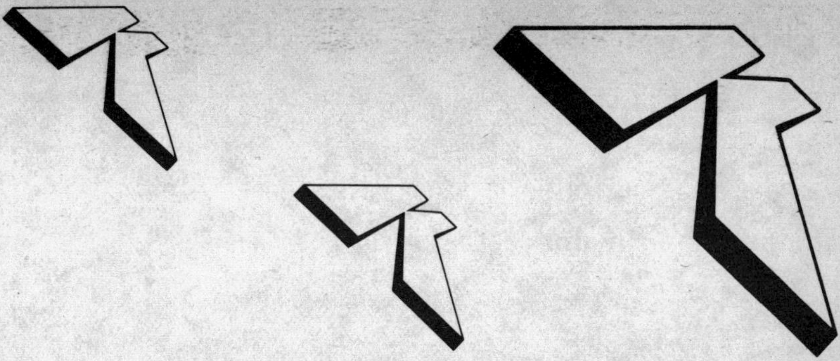

Keep My Grave Open ½

(1980) Color, 88 min. Director: S.F. Brownrigg.
Camilla Carr, Gene Ross. Twisted tale of a psychotic young woman who lures other young women to her remote mansion in order to sexually satisfy the lusts of her own imaginary lover. How's that again? Lots of gore.
(Unicorn Video) VC

Killing Kind, The ½

(1973) Color, 95 min. Director: Curtis Harrington.
John Savage, Ruth Roman, Cindy Williams, Ann Sothern. Mama's boy turns psychopathic killer in this odd variation on a *Psycho* theme. Taut thriller, well performed, with Savage particularly good as the neurotic young man, a role he could just about patent.
(Unicorn Video) VC

King Kong

(1933) B&W, 100 min. Director: Ernest B. Schoedsack.
Fay Wray, Bruce Cabot, Robert Armstrong. Movie producer Armstrong encounters a giant ape while shooting a film on a remote south sea island, captures the beast, then puts it on exhibit in New York as the Eighth Wonder of the World. Naturally, it escapes. One of the absolute best fantasy/adventure films ever made.
(Nostalgia Merchant, King of Video, RCA VideoDisc) VC, CED

King Kong

(1977) Color, 135 min. Director: John Guillermin.
Jeff Bridges, Charles Grodin, Jessica Lange. Lavish, Dino De Laurentiis remake of the 1933 classic which sacrifices all elements of fantasy that made the original so much fun. Here, Skull Island looks just like Hawaii, and Kong himself looks and acts just like a real gorilla. Not entirely worthless, but definitely without charm.
(Paramount Home Video) VC, LV

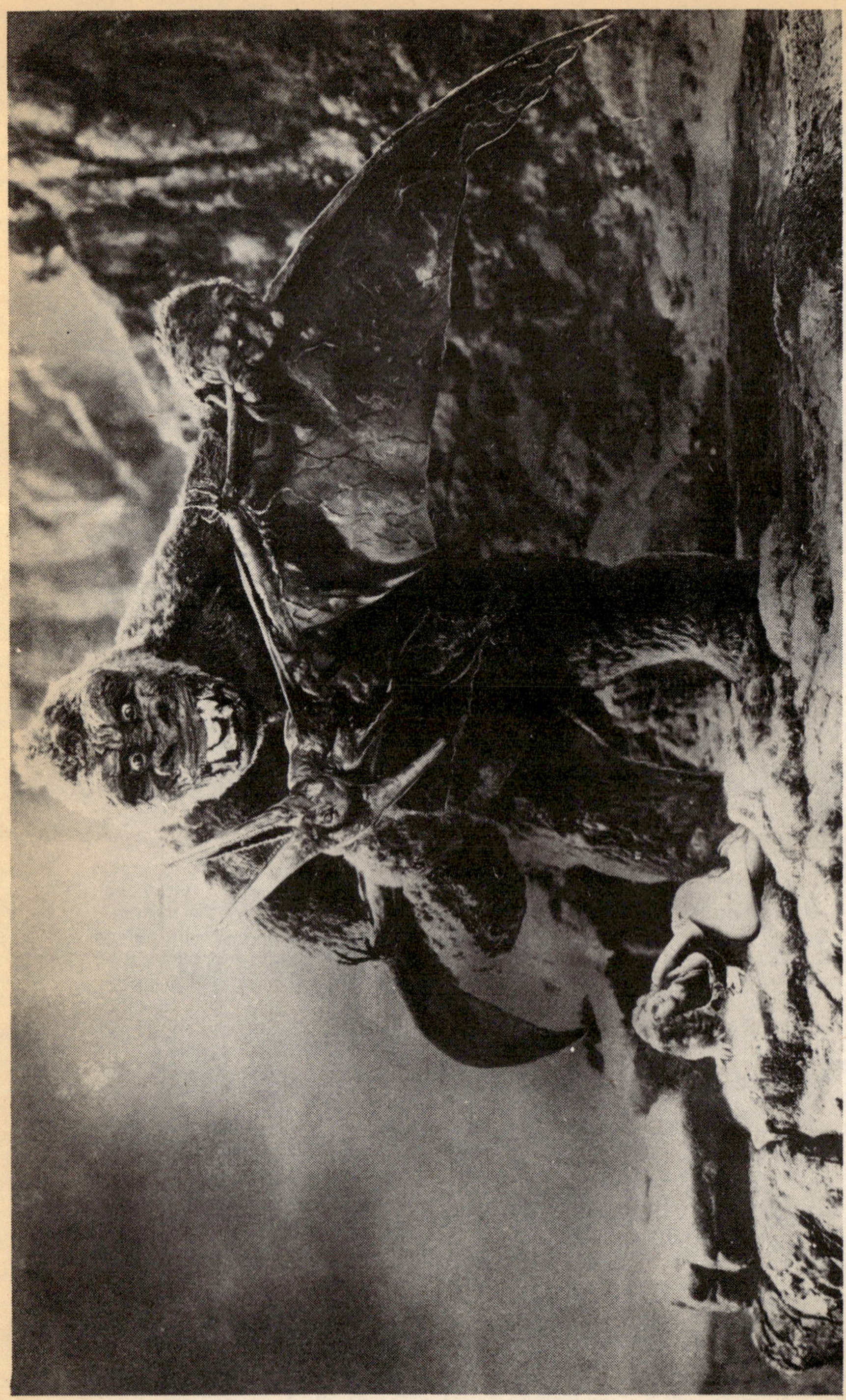

King Kong (1933)

King of Kong Island

(1968) Color, 92 min. Director: (?)
Brad Harris, Marc Lawrence. Mad scientists on a South Pacific atoll plant devices in the skulls of gorillas that turn them into remote-control killer robots. But a descendant of the original Kong comes to the rescue to stop all this monkeying around with his relatives' behavior.
(Video Communications) VC

King of the Zombies

(1941) B&W, 76 min. Director: Jean Yarbrough.
Dick Purcell, Joan Woodbury, Mantan Moreland, Henry Victor. An evil scientist creates a race of zombies to serve as tools of foreign agents during the war. Far-fetched enough for you?
(Video Archive) VC

King Solomon's Mines

(1937) B&W, 80 min. Director: Robert Stevenson.
Paul Robeson, Cedric Hardwicke, Roland Young, John Loder, Anna Lee. A varied group of adventurers goes in search of the legendary lost diamond mine of King Solomon, accompanied by a mysterious African chieftain (Robeson) who holds the key to the treasure's whereabouts. Exciting romantic fantasy faithfully adapted from the classic H. Rider Haggard novel.
(Embassy Home Entertainment) VC

Kingdom of the Spiders ½

(1977) Color, 94 min. Director: John "Bud" Cardos.
William Shatner, Tiffany Bolling, Woody Strode. Hordes of tarantulas descend upon an Arizona desert town, and scientist Shatner must deal with them. The problem is, the tarantulas have been stirred up because the local farmers have been overdosing them with pesticides. Predictable, environmental horror film.
(Video Communications) VC

Kiss Me Monster

(1968) Color, 77 min. Director: Jesus Franco.
Janine Reynaud, Rossano Yanni, Adrian Hoven, Chris Howland, Carlos Mendi. Evil scientist experiments with humans and animals on a remote Caribbean island. Shades of *The Island of Dr. Moreau.* A.k.a. *Besame, Monstruo.*
(Value Video) VC

Kronos

(1957) B&W, 78 min. Director: Kurt Neumann.
Jeff Morrow, Barbara Lawrence, John Emery, Morris Ankrum, Robert Shayne. An alien space ship crashes in the ocean off the California coast. From it emerges a giant, robotically controlled death machine, which descends upon Los Angeles, sucking up energy wherever it goes. Poor special effects, but the premise, despite the way it may sound, isn't all that bad.
(Nostalgia Merchant) VC

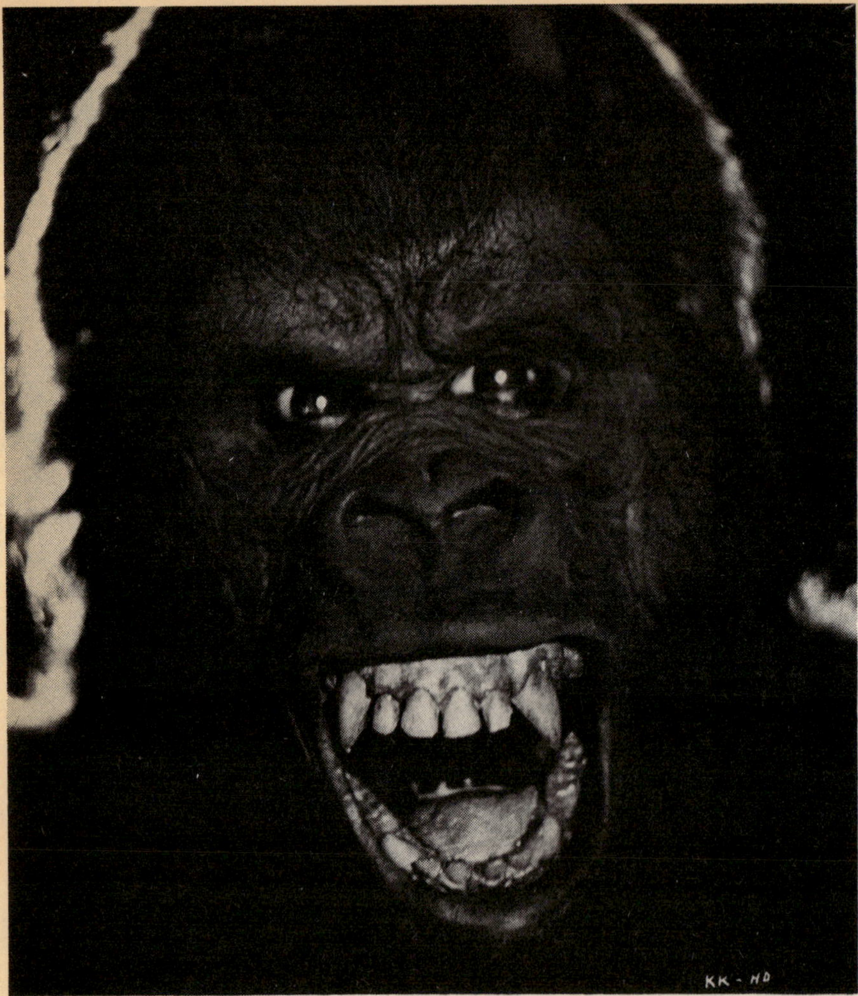

King Kong (1977)

". . .without charm."

Land of the Minotaur

(1976) Color. 94 min. Director: Costa Carayiannis.
Peter Cushing, Donald Pleasence, Luan Peters, Nikos Verlakis, Vanna Revilli, Costas Skouras. Minoan devil cult leader Cushing kidnaps tourists to use as offerings in his bizarre ritualistic sacrifices. Pleasence is the minister out to stop him. Cushing and Pleasence must have badly needed the bucks to have gotten involved in this one.
(Video Communications) VC

Laserblast ½

(1979) Color. 85 min. Director: Michael Rae.
Kim Milford, Keenan Wynn, Cheryl Smith, Roddy McDowall. A constantly victimized teenager stumbles upon a strange weapon which has been left almost on his doorstep by a lizard-like alien, and he uses it to get revenge on all those who've been kicking sand in his face over the years. Every teenager's high school fantasy.
(Media Home Entertainment) VC

Last House on Dead End Street

(1981) Color. 90 min. Director: Victor Juno.
A lot of people have accused splatter movies of being little more than fantasy snuff films—some have even gone so far as to accuse a few of them of being real snuff films. *Last House on Dead End Street* is a sick little piece of junk that virtually invites people to make the comparison. It's about a bunch of sleazoid filmmakers who make snuff films which their distributor doesn't know are snuff films—until the filmmakers slaughter the distributor and some other filmmakers and put those scenes in a new snuff film. Pointless, ugly and amateurish.
(Sun Video) VC

Last Wave, The

(1978) Color. 103 min. Director: Peter Weir.
Richard Chamberlain, David Gulpilil, Olivia Hamnett. An Australian lawyer (Chamberlain) takes on the defense of aboriginal tribesman accused of murder and finds himself drawn into a web of occult mysticism where illusion and reality blend and in which he plays a pivotal role as the reincarnation of a long dead deity whose reappearance spells doom to the world. An engrossing, hypnotic, occult drama, directed to perfection by a modern master of the form.
(Warner Home Video) VC

Legend of the Loch Ness, The ½

(1976) Color, 92 min. Director: Richard Martin.
Documentary which follows a modern research team using the latest technology to hunt down and capture the world's most famous sea monster. Scenic photography of the Scottish lake region.
(Video Communications) VC

Legend of Sleepy Hollow, The

(1980) Color, 100 min. Director: Henning Schellerup.
Jeff Goldblum, Dick Butkus, Paul Sand, Meg Foster. Made-for-TV version of Washington Irving's classic tale of quivering Ichabod Crane and his adventures with the redoubtable Headless Horseman. Goldblum is the embodiment of Irving's description of Crane, but the rest of the telefilm is just average.
(Video Communications) VC

Legend of Spider Forest, The

(1971) Color, 91 min. Director: Peter Sykes.
Simon Brent, Neda Arneric, Derek Newark, Sheila Allen. Nazi war criminals developing a nerve drug made of spider venom with which they intend to conquer the world devise legend of a spider goddess whose kiss brings death as a ruse to keep the nosey away from their forest hideaway.
(Wizard Video) VC

Legend of the Werewolf ½

(1975) Color, 90 min. Director: Freddie Francis.
Peter Cushing, Ron Moody, Hugh Griffith, David Rintoul. An orphan raised by wolves is adopted by Griffith's wayward circus, which puts him on display as a "wolfboy." When the boy grows up, he naturally becomes a wolfman—of the pointy-toothed, full moon variety. Coroner Cushing discovers his secret and helps to put him out of his misery. Low-keyed horror in the tradition and image of Hammer Films' 1961 *Curse of the Werewolf.*
(Electric Video) VC

Lemora, Lady Dracula

(1975) Color, 90 min. Director: Robert Blackburn.
Lesley Gilb, Cheryl Smith, William Whitton, Maxine Ballantyne, Hy Pike. Virginal young girl (Smith) is introduced to the world of sensuousness (and nonsense) by the lady vampire of the title as well as other assorted decadent monster types. Weird comic horror film that seems to be trying to say something—though what that something is, I, for one, have absolutely no idea. A.k.a. *Lemora—A Child's Tale of the Supernatural.*
(Demonique Video) VC

Leonor

(1977) Color, 100 min. Director: Juan Bunuel.
Liv Ullmann, Michel Piccoli, Ornella Muti, Angel Del Pozo. The dead wife (Ullmann) of a 14th century nobleman is resurrected by the devil so that she may claim the lives of a community's children. Mysterious, convoluted drama that could be a vampire tale, but then again. . .well, your guess is as good as mine. Bunuel is the son of surrealist director Luis Bunuel. Judging from this he shares his father's penchant for the bizarre, but little of his cinematic genius.
(CBS/Fox Video) VC

Leopard Man, The

(1943) B&W, 66 min. Director: Jacques Tourneur.
Dennis O'Keefe, Margo, Jean Brooks, James Bell, Isabel Jewell. A nightclub singer's pet leopard escapes, sending a wave of panic through a small New Mexican town. First a little girl is killed, then there are other victims of the leopard. Or are some of these other killings the work, perhaps, of a much more sinister killer? This atmospheric murder mystery with supernatural overtones from producer Val Lewton works very effectively right up to the denouement, then falls completely flat. Still worth seeing, though.
(Nostalgia Merchant) VC

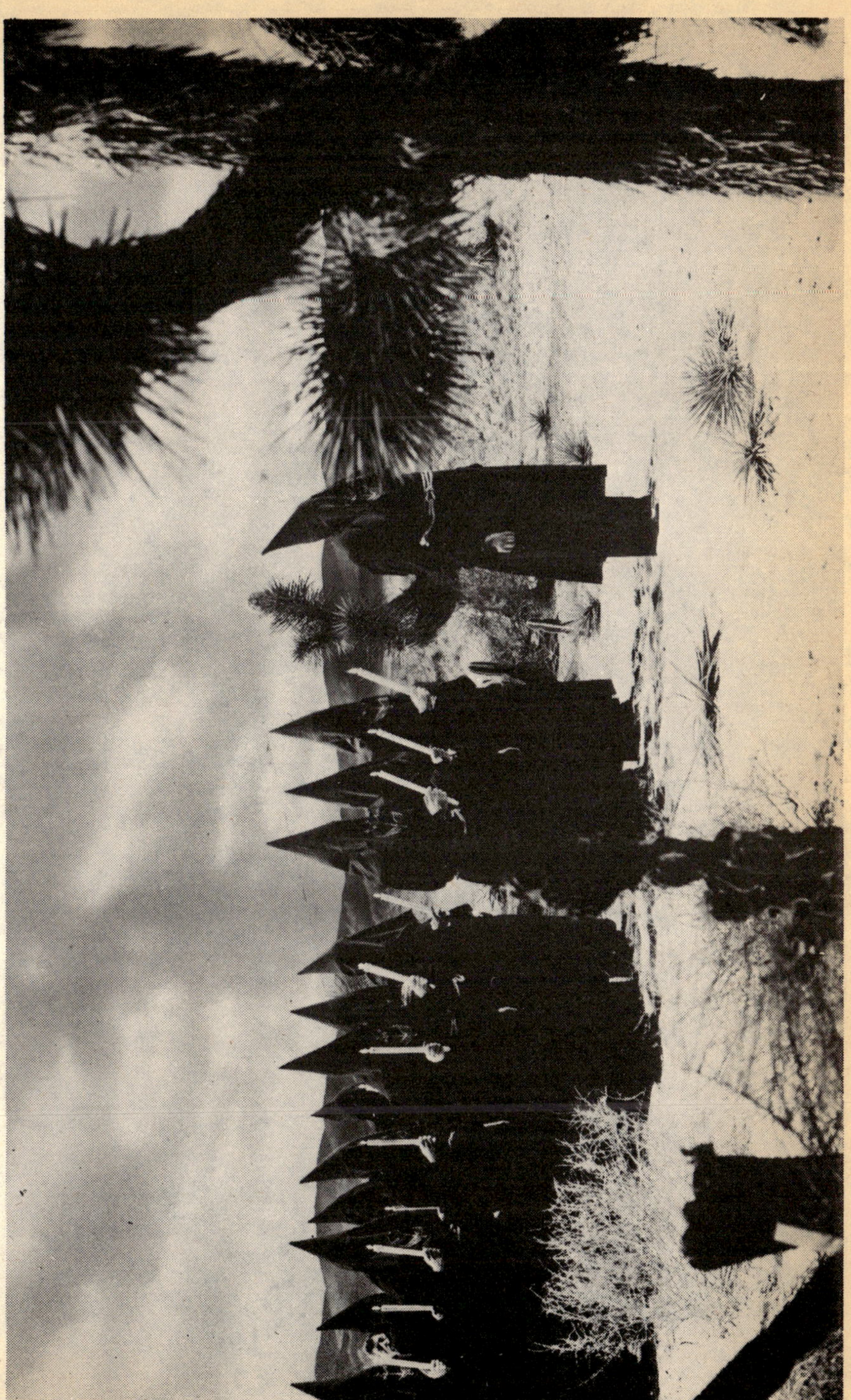

The Leopard Man (1943)

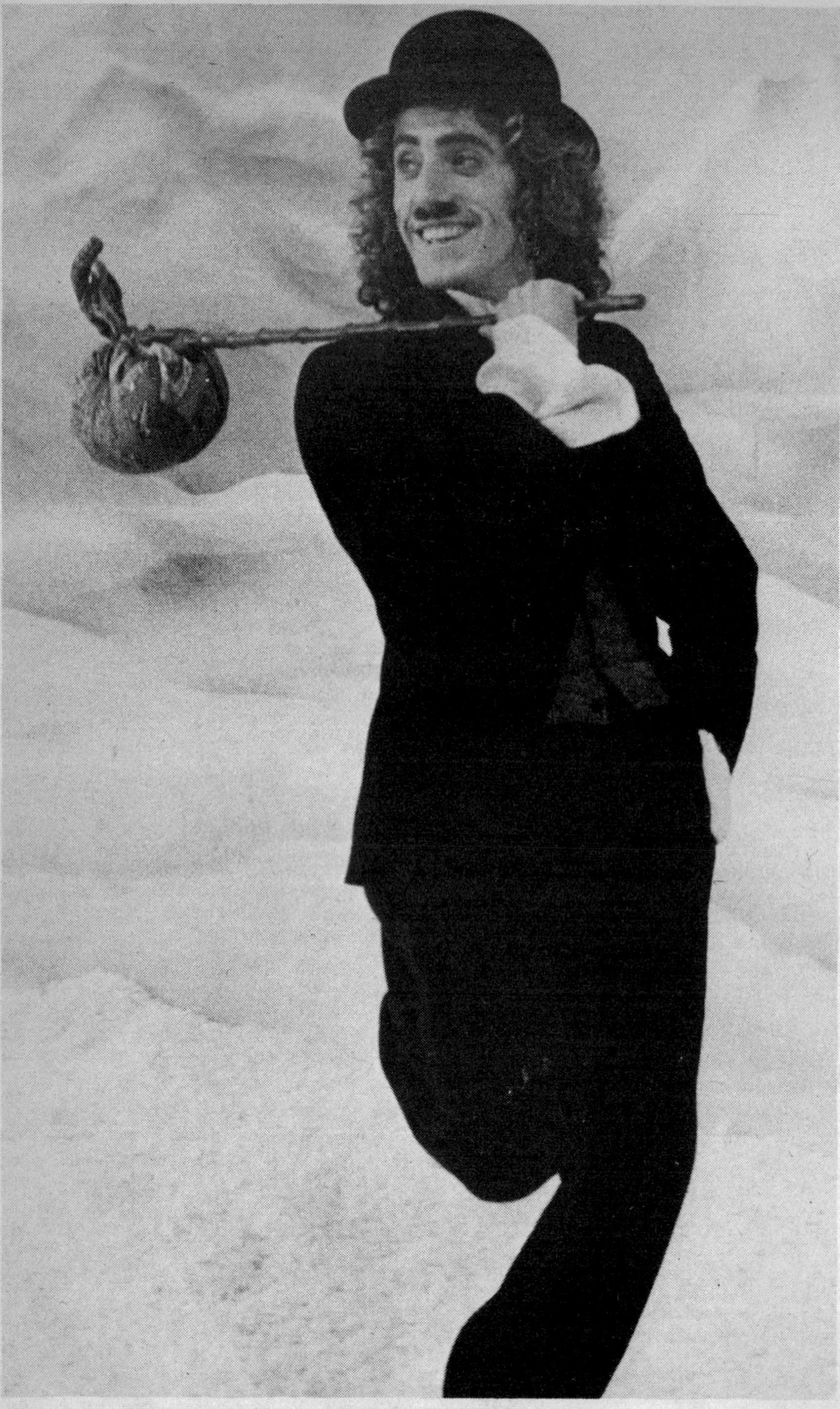

Lisztomania (1975)

Life of Brian ✪✪

(1979) Color, 90 min. Director: Terry Jones.

Graham Chapman, John Cleese, Terry Gilliam, Eric Idle, Terry Jones, Michael Palin. Brian (Chapman) is born at the exact same time and virtually in the same manger as the baby Jesus, and goes on to confuse his own role in life with that of the Savior's. Confusion is definitely the operative word here, though some of the Python troupe's bits are quite funny, particularly Palin's scenes as a lisping Pontius Pilate.

(Warner Home Video) VC

Lisztomania ✪✪✪✪

(1975) Color, 105 min. Director: Ken Russell.

Roger Daltrey, Sara Kestelman, Paul Nicholas, Fiona Lewis, Ringo Starr, Rick Wakeman. A flamboyant fantasy-musical based on the life of 19th century pianist-composer Franz Liszt (Daltrey), which presents Liszt as music's first pop superstar. Many critics originally dismissed this film as an example of Russell-mania at its most excessive. But despite its eye-popping imagery and frantic pacing, it's really a very subtle work about a passionate artist's undoing of himself and betrayal of his genius. A challenging and remarkable work by one of the most original filmmakers of our time.

(Warner Home Video) VC

Little Prince, The ✪✪

(1974) Color, 88 min. Director: Stanley Donen.

Richard Kiley, Steven Warner, Bob Fosse, Gene Wilder. Aviator Kiley crash lands in the desert and there encounters Warner, a lost little prince from another planet who teaches him the meaning of life, love and courage. Antoine de Saint-Exupery's very popular—and quite charming—fable is transformed here into a very dull musical despite the efforts of a lot of high-powered talent, including Lerner & Lowe, who wrote the score. Wilder overdoes it, as usual. But choreographer-director Fosse shines in his cameo as a snake.

(Paramount Home Video) VC

Little Shop of Horrors, The ✪✪✪

(1960) B&W, 70 min. Director: Roger Corman.

Mel Welles, Jackie Joseph, Jonathan Haze, Dick Miller, Jack Nicholson. This movie will strike you either as an hysterically funny spoof of horror movies (among other things) or as an exercise in total witlessness, depending on your mood at the time. My reaction has always been the former, but I can understand the latter because this movie really is *stupid.* Nerd Haze, who works in a flower shop, invents a new kind of plant to impress girlfriend Joseph. He even names it after her—Audrey, Jr. One problem though: the plant thrives on human blood. Nicholson's youthful cameo as a masochistic dental patient, Dick Miller's flower-eating "Mr. Yellow-Vest," and Welles' overbearing Gravis Mushnik, the "Bloom Tycoon," must tickle your funny bone at one point or another, however, no matter what your mood. Reportedly, Corman shot the film in a record two days!

(Budget Video) VC

Living Dead, The ✪✪

(1934) B&W, 65 min. Director: Thomas Bentley.

Gerald Du Maurier, George Curzon, Leslie Perrins, Belle Chrystal. Early British talkie-whodunit about a mad scientist who invents a serum that turns his victims catatonic. Based on a stage play by Wallace Geoffrey. A.k.a. *Scotland Yard Mystery.*

(Thunderbird Films) VC

Living Head, The ★

(1964) B&W, 75 min. Director: Chano Urueta.
Ana Luisa Peluffo, Abel Salazar, Mauricio Garces, German Robles. Archaeologists discover the preserved severed head of an ancient Aztec warrior named Acatl, and, despite the curse which warns them not to do so, steal it from the shrine in which it is kept to take back to the museum with them. Needless to say, all hell breaks loose. Mexican horror movie superstars Salazar and Robles team up for yet another dog—er, *perro.*
(Video Yesteryear) VC

Lodger, The ★★½

(1926) B&W, 75 min. Director: Alfred Hitchcock.
Ivor Novello, Malcolm Keen, Arthur Chesney, Marie Ault. A Jack the Ripper-style murderer calling himself the Avenger terrorizes all of London, but remains uncaught, his identity unknown. Suspicion eventually falls on Novello, a mysterious young man who has just moved into a rooming house near the scenes of the various crimes. Atmospheric, technically ingenious adaptation of the oft-filmed Marie Belloc-Lowndes novel which marked Hitchcock's debut as the screen's Master of Suspense. Dated, but nicely done.
(Video Dimensions) VC

Logan's Run ★

(1976) Color, 120 min. Director: Michael Anderson.
Michael York, Richard Jordan, Peter Ustinov, Jenny Agutter, Farrah Fawcett. York is a futuristic policeman who hunts down lawbreakers called "runners," people who are trying to escape society's mandate to terminate all those who are over the age of 30. An ingenious and provocative idea literally drowned in a sea of mindless special effects. Overlong, over *everything.*
(MGM/UA Home Video) VC

Looker ★½

(1981) Color, 93 min. Director: Michael Crichton.
Albert Finney, James Coburn, Susan Dey, Leigh Taylor-Young. A plastic surgeon uses some of the world's most beautiful models as deadly weapons through a unique method of mind and body control. Glittery, but empty-headed sci-fi.
(Warner Home Video) VC

Looney, Looney, Looney Bugs Bunny Movie, The ★★★

(1981) Color, 79 min. Director: Friz Freleng.
Bugs Bunny, Daffy Duck, Elmer Fudd, Porky Pig, et al. Sequel of sorts to *The Bugs Bunny/Road Runner Movie*, Warner Brothers' 1979 compilation of hilarious moments from some of its most famous cartoons by Chuck Jones. This time around, it's director Friz Freleng's turn. The film itself is on a par with the previous compilation—meaning it's packed with very funny clips, but it's also hampered by some rather dull, newly animated narration sequences featuring Bugs himself.
(Warner Home Video) VC

Lord of the Rings, The ★★★

(1978) Color, 133 min. Director: Ralph Bakshi.
Animated adaptation of the second of J.R.R. Tolkien's series of books about Middle Earth and the wizards and elves who live there—including Frodo the Hobbit, Gandalf the Wizard, and the evil Sauron. A spectacular fantasy with some very impressive animation, but the film ends abruptly, suggesting a sequel, but as yet there hasn't been one.
(Thorn/EMI Video, RCA VideoDisc) VC, CED

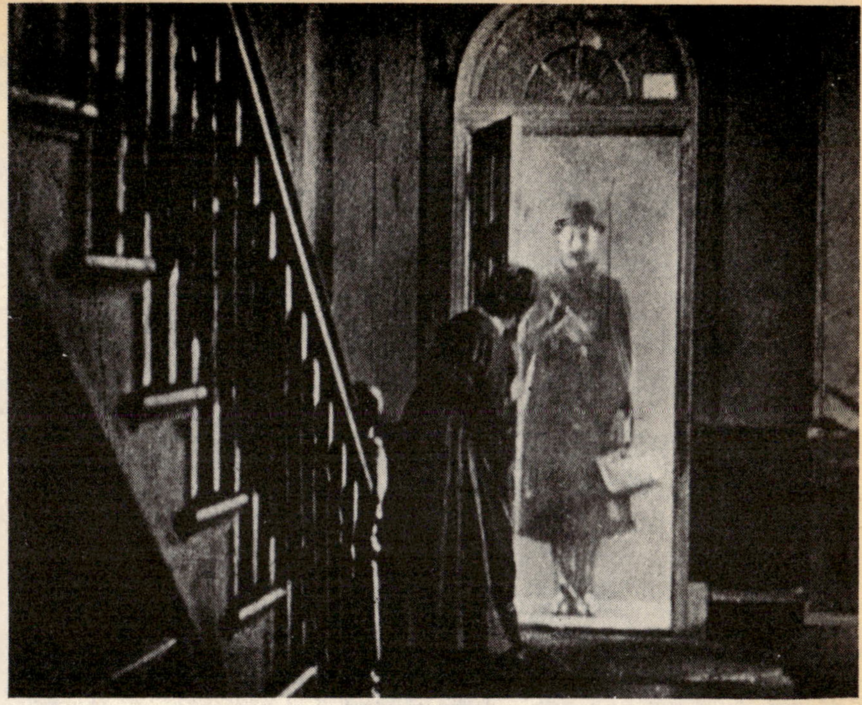

The Lodger (1926)

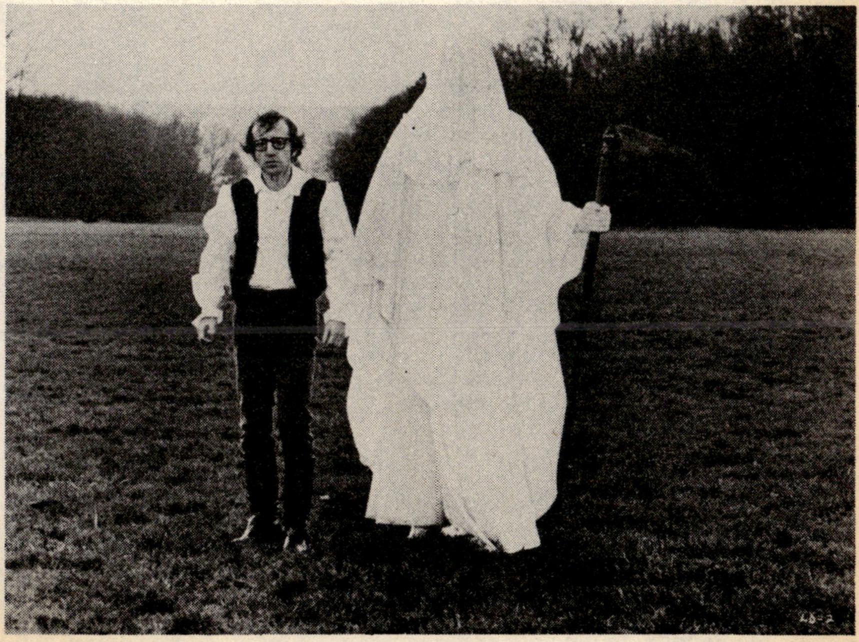

Love and Death (1975)

Lost Horizon ★★★

(1937) B&W, 118 min. Director: Frank Capra.

Ronald Colman, Sam Jaffee, Edward Everett Horton, Jane Wyatt, Thomas Mitchell, Margo, H.B. Warner, Isabel Jewell. The movie that transformed the word Shangri-La into a synonym for ultimate peace and happiness. Colman and four others, escaping from a revolution-torn country, are kidnapped and taken to a mountain paradise beyond the Himalayas where there is no war and no growing old. Haunting fantasy based on the novel by James Hilton.

(Video Communications) VC

Lost World, The ★★★

(1925) B&W, 60 min. Director: Harry Hoyt.

Wallace Beery, Bessie Love, Lewis Stone, Lloyd Hughes, Bull Montana. Love's father, Professor Maple White, disappears while exploring a strange, forbidding plateau in the heart of Peru, so she enlists Professor Challenger (Beery) to mount another expedition to go in search of him. What they find, of course, is a prehistoric land where dinosaurs still roam at large. A wonderful fantasy-adventure based on the novel by Sir Arthur Conan Doyle which boasts some amazing pre-*King Kong* model animation effects by *Kong* master magician Willis O'Brien. Unfortunately, the film no longer seems to exist in its original 10-reel (approximately 100 minute) length. A shame.

(Thunderbird Films) VC

Love and Death ★★★★

(1975) Color, 85 min. Director: Woody Allen.

Woody Allen, Diane Keaton, Harold Gould, Frank Adu. This is either Allen's most serious comedy, or his funniest drama, depending upon how you look at it, but either way, it's a gem. Allen plays a cowardly Russian peasant during the Napoleonic Wars, who gets involved in a romance with Keaton as well as a conspiracy to assassinate Napoleon. Along the way, director Allen pokes fun at everything from the films of Sergei Eisenstein and Ingmar Bergman to the novels of Leo Tolstoy and Dostoevsky. My favorite line, spoken by Allen on the eve of his execution: "There are worse things than death. If you've ever spent an evening with an insurance salesman, you know what I mean."

(CBS/Fox Video) VC

Love at First Bite ★★

(1979) Color, 96 min. Director: Stan Dragoti.

George Hamilton, Susan Saint James, Richard Benjamin, Dick Shawn, Arte Johnson. Dracula (Hamilton) abandons Transylvania for the Big Apple and finds the life-style there a little too weird even for his taste. Saint James is the girl he decides he wants to spend all of eternity with. Benjamin, a descendant of vampire killer Van Helsing, is the boyfriend who's vying for her hand—er, neck. A few funny moments, but overall quite anemic.

(Warner Home Video, RCA VideoDisc) VC, CED

Love Bug, The ★★★

(1969) Color, 108 min. Director: Robert Stevenson.

Dean Jones, Michele Lee, Buddy Hackett, David Tomlinson. Jones discovers that his brand new Volkswagen bug is more than a little unusual, for it can fly, do somersaults, fend off villains and even play matchmaker. Cute Disney comedy, which spawned two lesser, but still entertaining sequels—*Herbie Rides Again* and *Herbie Goes Bananas.*

(Walt Disney Home Video, RCA VideoDisc) VC, CED, LV

Lucifer Complex, The ☞

(1978) Color, 94 min. Director: David L. Hewitt.

Robert Vaughn, Keenan Wynn, Aldo Ray, Lynn Cartwright. Precursor of *The Boys from Brazil* in which renegade Nazis who escaped justice after World War II carry on their plans for world domination by sending out clones of Hitler to build a new Reich. Low budget sci-fi thriller that uses lots of stock WWII war footage for its major action sequences.

(Video Communications) VC

Lust for a Vampire ☞½

(1970) Color, 95 min. Director: Jimmy Sangster.

Ralph Bates, Michael Johnson, Suzanna Leigh, Yutte Stensgaard. Johnson falls in love with a gorgeous student (Stensgaard) at the plush girls' school where he teaches. But true love runs afoul when she turns out to be a vampire. Dull gothic horror thriller from England's Hammer Films.

(Thorn/EMI Video) VC

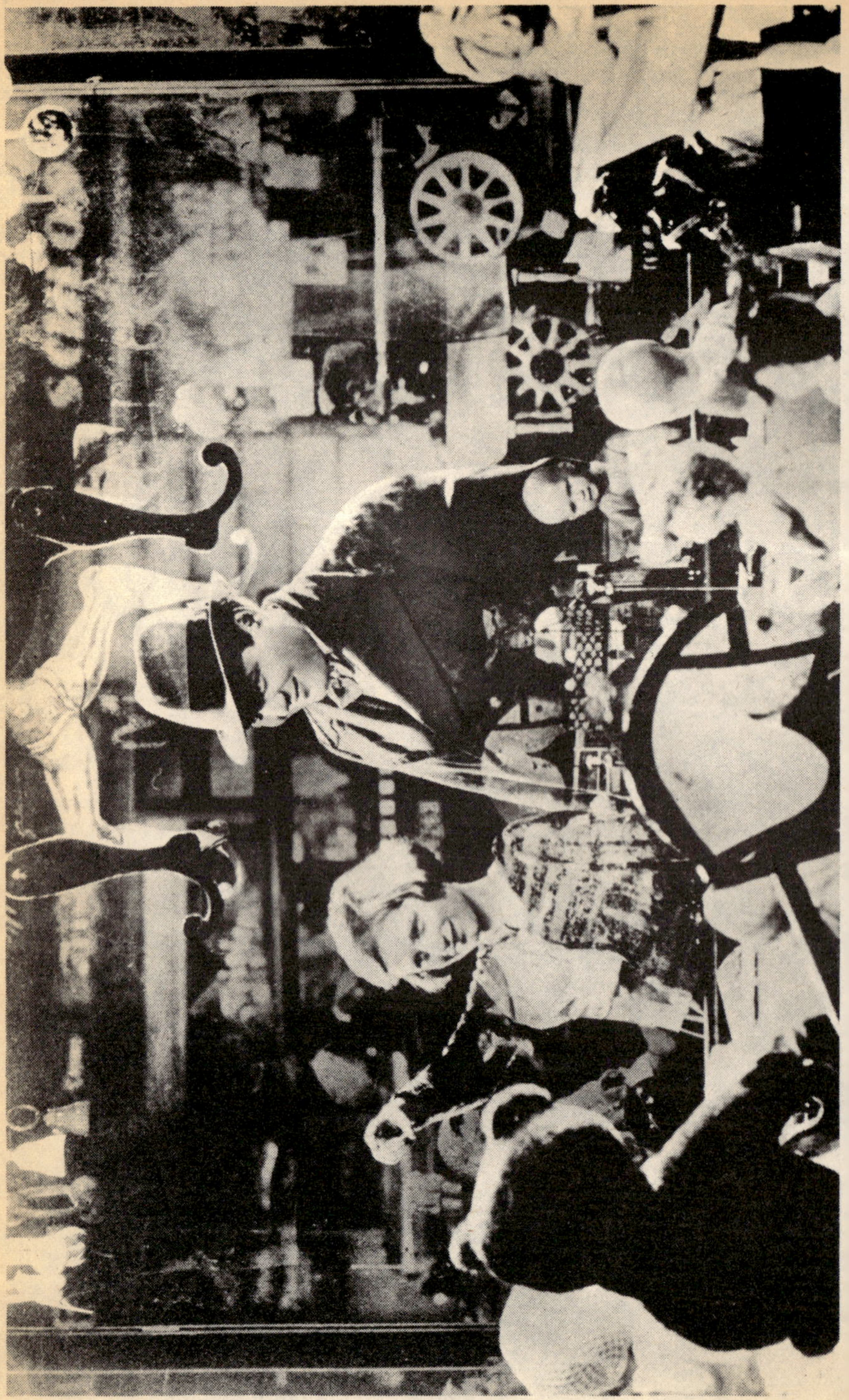

M (1931)

M ½

(1931) B&W, 99 min. Director: Fritz Lang.
Peter Lorre, Ellen Widmann, Inge Landgut, Gustav Grundgens. Lorre's powerhouse film debut as the child killer of Dusseldorf, who is hunted down and tried by the city's criminal element because his crimes are too heinous even for them. Today this landmark combination of German Expressionism and criminal pathology may seem a bit slow moving and stagey, but it's a strong film nevertheless, and Lorre's performance is spellbinding.
(Budget Video) VC

Mad Bomber, The

(1972) Color, 95 min. Director: Bert I. Gordon.
Vince Edwards, Chuck Connors, Neville Brand, Hank Brandt, Cristina Hart. Madman Connors terrorizes a city by placing explosives in public places, then setting them off, all part of a plot to get even with the world. Edwards is the cop who hunts him down. Based on a real case, but plays fast and loose with the facts.
(King of Video) VC

Mad Butcher, The ½

(1972) Color, 85 min. Director: Guido Zurli.
Victor Buono, Karen Field, Brad Harris, John Ireland. Buono does away with his victims' bodies by grinding them up into tasty sausages, which he then sells to the police. Cute. Variation on the story of Sweeney Todd.
(Astro Video) VC

Mad Monster

(1942) B&W, 77 min. Director: Sam Neufeld.
Johnny Downs, Anne Nagel, George Zucco, Glenn Strange, Henry Hall.
Mad doctor Zucco invents a serum that turns Strange into a werewolf. Nothing strange about that.
(Video Archive) VC

Madame Sin ✪✪½

(1972) Color, 73 min. Director: David Greene.

Bette Davis, Robert Wagner, Catharine Schell, Denholm Elliott, Roy Kinnear. Davis stars as the power behind a huge financial empire who uses super-sophisticated weapons that erase people's memories so that she may carry out her nefarious business schemes undetected. Made-for-TV movie.

(CBS/Fox Video) VC

Magic ✪

(1978) Color, 106 min. Director: Richard Attenborough.

Anthony Hopkins, Ann-Margret, Burgess Meredith, Ed Lauter. At the peak of his show business career, ventriloquist Hopkins skips town and returns to his Catskills roots where he looks up old flame Ann-Margret, now unhappily married to sullen Lauter. It appears Hopkins is suffering a mid-life as well as an identity crisis, both brought on by his wilfull and insufferable lookalike dummy. Hopkins' agent (Meredith) shows up to talk him out of his moroseness and is knifed for his trouble. A lot of high-powered talent is wasted in this weak reworking of the Michael Redgrave episode from the classic *Dead of Night.* Hopkins overacts.

(Embassy Home Entertainment) VC, LV

Magic Sword, The ✪

(1962) Color, 80 min. Director: Bert I. Gordon.

Basil Rathbone, Estelle Winwood, Gary Lockwood, Anne Helm, Liam Sullivan. Low-budget "extravaganza" about the fabled St. George and his bout with the equally fabled dragon. Also thrown in for good measure are bouts with ogres and vampires. Weak.

(Video Yesteryear) VC

Magical Mystery Tour ✪✪

(1969) Color, 60 min. Directors: The Beatles.

The Beatles. Amateurish psychedelic something-or-other concocted by the Beatles for showing on British TV. The album of the same name is a lot better.

(Media Home Entertainment) VC

Making of Star Wars, The S.P.F.X. The Empire Strikes Back ✪✪✪

(1980) Color, 100 min. Director: George Lucas.

Mark Hamill, Carrie Fisher, Harrison Ford. Fascinating behind-the-scenes look at the making of these two blockbuster space epics. Included are sequences revealing how R2-D2, C-3PO and Yoda were created, plus scenes of many of Hollywood's master magicians at work manipulating all sorts of live-action models, matte paintings, and other special effects in an effort to bring Lucas' space saga to life. Both films originally aired on network television.

(CBS/Fox Video) VC, LV, CED

Man in the White Suit, The ✪✪✪

(1952) B&W, 84 min. Director: Alexander Mackendrick.

Alec Guinness, Cecil Parker, Joan Greenwood, Michael Gough, Ernest Thesiger. Naive inventor Guinness comes up with a fabulous new material for making suits that resist wear and tear and throws the British garment industry into a panic. Amusing fantasy/satire.

(Thorn/EMI Video) VC

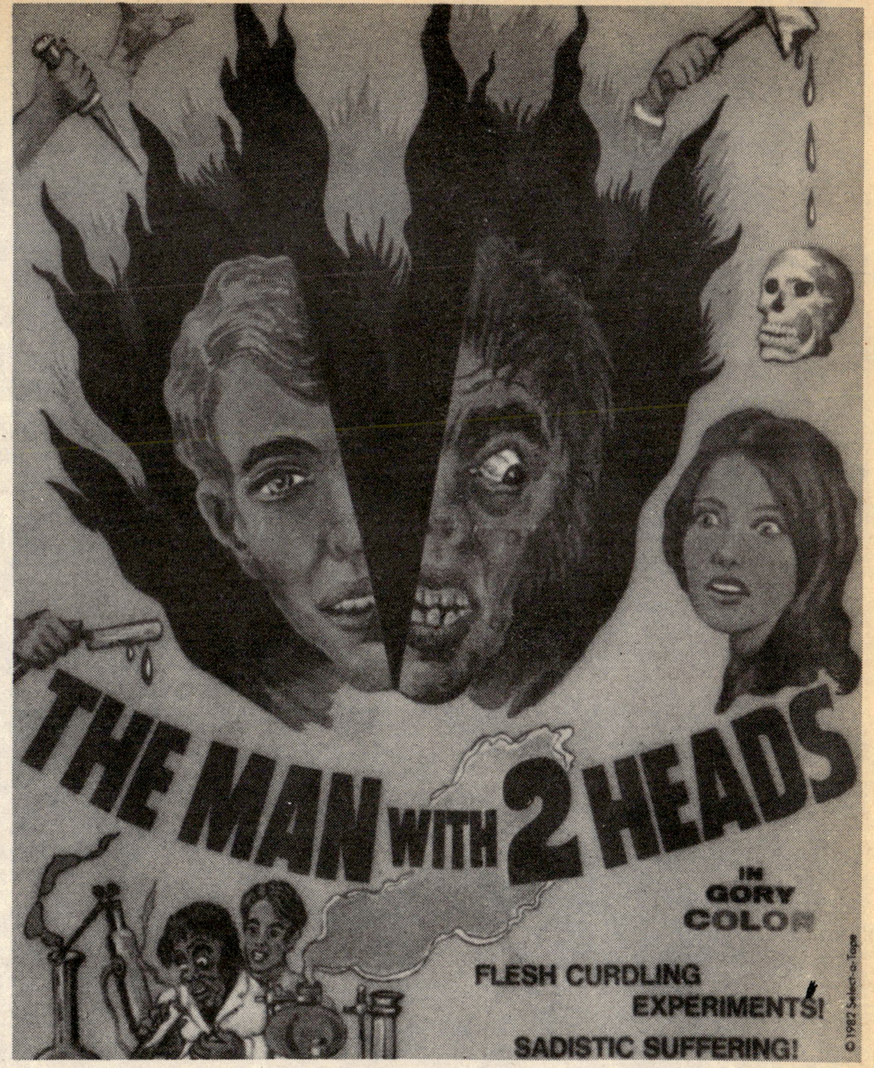

The Man with Two Heads (1972)

". . .made for about a buck and a half."

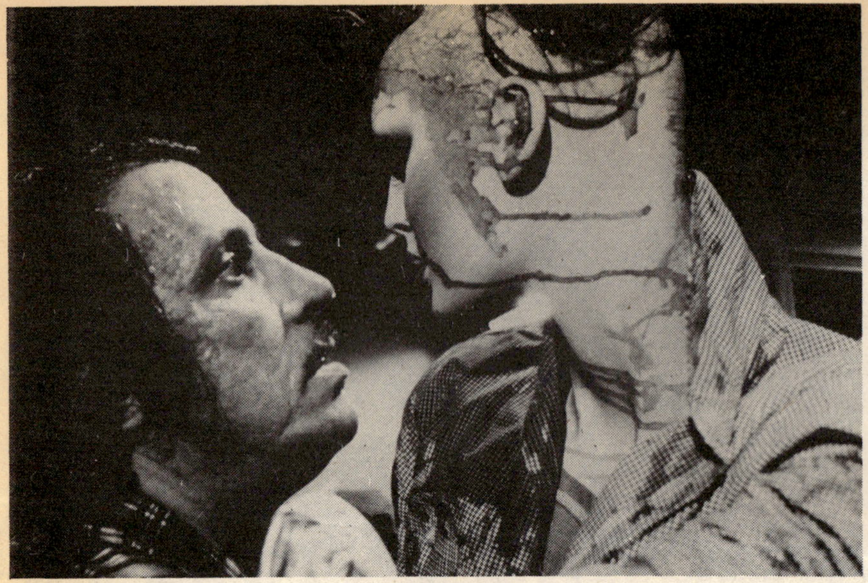

Maniac (1981)

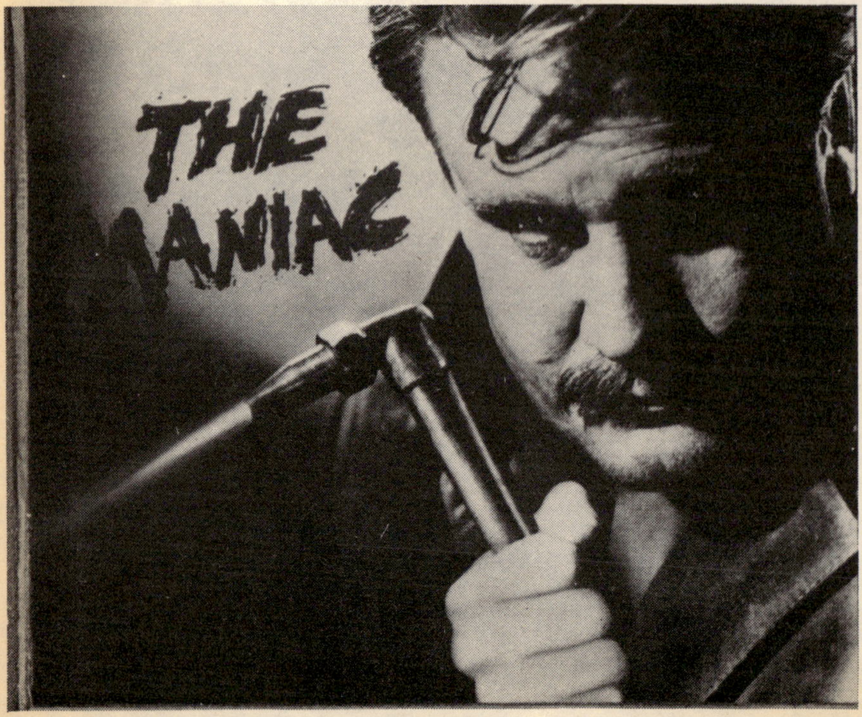

The Maniac (1962)

Man Who Fell to Earth, The ★★½

(1976) Color, 118 min. Director: Nicolas Roeg.
David Bowie, Rip Torn, Candy Clark, Buck Henry, Bernie Casey. An alien from another world lands on earth to find water for his dying planet and becomes enmeshed in the politics of a multinational conglomerate. The plot description may sound ridiculously far-fetched, which it is, but the film is a very unusual bit of sci-fi, crammed with ideas and full of wondrously imaginative special effects. Originally the film ran 140 minutes; this is the truncated American release version, and suffers because of it.
(Columbia Pictures Home Entertainment) VC

Man Who Haunted Himself, The ★★

(1970) Color, 94 min. Director: Basil Dearden.
Roger Moore, Hildegard Neil, Alastair MacKenzie, Hugh MacKenzie. Moore survives a car crash only to find himself being dogged by his doppelganger, who is assuming his identity by showing up at his job, etc. Interesting premise falls flat at the end. Besides, two Roger Moores are definitely tough to take.
(Thorn/EMI Video) VC

Man with Two Heads, The ★

(1972) Color, 80 min. Director: Andy Milligan.
Denis DeMarne, Julia Stratton, Berwick Kaler, Jacqueline Lawrence. Umpteenth re-telling of the familiar R.L. Stevenson story of Dr. Jekyll and you-know-who. What sets this one apart is that it was made for about a buck and a half. In this version, Dr. Jekyll downs his famous potion and turns into the appropriately named Mr. Blood. Made in England. A.k.a. *Dr. Jekyll and Mr. Blood.*
(Midnight Video) VC

Maniac ★

(1981) Color, 91 min. Director: William Lustig.
Joe Spinell, Caroline Munro. Spinell is psycho who murders young girls in all sorts of graphically horrible ways, scalps them, then uses their scalps to adorn the bald heads of female department store mannequins that he uses for sex at home. A roller coaster ride of pathology and splatter that gives new meaning to the word *sleaze.*
(Media Home Entertainment) VC

Maniac, The ★★

(1934) B&W, 60 min. Director: Dwain Esper.
Bill Woods, Horace Carpenter. A mad doctor's assistant kills his mentor, then walls him up, but a cat gives away the crime. Loosely based on Edgar Allen Poe's *The Black Cat.* A.k.a. *Sex Maniac.*
(Thunderbird Films) VC

Maniac, The ★★½

(1962) B&W, 86 min. Director: Michael Carreras.
Kerwin Mathews, Donald Houston, Nadia Gray. While vacationing in France, artist Mathews falls for a girl whose unbalanced father is locked up in the local mental asylum. At the height of their romance, "Dad" escapes and starts killing people with a blow torch, his murderous sights, of course, set upon Mathews. One of Hammer Films' *Psycho* imitations of the early sixties. Jimmy Sangster's script boasts a neat surprise twist at the conclusion.
(Columbia Pictures Home Entertainment) VC

Manitou, The ★

(1978) Color, 105 min. Director: William Girdler.
Susan Strasberg, Tony Curtis, Michael Ansara, Stella Stevens, Ann Sothern. Strasberg develops a growth on her neck, goes to the doctor and learns that inside the growth there is a developing fetus. Turns out that she's in the process of giving birth to the reincarnated spirit of an evil Indian sorcerer who is bent on wreaking havoc throughout the world. Curtis is the phoney spiritualist who tries to help rid her of the ugly pain in the neck. The actors try hard, but the script is just too awful for them to overcome.
(CBS/Fox Video) VC

Mary Poppins ★★★

(1964) Color, 139 min. Director: Robert Stevenson.
Julie Andrews, Dick Van Dyke, Glynis Johns, David Tomlinson. Andrews lost the part of Eliza Doolittle in the film version of *My Fair Lady* to Audrey Hepburn, so she made her film debut instead in this whimsical Disney film about an English nanny with magical powers. Ironically, she then won the Oscar as Best Actress, beating out competitor Hepburn. Apparently, there is justice after all. A delightful film for everyone, not just kids. Based on the novel by P.L. Travers.
(Walt Disney Home Video, RCA VideoDisc) VC, CED

Massacre at Central High ★★

(1980) Color, 90 min. Director: Renee Daalder.
Derrel Maury, Andrew Stevens, Robert Carradine, Kimberly Beck. Students at a California high school are being methodically murdered. Suspense film that also strives for significance by making the murder plot and the surviving students' subsequent desire for protection a parable of how easily fascism can take root in the minds of the young. Interesting, but not entirely successful.
(Electric Video) VC

Master Race ★★★

(1944) B&W, 96 min. Director: Herbert J. Biberman.
George Coulouris, Lloyd Bridges, Osa Massen, Nancy Gates. A high-ranking Nazi officer flees Hitler's crumbling empire at the close of the war with a plan to continue Hitler's efforts to achieve a master race even if it means starting World War III. Interesting speculative drama.
(King of Video) VC

Medusa Touch, The ★★

(1978) Color, 109 min. Director: Jack Gold.
Richard Burton, Lee Remick, Lino Ventura. Burton is born with the ability to will disasters with his mind. As a boy he slayed his hated parents and nanny with his talent. Now a grownup, he finds himself being driven to will even greater destruction. Frequently effective little thriller in the restrained British manner. But Burton overplays his anguish (as usual) and the repeated shots of him staring into the camera lens with his temples throbbing seem endless.
(CBS/Fox Video) VC

Megaforce ★

(1982) Color, 99 min. Director: Hal Needham.
Barry Bostwick, Persis Khambatta, Michael Beck, Edward Mulhare, George Furth, Henry Silva. Futuristic action movie vaguely along the lines of *Mad Max* (though without the grit) with Bostwick a superhero cop out to stop the "bad guys." Ex-stuntman Needham is without a doubt one of the worst directors in Hollywood and this dog proves it.
(CBS/Fox Video) VC

Meteor ★½

(1979) Color, 105 min. Director: Ronald Neame.
Sean Connery, Natalie Wood, Brian Keith, Karl Malden, Martin Landau, Trevor Howard, Henry Fonda. A five-mile wide meteor moving at an awesome rate of speed is but six days from colliding with the earth. What to do? Call in the cavalry—in the form of Sean Connery, who, together with the Russians, devises a scheme to use some spectacular nuclear weapons to blow the meteor up. Nice special effects, but an ultra-superficial plot and cast of characters. Landau overacts outrageously.
(Warner Home Video) VC

Metropolis ★★★

(1926) B&W, 120 min. Director: Fritz Lang.
Rudolf Klein-Rogge, Brigitte Helm, Alfred Abel, Gustav Frohlich. Reportedly director Lang got the idea for this futuristic urban nightmare when he set his eyes on New York City for the first time. The metropolis of the title is an unnamed city full of towering skyscrapers, flashing lights, and elevated subways that is controlled by Frohlich's power hungry and insensitive father, but operated by a mass of worker/slaves who live beneath the city streets and beat time to a giant timeclock. Some of the performances are terribly hammy, but the film itself abounds with imagination, highlighted by a spectacular flood sequence that unites the workers against their oppressors above.
(Thunderbird Films, Budget Video, Video Yesteryear) VC

Mighty Joe Young ★★½

(1949) B&W, 94 min. Director: Ernest B. Schoedsack.
Terry Moore, Ben Johnson, Robert Armstrong. Moore nurses mini-ape Joe from a baby, so he's docile with her even when he reaches the size of a junior grade King Kong. Armstrong then persuades her to let him use Joe in a nightclub act. Joe gets drunk, and the fun and breakage begin. *Kong* producer Merian C. Cooper and director Schoedsack try to rework the old magic, but the original's strong story line and powerful sense of fantasy simply aren't here. The special effects are marvelous, though, due to *Kong* master magician Willis O'Brien's (and assistant Ray Harryhausen's) superb craftsmanship, for which he deservedly won an Oscar. Definitely a mixed bag, but worth seeing.
(Nostalgia Merchant, King of Video) VC

Missile to the Moon ★

(1958) B&W, 78 min. Director: Richard Cunha.
Richard Travis, Gary Clarke, Cathy Downs, Laurie Mitchell, Nina Bara, Michael Whalen. Man's first rocketship expedition to the moon is beset by all kinds of problems. For example, there are two escaped convicts on board. Pretty soon everybody has to start getting along, however, when the ship's landing on the moon reveals a race of rock monsters, giant spiders, and—well, this one isn't too bad—glamorous moon maidens. A far cry from *2001*.
(Nostalgia Merchant) VC

Mission Galactica/Cylon Attack ★★

(1980) Color, 94 min. Director: Vince Edwards.
Lloyd Bridges, Ann Lockhart, Lorne Greene. Theatrical feature drawn from two episodes of the *Battlestar Galactica* TV series, *The Living Legend* and *Fire in Space*, in which a legendary Battlestar commander launches an all-out attack on the warring Cylons for the crimes they committed against his home planet. Good special effects, but the film's TV origins are sorely revealed by the weak scripting and acting.
(MCA Videocassette and Disc) VC, LV

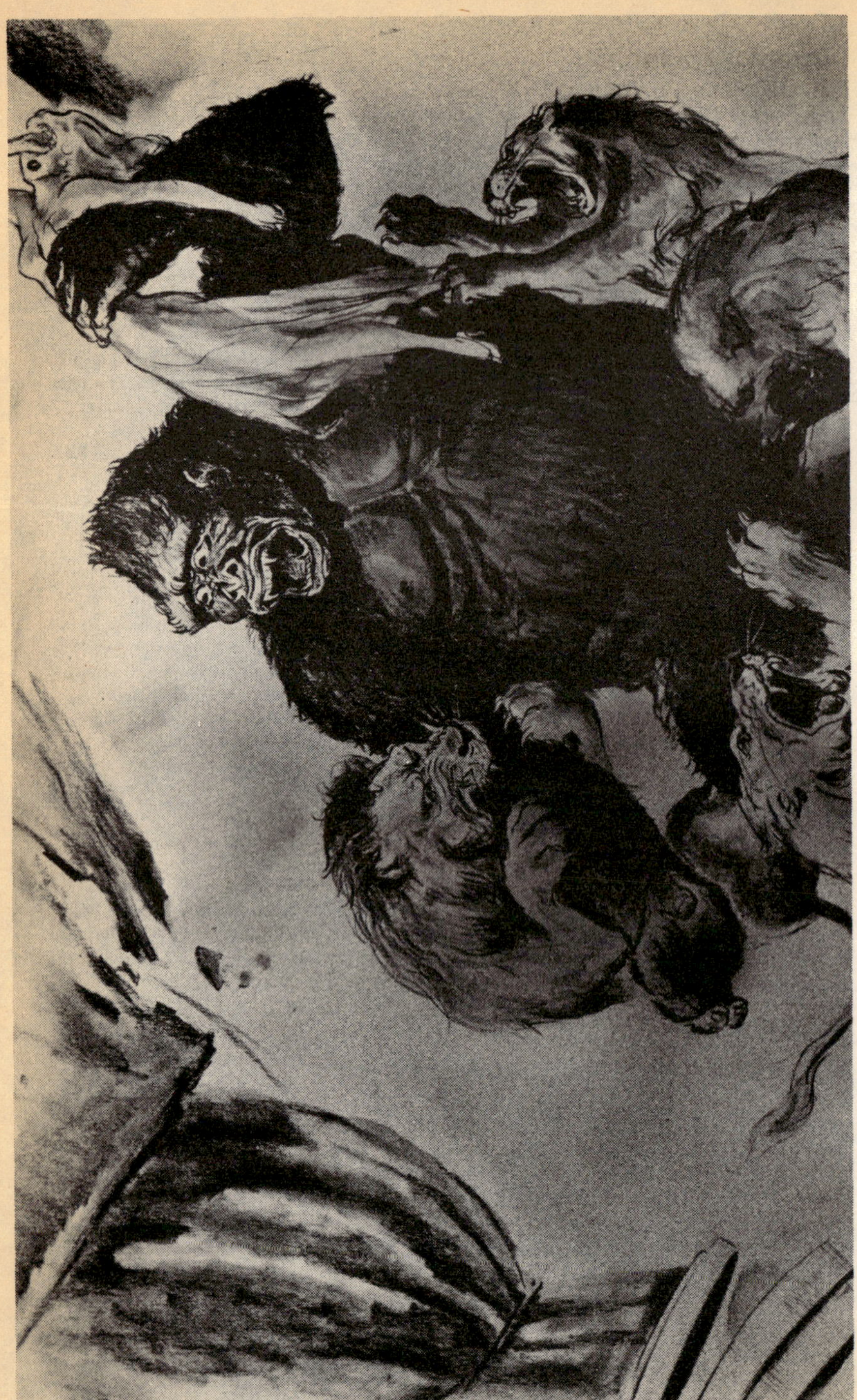

Mighty Joe Young (1949)

Mondo Trasho ☆

(1969) B&W, 95 min. Director: John Waters.

Mary Vivian Pearce, Divine, David Lochary, Mink Stole. Waters' first feature film (made for $2,000!) follows Pearce's exploits through Baltimore's underbelly. Along the way she meets a foot fetishist, gets run over by a Jayne Mansfield lookalike (Divine), gets committed to an insane asylum, gets wounded in a knife fight and winds up dying in a pig pen. Offbeat enough for you? A self-described "gutter film."

(Wizard Video) VC

Monster, The ☆☆

(1925) B&W, 80 min. Director: Roland West.

Lon Chaney, Gertrude Olmstead, Edward McWade, Walter James. Chaney plays a Dr. Moreau-like vivisectionist who obtains human victims for his experiments by arranging for motor accidents to occur near his secluded laboratory. Creaky vehicle for the "man of a thousand faces" that is more melodramactic than horrific. From a play by Crane Wilbur.

(Classic Video Cinema Collector's Club) VC

Monster from Green Hell, The ☆½

(1958) B&W, 71 min. Director: Kenneth Crane.

Jim Davis, Barbara Turner, Robert E. Griffin, Eduardo Cianelli. An experimental rocket containing radiation-contaminated wasps crashes in the African jungle. Scientists Davis and Turner rush to the scene and are most distressed to find that not only has their rocket turned to scrap metal, but their wasps have turned into giants. Must be the air. Dull.

(Nostalgia Merchant) VC

Monster Walks, The ☆

(1932) B&W, 67 min. Director: Frank Strayer.

Rex Lease, Vera Reynolds, Mischa Auer, Sheldon Lewis, Willie Best. Quasi-horror/whodunit that takes place in—where else?—a haunted house. There's a storm outside, lots of bodies piling up inside, weird servants, unsavory cripples, and, to put the frosting on the cake, a howling gorilla, which may, in fact, be the murderer—but don't you believe it! Not just the doors creak in this one.

(Video Yesteryear) VC

Monty Python and the Holy Grail ☆☆☆

(1974) Color, 90 min. Directors: Terry Gilliam, Terry Jones.

Graham Chapman, Eric Idle, Michael Palin, Terry Jones, Terry Gilliam, John Cleese. Lunatic retelling of the legend of King Arthur by England's most celebrated gang of comic crazies. Uneven but frequently hilarious (and bloody) spoof. Visually gorgeous.

(Columbia Pictures Home Entertainment) VC

Morgan! ☆☆☆

(1966) B&W, 97 min. Director: Karel Reisz.

David Warner, Vanessa Redgrave, Robert Stephens. Artist Warner goes bonkers when wife Redgrave decides to leave him and lapses into a fantasy life in which he plays King Kong to her Fay Wray. Offbeat comedy/fantasy about the perils of mental illness that doesn't make a lot of sense, but probably isn't supposed to. It's amusing nonetheless.

(Thorn/EMI Video) VC

Most Dangerous Game, The ☆☆☆

(1932) B&W, 63 min. Directors: Ernest B. Schoedsack, Irving Pichel.

Joel McCrea, Fay Wray, Leslie Banks, Robert Armstrong. Count Zaroff (Banks) lures passing ships to their doom, rescues the survivors, nurses them back to health at his island hideaway, then releases them so that he can hunt them down for sport. McCrea is his latest shipwrecked victim, a big game hunter who finally gives old Zaroff a run for his money. Shot back-to-back with *King Kong* by the same production team and utilizing many of the same sets and actors. Exciting adventure based on a short story by Richard Connell.

(Media Home Entertainment, Budget Video) VC

Multiple Maniacs ★½

(1970) B&W, 90 min. Director: John Waters.

Divine, David Lochary, Mary Vivian Pearce, Mink Stole, Edith Massey. Baltimore's redoubtable John Waters concocted this picaresque tale of a traveling freak show called the Cavalcade of Perversion. Run by the psychotic Divine, the show serves as a front for a gang of drug crazed killers which bears a striking resemblance to the Manson family. Film's climax has Divine raped by a giant lobster. Total lunacy.

(Wizard Video) VC

Murder at the Baskervilles ★★½

(1937) B&W, 67 min. Director: Thomas Bentley.

Arthur Wontner, Lyn Harding, Ian Fleming, Judy Gunn, Lawrence Grossmith. Sherlock Holmes (Wontner) gets an invite from old pal Sir Henry Baskerville (Grossmith) to spend a relaxing few days at Baskerville Hall. But Holmes' vacation is interrupted when one of Sir Henry's prize race horses, Silver Blaze, is stolen and the horse's keeper is murdered. And the game's afoot for Holmes and Watson (Fleming). I might also add that the nefarious Professor Moriarty (Harding) is not exactly sitting idle either. Subdued British mystery based on *Silver Blaze* and other stories by Sir Arthur Conan Doyle.

(Blackhawk) VC

Murder by Death ★★

(1976) Color, 95 min. Director: Robert Moore.

Peter Falk, Peter Sellers, Maggie Smith, Sir Alec Guinness, Nancy Walker, Truman Capote. Lame Neil Simon spoof of detective movies in which some of moviedom's most famous supersleuths—or caricatures thereof—gather at Capote's mansion for an evening of murder, mayhem and out-guessing each other as to whodunit. Falk's take-off on Bogart's Sam Spade is funny at first, but wears thin after awhile, and Sellers' overly broad Charlie Chan doesn't produce a smile. But mute servant Nancy Walker's "silent scream" is a comic high point.

(Columbia Pictures Home Entertainment) VC

Murder by Decree ★★★

(1978) Color, 120 min. Director: Bob Clark.

Christopher Plummer, James Mason, David Hemmings, Susan Clark, Genevieve Bujold, Anthony Quayle, Sir John Gielgud. Sherlock Holmes (Plummer) and Watson (Mason) determine to unmask the elusive killer known as Jack the Ripper, and the trail of clues leads them all the way to the throne of England. Conan Doyle's fictional detective is used here as a mouthpiece through which the filmmakers attempt to pose their own solution to this most famous of all unsolved murder mysteries. Plummer overdoes the earnesty bit, occasionally lapsing into the maudlin. But Mason, who is admittedly a tad too old for the part, plays Watson to perfection. Fascinating, and thought provoking.

(CBS/Fox Video) VC, LV

Murder by Television ★

(1935) B&W, 60 min. Director: Clifford Sanforth.

Bela Lugosi, June Collyer, Huntley Gordon, George Meeker. The story of what the major networks have been doing to us for years. Actually, it's a murder mystery in which a television camera is made to commit murder through remote control; its signal is turned into a lethal death ray. You've gotta give it one thing. It was years ahead of its time.

(Video Yesteryear) VC

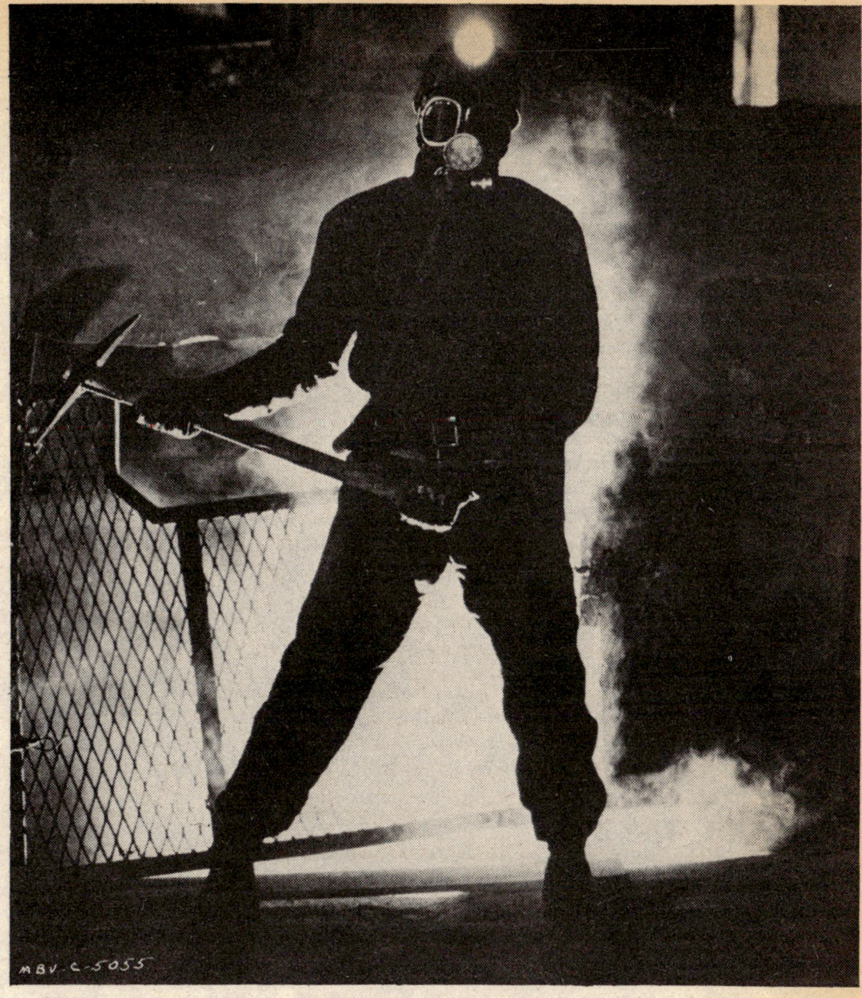

My Bloody Valentine (1981)

". . .lots of slash and drip."

Murder Clinic, The ☐

(1968) Color, 86 min. Director: Elio Scardmaglia.

William Berger, Francoise Prevost, Mary Young, Barbara Wilson. Surgeon attempts to restore the face of a woman he accidentally disfigured—or thinks he did. The locale of the operation is an out-of-the-way clinic for the incurably eccentric. As the doc works on the face, a hooded killer roams the corridors in search of someone to stick a knife in. Eccentric is right. Based on the novel *The Knife in the Body* by Robert Williams. A.k.a. *The Blade in the Body, Night of Terrors, The Murder Society* and *Revenge of the Living Dead.*

(Video Communications) VC

Muppet Movie, The ☐☐½

(1979) Color, 98 min. Director: James Frawley.

The Muppets, Charles Durning, Steve Martin, Mel Brooks. The Muppets head for Hollywood in search of stardom on the big screen. Cute musical/fantasy featuring television's most lovable characters in their feature film debut.

(CBS/Fox Video, RCA VideoDisc) VC, CED, LV

My Bloody Valentine ☐½

(1981) Color, 91 min. Director: George Mihalka.

Paul Kelman, Lori Hallier, Neil Affleck. A psychotic miner terrorizes the Canadian town of Valentine Bluffs on guess what day? His motive: revenge for a mining disaster that took place twenty years ago. Typical splatter movie with lots of slash and drip.

(Paramount Home Video) VC

My Sister, My Love ☐☐

(1980) Color, 99 min. Director: (?)

Lee Grant, Carol Kane. Odd spin-off of Polanski's *Repulsion* which introduces incest and lesbianism to the proceedings. The strain of Grant's having to take care of her mentally disturbed sister Kane, while at the same time trying to maintain a normal life, finally takes its toll when a co-worker presses his romantic attentions and the pair murders him. A sickie.

(Wizard Video) VC

Mysterians, The ☐½

(1958) Color, 89 min. Director: Inoshiro Honda.

Kenji Sahara, Yumi Shirakawa, Akihiko Hirata. Denizens of the planet Mysteroid discover that the population seems to be too heavily weighted with males and not enough females. The reason: the female population is dwindling. The solution: attack earth and steal its women. So the Mysterians set off for the moon, from which they barrage earth with deadly rays and an army of robots in spaceships. All's well that ends well though, and, mercifully, this movie *does* end.

(Video Communications) VC

Mysteries from Beyond Earth ☐☐

(1975) Color, 95 min. Director: George Gale.

Charles Hickson, Dr. Thelma Moss, Major Donald Kehoe, James McDivitt. Host/narrator, Lawrence Dobkin. Documentary look with lots of interviews at such bizarre phenomena as UFOs, the Bermuda Triangle mystery, ESP, Kirlian photography, etc.

(Video Communications) VC

Mysteries from Beyond the Triangle ☐☐

(1977) Color, 94 min. Director: William Miller.

Chet Curtis, Ann Swain. Documentary investigation of the disappearances of planes and ships in the mysterious Bermuda Triangle area. Plenty of theories, no conclusions.

(Video Communications) VC

Mysterious Island ✪✪✪

(1961) Color, 101 min. Director: Cy Endfield.
Michael Craig, Michael Callan, Joan Greenwood, Gary Merrill, Herbert Lom. A group of Confederate prisoners breaks out of a Union stockade and escapes aloft in a giant balloon. A storm blows up and whisks them off to a strange island inhabited by giant crabs and chickens—products of an experiment by the visionary Captain Nemo (Lom) to increase the world's food supply. Ray Harryhausen's marvelous model animation effects and a rousing score by Bernard Herrmann highlight this exciting adventure based on a novel by Jules Verne.
(Columbia Pictures Home Entertainment) VC

Mysterious Mr. Wong ✪ ½

(1935) B&W, 60 min. Director: William Nigh.
Bela Lugosi, Wallace Ford, Arline Judge, Lee Shumway, Lotus Lang. Oriental hatchetman Lugosi (Oriental? With *that* accent?) unleashes a reign of terror on San Francisco's Chinatown in pursuit of the twelve coins of Confucius, ownership of which means being able to rule China. Lots of torture in this one—especially sitting through it. Based on the novel *The Twelve Coins of Confucius* by Harry Stephen Keeler.
(Thunderbird Films) VC

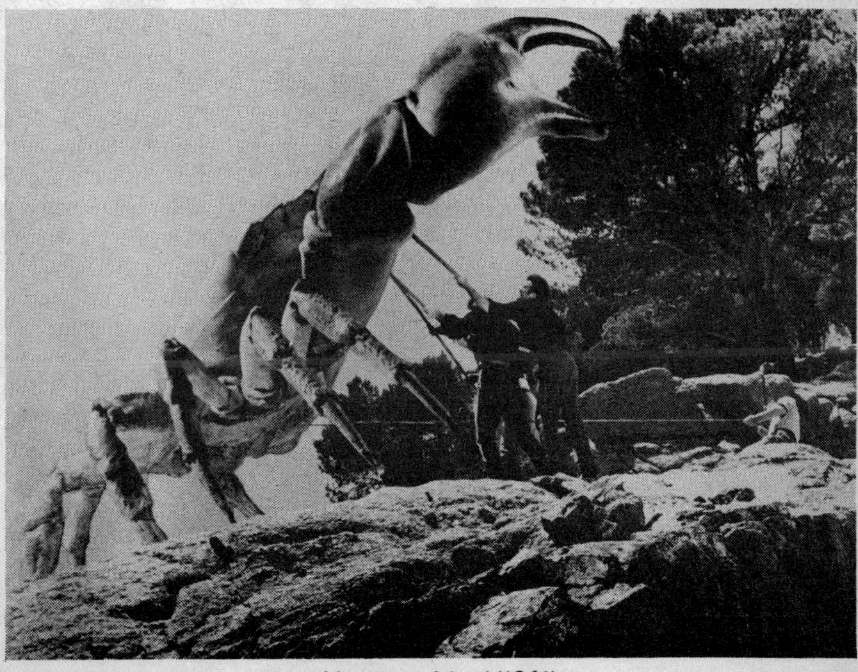

Mysterious Island (1961)

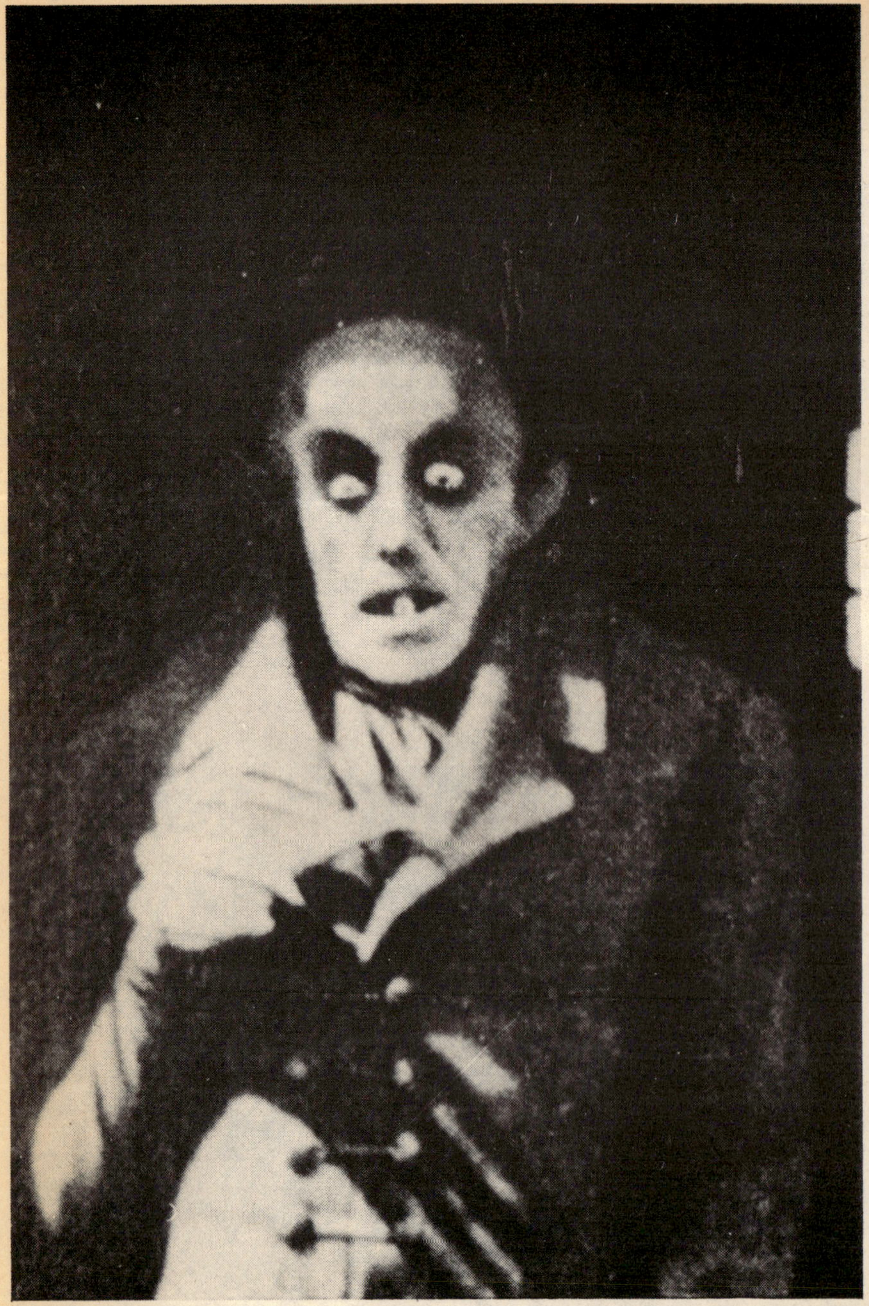

Nosferatu (1922)

N

New Year's Evil ½

(1980) Color, 85 min. Director: Emmett Alston.

Roz Kelly, Kip Niven, Grant Cramer. Psychopathic killer goes on a cross-country murder spree, timing each of his orgies of blood-letting to coincide with local TV coverage of the evening's New Year's Eve celebrations around the country. Talk about a fast worker!

(Paragon Video) VC

Night Creature

(1978) Color, 83 min. Director: Lee Madden.

Donald Pleasence, Nancy Kwan, Ross Hagen, Lesly Fine, Claire Hagen, Jennifer Rhodes. Pleasence, a world-famous writer and hunter in the Hemingway mould, determines to conquer his fear of a man-eating leopard which had once attacked and almost killed him on a previous hunt. His daughters and granddaughter arrive for a vacation and are thrown into the terrors of the hunt along with him. Unsurprising thriller.

(Video Communications, Cult Video) VC

Night of the Living Dead

(1968) B&W, 90 min. Director: George A. Romero.

Duane Jones, Judith O'Dea, Karl Hardman, Russell Streiner. Produced on a shoestring over a long series of weekends by a crew of filmmaking unknowns, this ghoulishly clever splatter movie became a minor cause celebre on its initial release. Much of that furor has since died down and the film is now considered to be a classic. Its plot is very straightforward: all manner of corpses come back from the dead as the result of a freak, but undefined outer space accident, and begin feeding on the living. Despite its many imperfections, this low-budget shocker really delivers the goods.

(Media Home Entertainment, Budget Video, Direct Video, Nostalgia Merchant) VC

Night Stalker, The ½

(1971) Color, 74 min. Director: John Moxey.

Darren McGavin, Simon Oakland, Barry Atwater. A newspaper reporter (McGavin), investigating a series of unsolved murders in Las Vegas, uncovers evidence that the killings are the work of a modern day vampire. But no one will believe him, especially his irascible editor (Oakland), who thinks he's finally cracked. Soon the vampire starts stalking McGavin. This made-for-TV monster movie has a lot more bite than most due to some very violent (for television) action sequences sharply directed by Moxey, and two very energetic performances by McGavin and Oakland.

(CBS/Fox Video) VC

Night Visitor, The ½

(1970) Color, 106 min. Director: Laslo Benedek.

Max von Sydow, Liv Ullmann, Trevor Howard, Per Oscarsson. Von Sydow is committed for having killed someone with an axe—an act of passion rather than premeditated murder. But then, one by one, those who convicted him start getting axe-murdered too. Is he the guilty party this time? And if so, how did he get out of prison to commit the crimes?

(Video Communications) VC

Nightmare ½

(1981) Color, 97 min. Director: Romano Scavolini.

Baird Stafford, Sharon Smith, C.J. Cooke, Mik Cribben. Convict Stafford is given a test drug to curb his appetite for violence. When it appears to be a success, he is released, after which he promptly goes on a murder spree, killing and mutilating women from New York City to Florida. Lurid schocker with liberal doses of splatter.

(Planet Video) VC

Nightmare Castle

(1966) B&W, 90 min. Director: Allan Grunewald.

Barbara Steele, Paul Mueller, Helga Line, Lawrence Clift. Mad scientist kills his wife and her lover, but they come back from the dead to collect revenge. Typical.

(Budget Video) VC

Nightmare in Wax ½

(1969) Color, 91 min. Director: Bud Townsend.

Cameron Mitchell, Anne Helm, Scott Brady, Barry Kroeger, Johnny Cardos. A screen make-up man who is disfigured in a freak accident caused by a movie producer opens a wax museum, killing people and embalming them in wax to use as his exhibits. Obvious rip-off of *House of Wax*.

(Video Communications) VC

1941

(1979) Color, 120 min. Director: Steven Spielberg.

John Belushi, Dan Ackroyd, Ned Beatty, Nancy Allen, Christopher Lee. Los Angeles goes invasion-crazy in the chaotic days following the Japanese bombing of Pearl Harbor. This overblown, over-produced, *over-everything* "comedy" is based on an actual historical incident—anecdote, really. Some sequences in the film are among the best Steven Spielberg has directed, but overall, the film is a witless elephant, full of mindless destruction.

(MCA Videocassette and Disc) VC, LV

Nocturna

(1979) Color, 83 min. Director: Harry Tampa.

John Carradine, Yvonne DeCarlo, Brother Theodore, Adam Keefe. Soft core porno-horror-comedy with a disco beat in which Dracula (Carradine) follows his nubile granddaughter Nocturna to the flesh pots of the Big Apple for some skin and excitement. Awful.

(Media Home Entertainment) VC

Nosferatu ★★★

(1922) B&W, 63 min. Director: F.W. Murnau.

Max von Schreck, Alexander Granach, Gustav von Wangenheim, Greta Schroeder. This may not be the scariest film version of *Dracula* ever made, nor even the best, but it is undeniably the first. Murnau and screenwriter Henrik Galeen pirated the plot of Stoker's novel, changed the names of the characters and added a few other touches of their own, made the film and were immediately sued for plagiarism by Stoker's widow. Prints of the film were confiscated and destroyed. For many years, historians thought the film had been irretrievably lost. They were wrong, but while prints of Murnau's film have survived, no two of them are alike, including the versions on these two videocassettes. As to the film itself: yes, it is a bit heavy-handed and even primitive at times, but much of it still works—especially Schreck's performance as the ugliest Dracula ever.
(Thunderbird Films, Blackhawk Films) VC

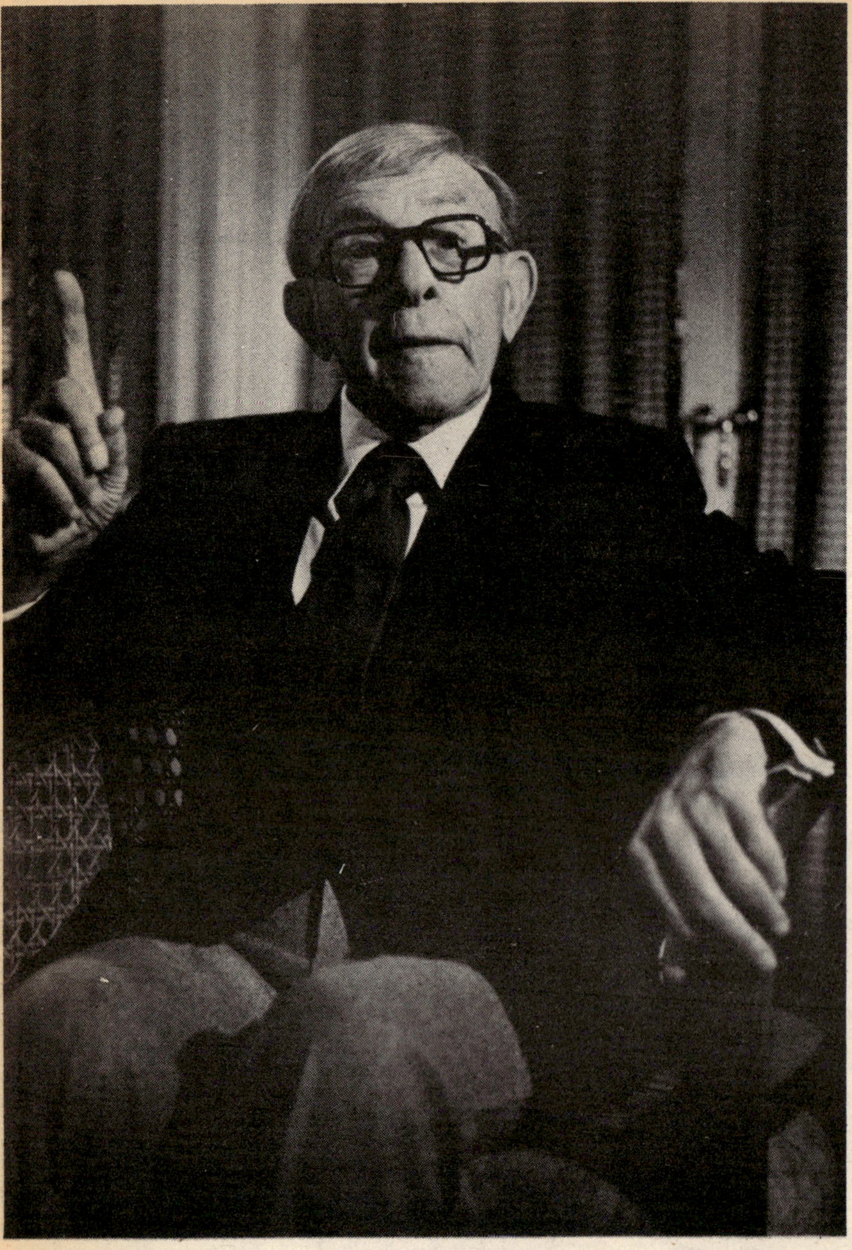

Oh God! Book II (1980)

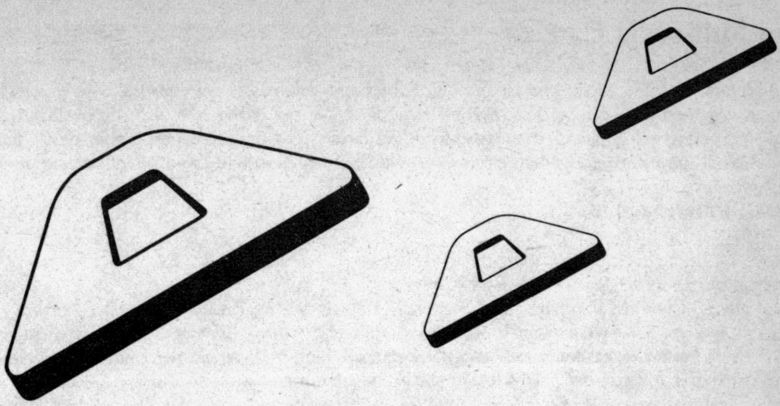

Oh, God! ½

(1977) Color, 104 min. Director: Carl Reiner.
George Burns, John Denver, Terri Garr, Paul Sorvino. Disgusted with the way things are going in the world, God (Burns) makes Himself visible to everyman Denver, commissioning him to spread His word to a doubting populace. Naturally, the populace thinks Denver is nuts. Amusing fantasy/comedy in the Frank Capra tradition. Denver is good, Burns even better.
(Warner Home Video) VC

Oh, God!—Book II ½

(1980) Color, 94 min. Director: Gilbert Cates.
George Burns, Suzanne Pleshette, David Birney, Louanne. Pointless sequel in which Burns enlists the aid of child Louanne to help bring His message of Love to the world. Terminally cute.
(Warner Home Video) VC

Omen, The

(1976) Color, 111 min. Director: Richard Donner.
Gregory Peck, Lee Remick, David Warner, Billie Whitelaw. Peck is the U.S. ambassador to the Court of St. James, whose newborn son is switched at birth by a group of satanists and replaced with the devil's spawn. Little Damien grows into a very nasty little toddler indeed, causing murder and mayhem wherever he goes. Gruesome, but well made.
(CBS/Fox Video) VC, LV, CED

On the Beach ½

(1959) B&W, 133 min. Director: Stanley Kramer.
Gregory Peck, Ava Gardner, Fred Astaire, Anthony Perkins. A diversity of people, lone survivors of a nuclear holocaust, comes together in Australia to await its doom as the result of the fallout. Stock disaster movie situations and characters plus Kramer's customary heavy hand with a message prevent this cautionary tale of the perils of the nuclear arms race from achieving much of its potential power. Still, the message is a sober one and cannot be made too often.
(CBS/Fox Video) VC

One Million B.C. ★★

(1940) B&W, 80 min. Directors: Hal Roach, Hal Roach, Jr., D.W. Griffith.
Victor Mature, Carole Landis, Lon Chaney, Jr. Fantasy-adventure set in prehistoric days in which muscular cavemen and scantily clad cavegirls struggle to survive in the face of many obstacles, including erupting volcanos and man- (and woman-) beasts. The special effects are far below those of the original *King Kong,* but Mature makes a suitably beefy hero and Landis is quite cute in her prehistoric sun suit.
(Nostalgia Merchant) VC

Orca ★

(1977) Color, 92 min. Director: Michael Anderson.
Richard Harris, Charlotte Rampling, Will Sampson, Keenan Wynn, Bo Derek. Whaler Harris catches a pregnant killer whale, which proceeds to give birth on the deck of his ship. Both mama and the baby die, however, and papa, who has been watching from anear, determines to revenge himself on Harris and company. This totally absurd adventure film was made by producer Dino De Laurentiis with but one goal in mind: to capitalize on the success of *Jaws.* Derek has a small part in which, as one of the victim's of Orca's wrath, she sheds one of her legs instead of her clothes.
(Paramount Home Video) VC, LV

Orpheus ★★★

(1950) B&W, 95 min. Director: Jean Cocteau.
Jean Marais, Francois Perier, Maria Casares. Avant-garde retelling of the legend of Orpheus and Eurydice set in present day Paris. Full of imaginative touches.
(Video Yesteryear, Budget Video) VC

Outer Space Connection, The ★★

(1975) Color, 106 min. Director: Fred Warshofsky.
Narrated by Rod Serling. Speculative documentary which proclaims that earth was visited by extraterrestrials many millions of years ago and that they plan to return. Of late, this idea has been done to death in the documentary film form. Even the clips are getting to be redundant.
(Video Communications) VC

Outland ★½

(1981) Color, 109 min. Director: Peter Hyams.
Sean Connery, Peter Boyle, Frances Sternhagen. Connery is the newly installed federal marshal of a mining colony on one of Jupiter's moons, a forbidding place where overworked miners are developing acute cases of the crazies. Connery learns that the workers are being given lethal drugs that step up their productivity but drive them insane as well. He determines to stop the killing, but finds that he must stand alone. His final showdown against a trio of gunmen hired by company man Boyle to silence him is a total rip-off of the plot of *High Noon,* but is devoid of that film's suspense because none of the characters in this film display any real depth or motivation. A cynical, superficial attempt to take a worn out western movie theme and re-work (or rather re-hash) it in outer space.
(Warner Home Video) VC

P

Panda and the Magic Serpent ★★½

(1958) Color, 78 min. Directors: Taija Yabushita, Kazuhiko Okabe.
Animated Japanese feature based on an ancient Japanese fable about a little boy who finds a white snake in the family garden, but his parents won't let him keep it. Years later he discovers that the snake has metamorphosed into a beautiful maiden, who eventually rescues him from the clutches of an evil magician.
(Family Home Entertainment) VC

Parasite ★½

(1982) Color, 85 min. Director: Charles Band.
Robert Glaudini, Demi Moore, Luca Bercovici. Another spawn of *Alien* in which a malevolent creature rips its way in and out of people's bodies. Filmed in 3-D, but the effect doesn't quite come off.
(Wizard Video) VC

Patrick ★½

(1978) Color, 90 min. Director: Richard Franklin.
Susan Penhaligon, Robert Helpmann, Rod Mullinar, Julia Blake, Robert Thompson. Comatose young man possessed of telekinetic powers falls in love with his nurse (Penhaligon), kills her ambulatory suitor with his powers, then starts knocking off members of the hospital staff as well, including his evil doctor (Helpmann), who wishes to use the boy's powers for his own villainous ends. Dull Australian horror film.
(Unicorn Video, Harmony Vision) VC

Penalty, The ★★

(1920) B&W, 70 min. Director: Wallace Worsley.
Lon Chaney, Claire Adams, Kenneth Harlan, Charles Clary. When an operation performed on him by a careless surgeon robs him of his legs as a child, the Chaney character vows revenge against the surgeon and society at large. As an adult, he turns to a life of crime, becoming "king of the underworld." Standard crime drama with overtones of the bizarre due to Chaney's remarkable make-up and performance as the legless kingpin.
(Classic Video Cinema Collector's Club) VC

People Who Own the Dark, The ★½

(1980) Color, 86 min. Director: Leon Klimovsky.

Maria Perschy, Tony Kendall, Paul Naschy, A. de Mendoza, T. Gimpera. Spanish horror flick about a post-nuclear holocaust in which the surviving leads, followers of the Marquis De Sade, find the chaos that surrounds them very much to their liking. They get their comeuppance, though, when a decontamination team finds them, puts them to sleep, then buries them alive. Strives for significance, but is just unpleasant.

(Sun Video) VC

Persecution ★½

(1974) Color, 90 min. Director: Don Chaffey.

Lana Turner, Trevor Howard, Ralph Bates, Susan Farmer. Evil Turner becomes pregnant by Howard, who refuses to marry her. The son she gives birth to (Bates), she then proceeds to humiliate even into adulthood, at which time his mind finally snaps and he decides to give her her comeuppance. Empty horror thriller.

(Electric Video) VC

Pete's Dragon ★★½

(1977) Color, 129 min. Director: Don Chaffey.

Helen Reddy, Shelley Winters, Mickey Rooney, Jim Dale, Red Buttons, Sean Marshall. Orphan Marshall befriends a dragon named Elliot, a clutsy beast who delights in engaging in heroics. Sprightly live-action Disney fantasy-musical with some wonderful—and quite funny—animation sequences combining live actors with Elliot. Overlong, though.

(Walt Disney Home Video) VC, LV

Phantasm ★

(1977) Color, 90 min. Director: Don Coscarelli.

Michael Baldwin, Bill Thornsberry, Reggie Bannister. Two brothers investigate a mysterious house where a friend of theirs was recently murdered and encounter some very strange goings-on indeed. For example, a proliferation of ghouls and a flying silver disc, which, when hurled at its intended victim, sprouts a sharp blade for impalement. Ludicrous low-budget horror yarn that makes no sense at all.

(CBS/Fox Video) VC, LV

Phantom of the Opera, The ★★½

(1925) Color/B&W, 85 min. Director: Rupert Julian.

Lon Chaney, Sr., Norman Kerry, Mary Philbin. A mysterious creature terrorizes the Paris Opera House. Philbin is the new lead singer with whom he falls in love and whom he spirits off to his underground lair. This first filming of the oft-filmed tale boasts one of Chaney's most imaginative performances, as well as one of his most startling make-ups. But on the whole, except for him, it's a rather dull affair.

(Blackhawk) VC

Phantom Ship ★★

(1936) B&W, 80 min. Director: Denison Clift.

Bela Lugosi, Shirley Grey, Arthur Margetson, Dennis Hoey, Terence de Marney. An American ship called the Marie Celeste is found adrift in the Atlantic with no hands on board and no trace of them found afterward. The film goes on to suggest a solution to the mystery as Lugosi, a crazed deck hand, murders everyone, dumps their bodies overboard, then commits suicide by drowning himself. Lightweight early Hammer film. A.k.a. *The Mystery of the Marie Celeste.*

(Cable Films) VC

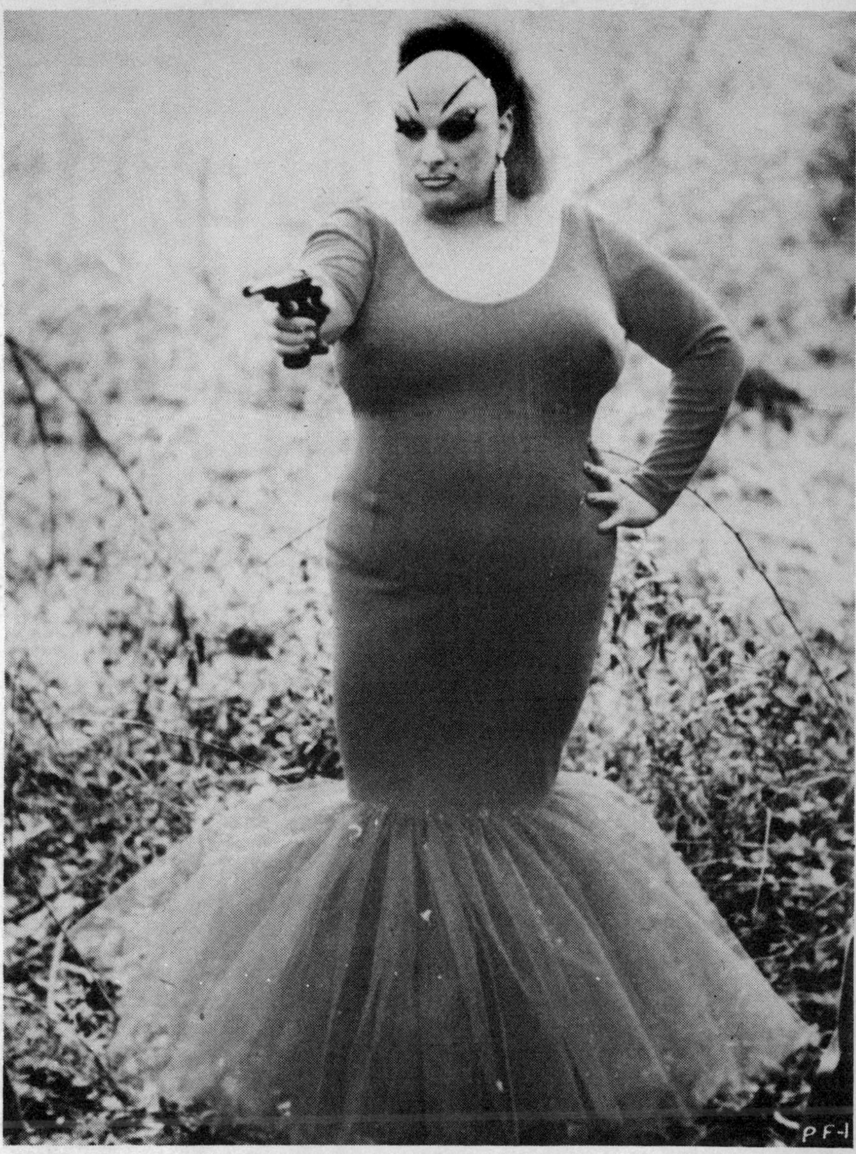

Pink Flamingos (1972)

"A genuinely rancid movie."

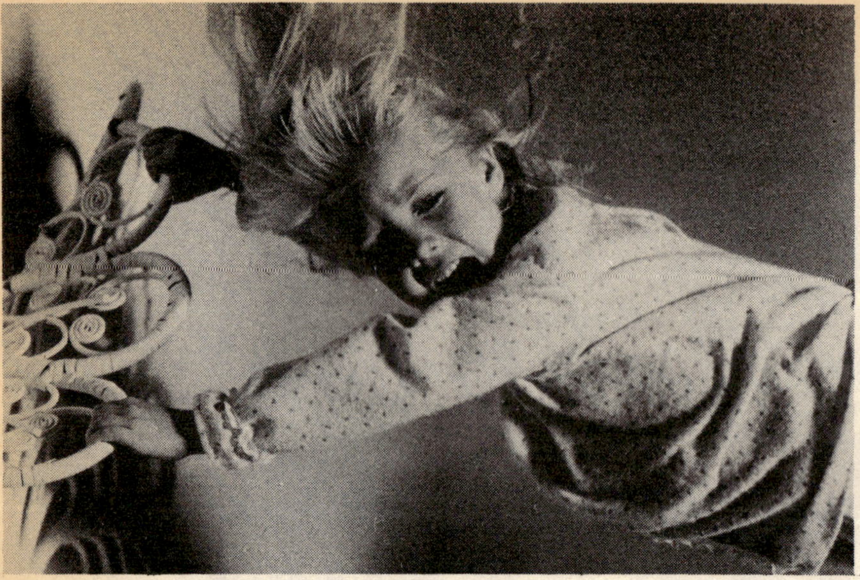

Poltergeist (1982)

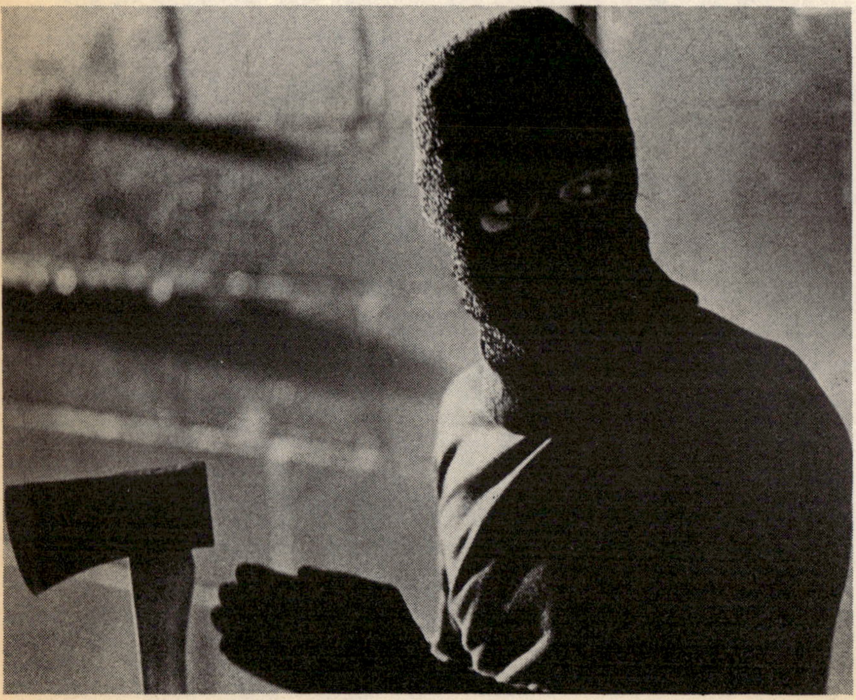

Prom Night (1980)

Phantom Tollbooth, The ½

(1970) Color, 90 min. Directors: Chuck Jones, Abe Levitow, David Monahan.
Butch Patrick; voices of Mel Blanc, June Foray, Hans Conreid, Daws Butler. Musical comedy-fantasy that combines live action with animation in which Patrick daydreams himself into the Kingdom of Wisdom by first going through a magical tollbooth.
(MGM/UA Home Video) VC, CED

Picnic at Hanging Rock

(1976) Color, 110 min. Director: Peter Weir.
Rachel Roberts, Dominic Guard, Anne Lambert, Helen Morse. A group of schoolgirls goes on an outing in the Australian outback on Valentine's Day 1900 and some never return. A search for them is mounted, but the film poses no straightforward solution to this mystery. Some of the girls are found, but the reason for the disappearance is never explained. Puzzling, esoteric, beautifully photographed and scored mood piece handled with consummate control by Weir. Confounding, but fascinating.
(Vestron Video) VC

Pink Flamingos

(1972) Color, 93 min. Director: John Waters.
Divine, David Lochary, Mary Vivian Pearce, Mink Stole, Edith Massey. Two groups of outcasts compete for the title of "The Filthiest People Alive" in this self-billed exercise in poor taste by the Baltimore director who could write a book on the subject—in fact, he has. There are some raunchily funny moments in the film, but overall it's just plain disgusting. Divine's parting shot, which wins her the title, is especially nauseating. A genuinely rancid movie.
(Wizard Video) VC

Pink Panther Strikes Again, The

(1976) Color, 103 min. Director: Blake Edwards.
Peter Sellers, Herbert Lom, Lesley-Anne Down, Colin Blakely, Burt Kwouk. This Inspector Clouseau (Sellers) comedy is pure fantasy. Lom reprises his role as the harried head of the Surete who is driven bonkers by Clouseau and gets sent to an asylum. He escapes and threatens to destroy the world with a ray gun unless Clouseau is given over to him for "justice." At times Lom almost seems to be parodying his starring role in Hammer's *Phantom of the Opera;* in any event, he's very funny, even managing to upstage Sellers. A delightful farce.
(CBS/Fox Video) VC, LV

Pinocchio in Outer Space

(1965) Color, 71 min. Director: Ray Goossens.
Voices of Arnold Stang, Conrad Jameson, Minerva Pious. Giant intergalactic spiders, scorpions and satellite-eating whales are only a few of the amazing creatures encountered by Pinocchio in this animated, space-age retelling of the classic children's story by Carlo Collodi.
(Columbia Pictures Home Entertainment) VC

Pit and the Pendulum, The ½

(1961) Color, 85 min. Director: Roger Corman.
Vincent Price, John Kerr, Barbara Steele, Luana Anders. Second in Corman's series of gothic thrillers based on stories by Edgar Allen Poe. In this one, which is set just after the Spanish Inquisition, Price is the son of a sadistic Inquisitor; when his mind snaps, he begins thinking he's dear old dad in more ways than one. A bit slow moving, but the finale makes up for it.
(Warner Home Video) VC

Plague ✪✪

(1978) Color, 87 min. Director: Ed Hunt.
Kate Reid, Celene Lomez, Daniel Pilon. Scientists develop a deadly new strain of virus by accident, which then proceeds to escape from the lab and threaten the world. Lifeless sci-fi in the tradition of *The Andromeda Strain.*
(VidAmerica) VC

Planet of the Apes ✪✪✪

(1968) Color, 112 min. Director: Franklin J. Schaffner.
Charlton Heston, Roddy McDowall, Kim Hunter, Maurice Evans. A team of American astronauts crashes on an alien planet some 2000 years in the future and discovers that on it the evolutionary history of earth has been reversed; apes are the civilized rulers and men are the beasts. Well done science-fiction thriller with a socko ending.
(CBS/Fox Video) VC, CED

Planet Outlaws ✪✪

(1953) B&W, 70 min. Directors: Ford Beebe, Saul A. Goodkind.
Buster Crabbe, Constance Moore, C. Montague Shaw, Jack Moran. Another compilation feature drawn from segments of the 1930s Buck Rogers serial.
(Thunderbird Films) VC

Plan 9 from Outer Space ✪

(1962) B&W, 78 min. Director: Edward D. Wood, Jr.
Bela Lugosi, Vampira, Lyle Talbot, Tor Johnson, Gregory Walcott. Here it is, folks, the film that invariably makes everybody's list of the ten worst films ever made—and usually cops the number one spot to boot. Having failed to conquer earth after eight previous attempts, a group of stumble bum aliens decides to give it one last shot—thus the title. Their plan this time involves resurrecting the dead and using them to destroy the living. Absolutely awful. But funny. A.k.a. *Graverobbers from Outer Space.*
(Nostalgia Merchant) VC

Play Misty for Me ✪✪✪

(1971) Color, 102 min. Director: Clint Eastwood.
Clint Eastwood, Jessica Walter, Donna Mills, John Larch. Eastwood is a low-keyed disc jockey at a small-time Carmel, California radio station. Walter is an ardent admirer who pursues him relentlessly until they become lovers. But she's the jealous, possessive type, so he dumps her, discovering afterward in her continued, relentless pursuit of him that she's dangerously psychotic as well. Eastwood's directorial debut is a genuine nail-biter with a performance by Walter that's almost in a class with Anthony Perkins' Norman Bates. Look for director Don Siegel in a small role as a bartender. Nicely done.
(MCA Videocassette and Disc) VC, LV

Poltergeist ✪✪✪

(1982) Color, 114 min. Director: Tobe Hooper.
JoBeth Williams, Craig T. Nelson, Beatrice Straight, Heather O'Rourke. Suburban home is beseiged by evil spirits emanating from the family TV set. The uninvited houseguests snatch the family's youngest daughter, then subject everyone to a reign of supernatural terror as mom and dad bring in parapsychology researchers and an eccentric spiritualist to reclaim their stolen tot. Turns out that a greedy land developer erected their house on land that was once a cemetery but didn't bother to relocate the dead. Nice combination of humor and horror that falters mid-stream due to an overabundance of razzle-dazzle lighting effects and seemingly endless mumbo jumbo about whether the missing little girl should go "near the light" or not. Otherwise, this Steven Spielberg production is solid fright fare.
(MGM/UA Home Video) VC

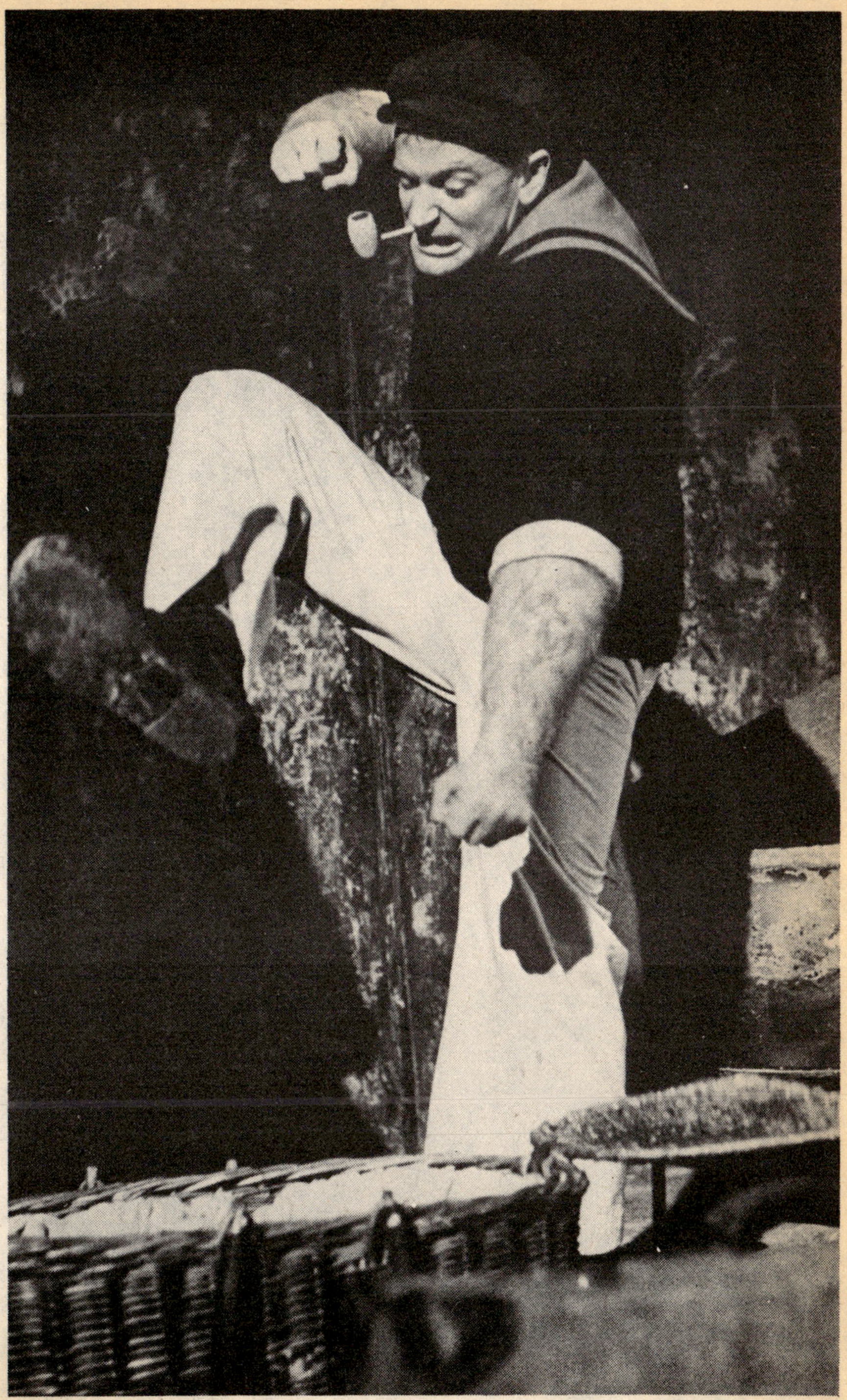

Popeye (1980)

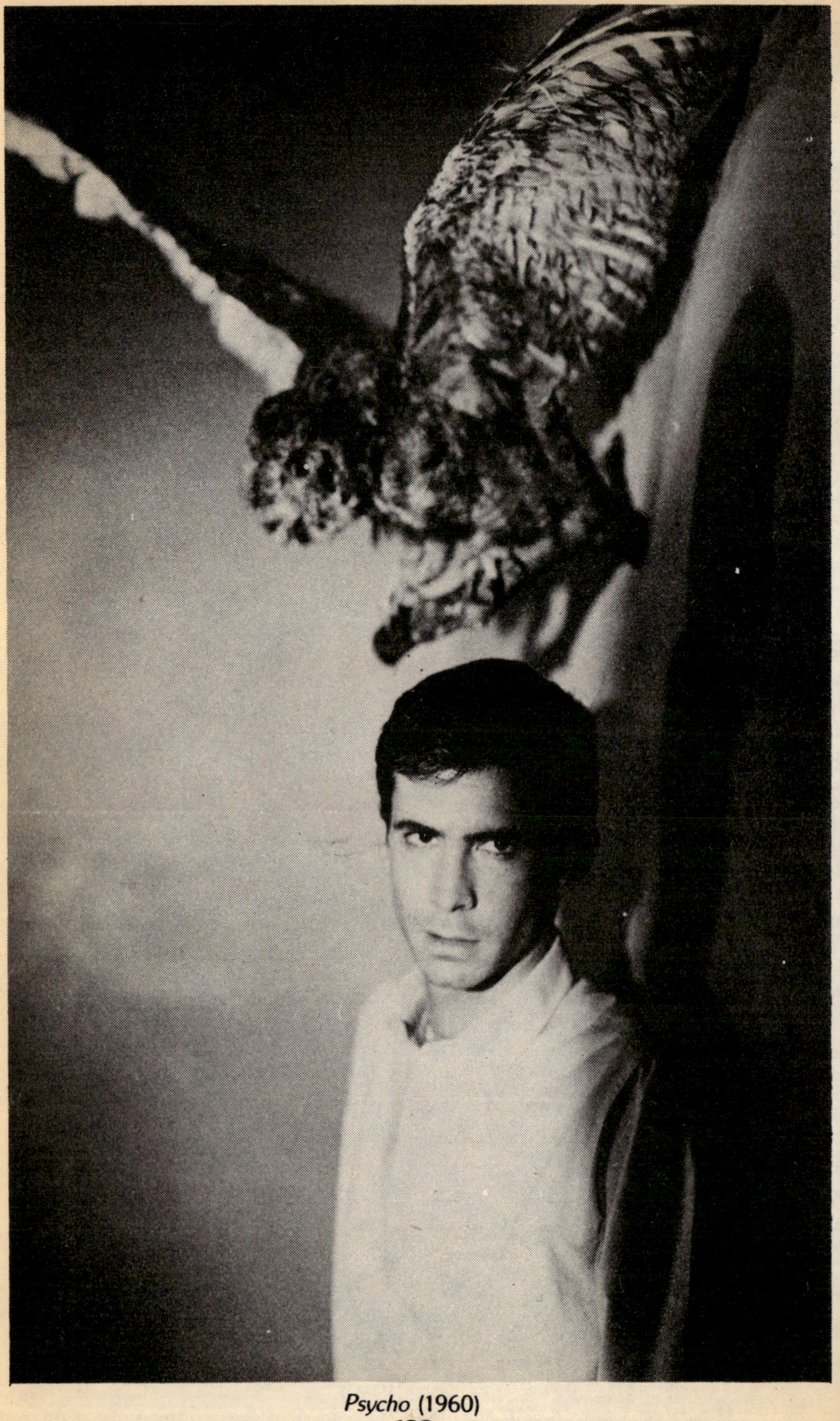

Psycho (1960)

Popeye

(1980) Color, 114 min. Director: Robert Altman.
Robin Williams, Shelley Duvall, Ray Walston, Paul Dooley. Williams and Duvall do consummate impressions of Popeye and Olive Oyl in this live-action musical-fantasy based on the famous comic strip. However, the songs aren't particularly memorable, the jokes aren't all that funny, and Altman's rambling technique slows down the action altogether. Ironically, this *Popeye's* greatest single achievement is to make one long for the real thing. Which, of course, is not real at all, but a cartoon.
(Paramount Home Video, RCA VideoDisc) VC, LV, CED

Prom Night

(1980) Color, 91 min. Director: Paul Lynch.
Jamie Lee Curtis, Leslie Nielsen. A masked killer stalks a group of high school kids on the night of their senior prom, as revenge for an accidental death caused by the careless teens six years earlier. Predictable thrillshow in the *Halloween* mould.
(MCA Videocassette and Disc) VC, LV

Prophecy ½

(1979) Color, 119 min. Director: John Frankenheimer.
Robert Foxworth, Talia Shire, Armand Assante, Victoria Racimo. Doctor Foxworth and pregnant wife Shire travel to backwoods Maine to investigate the effects of pollution from a local lumber mill on the area's flora and fauna. What they discover is a race of mutant giants, ugly critters which resemble a cross between Godzilla and a pizza. One or two good moments, but overall a tiresome affair.
(Paramount Home Video) VC

Prowler, The

(1981) Color, 91 min. Director: Joseph Zito.
Vicki Dawson, Christopher Goutman, Cindy Weintraub, Laurence Tierney, Farley Granger. Low-budget revenge shocker in the *Friday the 13th* mould in which couples are systematically butchered by a pitchfork-wielding maniac at a graduation dance, a reprise of similar events which occurred 35 years before at another graduation dance. Nothing new here except for Tom Savini's gore effects. A.k.a. *The Graduation.*
(Direct Video) VC

Psycho

(1960) B&W, 109 min. Director: Alfred Hitchcock.
Anthony Perkins, Janet Leigh, John Gavin, Martin Balsam, Vera Miles. Leigh steals $40,000 so that she and Gavin can run off, but during her getaway, she's caught in the rain and decides to spend the night at a rundown hotel run by Perkins and his slightly mad ma. The granddaddy of all modern horror films, which, despite its countless imitations since, still packs a suspenseful wallop.
(MCA Videocassette and Disc) VC, LV

Psychomania

(1973) Color, 95 min. Director: Richard Hilliard.
Lee Philips, Sheppard Strudwick, Jean Hale, Lorraine Rogers. A sex killer is loose on the campus of a girl's college and a former war hero is accused of the crimes and must clear himself. Gory.
(Budget Video) VC

Psychomania

(1973) Color, 89 min. Director: Don Sharp.
George Sanders, Beryl Reid, Nicky Henson, May Larkin, Robert Hardy, Patrick Holt. Off-the-wall mixture of comedy and horror in which Reid makes a deal with the devil to return her dead motorcycle gang leader son from the grave. In the end, she revokes the deal and turns into a toad.
(Media Home Entertainment) VC

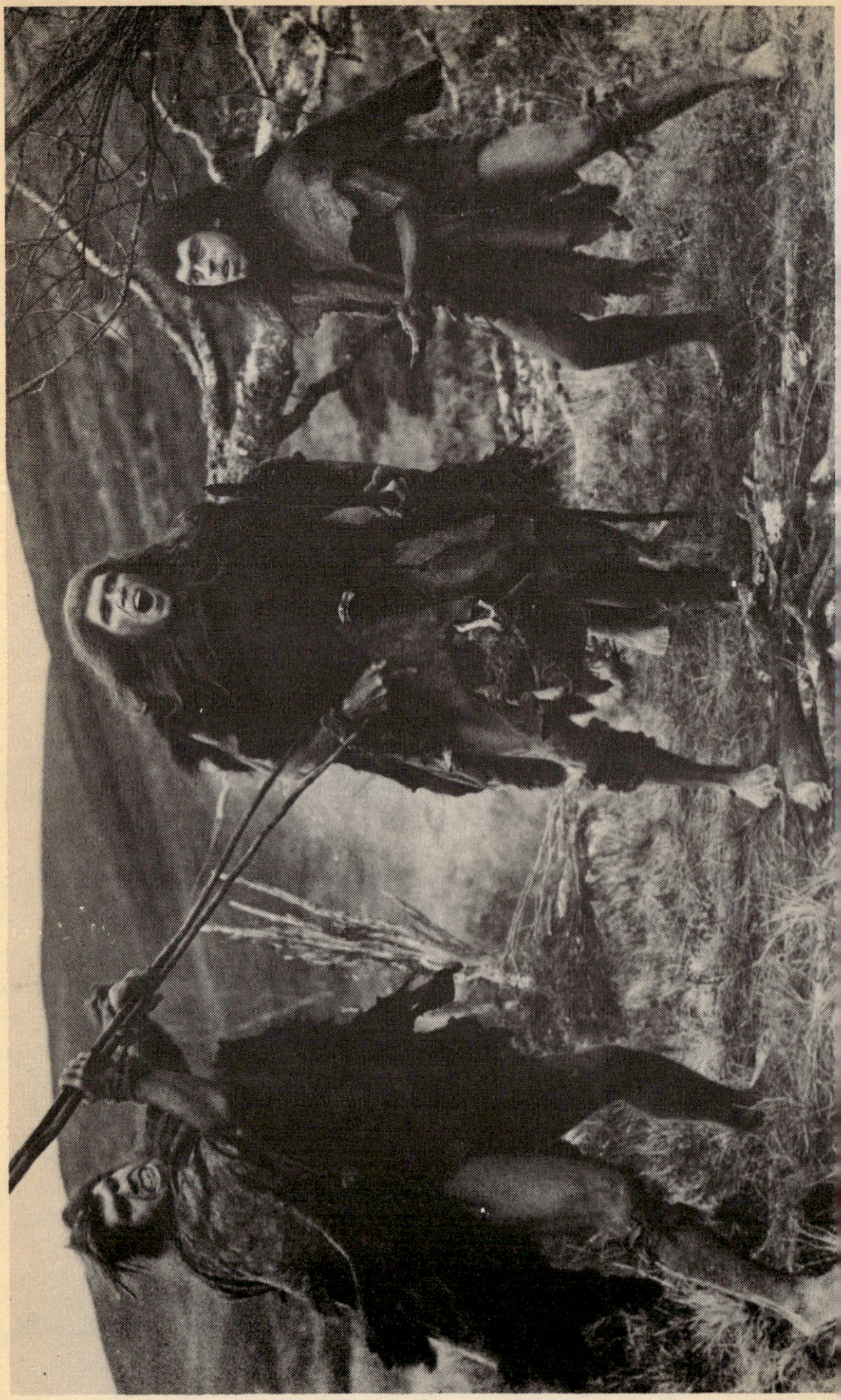

Quest for Fire (1981)

Quest for Fire ½

(1981) Color, 97 min. Director: Jean-Jacques Annaud.
Everett McGill, Rae Dawn Chong, Ron Perlman, Nameer El Kadi. Anthony Burgess devised the spoken language, Desmond Morris devised the body language, and Polanski collaborator Gerard Brach devised the screenplay for this dawn of man epic in which a group of cavemen loses its source of fire, sets out to reclaim it, and along the way discovers the missionary position. Brilliantly photographed, but Kubrick's dawn of man sequence in *2001* was better—if only because it was shorter.
(CBS/Fox Video) VC, CED

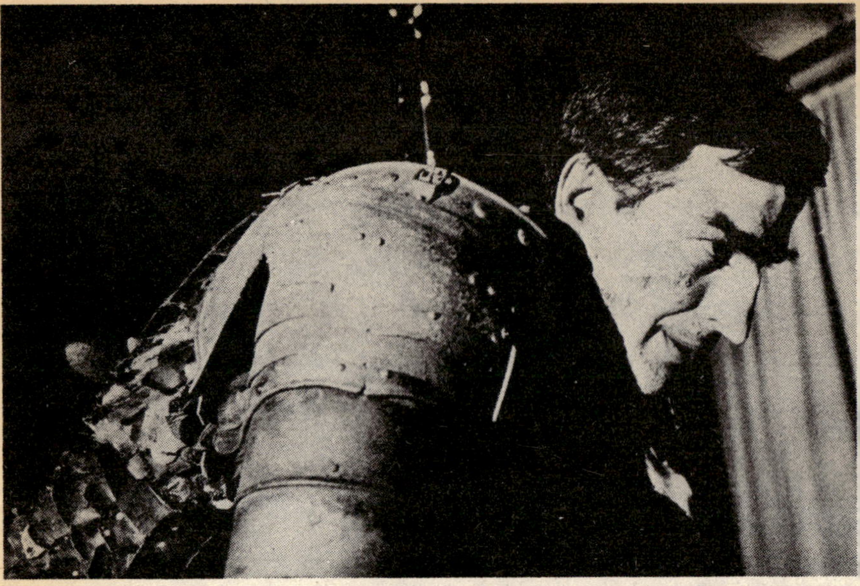

Rosemary's Baby (1968)

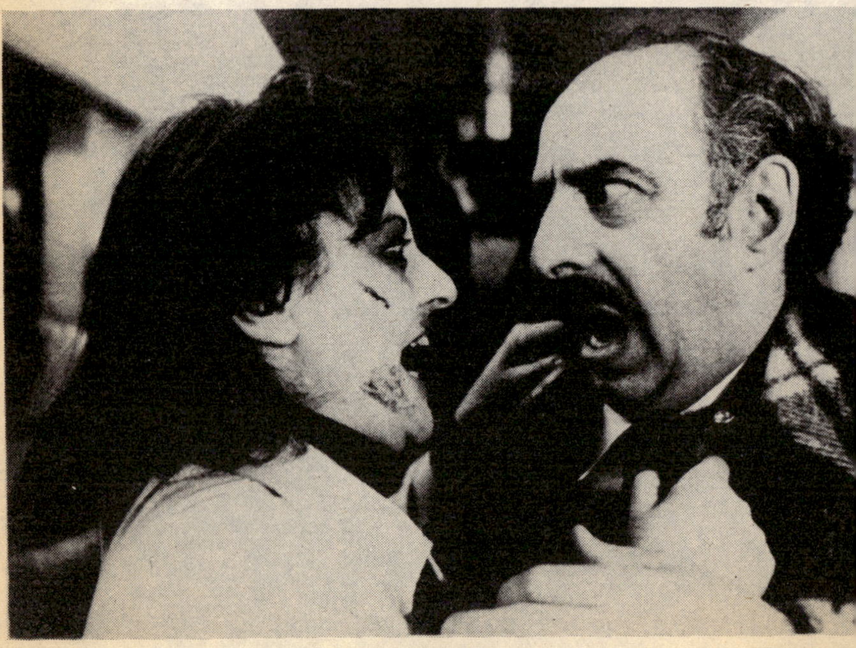

Rabid (1977)

Rabid ½

(1977) Color, 90 min. Director: David Cronenberg.
Marilyn Chambers, Joe Silver, Howard Ryshpan, Patricia Gage, Susan Roman, Frank Moore. Porno queen Chambers took time out from her X-rated romps to appear in this low-budget medical horror film in which she plays an accident victim who undergoes a skin grafting experiment that results in her turning into a sort of vampire. Instead of biting her victims in the neck, however, she lets her armpit do the work. How? Well, you'll just have to see. Writer-director Cronenberg is capable of much better things than this sad reprise of elements from *Night of the Living Dead.*
(Warner Home Video) VC

Raise the Titanic

(1980) Color, 112 min. Director: Jerry Jameson.
Richard Jordan, Anne Archer, Jason Robards. Adventurer Jordan is hired to head a salvage operation to raise the riches-laden Titanic from her icy grave. Turns out that there's more on board than just riches, however, as the Russians are mounting their own salvage operation. Clive Cussler's exciting best-seller is here given the superficial whammy. A leaden "thriller" that sinks under the weight of its own ponderousness. Dull, dull, dull.
(CBS/Fox Video) VC, LV, CED

Rats are Coming! The Werewolves are Here!, The

(1972) Color, 92 min. Director: Andy Milligan.
Hope Stansbury, Jacqueline Skarvellis, Berwick Kaler, Noel Collins. Apocalyptic nightmare (with a title like that, what else could it be?) about a family of werewolves and a deranged girl who raises man-eating rats. Quite a combo. You *know* the world's in trouble!
(Midnight Video) VC

Raven, The

(1943) B&W, 92 min. Director: Henri-Georges Clouzot.
Pierre Fresnay, Sylvie. A series of poison pen letters succeeds in tearing apart a small French town with suspicion and fear. Engrossing thriller, remade by Otto Preminger in 1951 as *The Thirteenth Letter.* A.k.a. *Le Corbeau.*
(Thunderbird Films) VC

Redeemer, The

(1978) Color, 83 min. Director: Constantine S. Gochis.
Michael Hollingsworth, Damien Knight, Gyr Patterson, T.G. Finkbinder, Nikki Barthen. Peculiar satanist drama about a strange young boy who materializes excalibur-style from a mountain lake to smite sinners. A.k.a. *Son of Satan.*
(Video Communications) VC

Repulsion

(1965) B&W, 105 min. Director: Roman Polanski.
Catherine Deneuve, Ian Hendry, John Fraser, Patrick Wymark, Yvonne Furneaux. Polanski's first feature film in English is a harrowing, meticulously detailed study of a beautiful Belgian girl's (Deneuve) descent into sexual psychosis. Deneuve is left alone in her seedy South Kensington flat when sister Furneaux and married boyfriend Hendry head off to Italy for a weekend. Alone, her madness festers. Soon a phantom rapist, a creature born of her own diseased imagination, begins stalking the flat; the walls begin to crack, and two men wind up murdered. Grim, but unforgettable.
(Video Dimensions) VC

Resurrection of Zachary Wheeler, The ½

(1971) Color, 100 min. Director: Bob Wynn.
Angie Dickinson, Bradford Dillman, James Daly, Leslie Nielsen. A presidential candidate is almost killed in a fiery car crash, but his body is transported to a mysterious, out-of-the-way clinic in New Mexico just in time for a cloning operation to be performed. He dies, yet he lives. Interesting and suspenseful, but the ending is weak.
(Video Communications) VC

Return, The

(1980) Color, 91 min. Director: Greydon Clark.
Jan-Michael Vincent, Cybill Shepherd, Martin Landau, Raymond Burr, Neville Brand. Vincent and Shepherd have a childhood close encounter with aliens. When they grow up, they meet again in the same town, fall in love, then re-encounter the same alien force. Ridiculous, confused, and pretentious science-fiction thriller from the director of the equally ridiculous but somehow more enjoyable *Without Warning.*
(Thorn/EMI Video) VC

Return of Chandu, The

(1934) B&W, 76 min. Director: Ray Taylor.
Bela Lugosi, Maria Alba, Clara Kimball Young, Lucien Prival. Feature film compilation drawn from the 12-part serial released the same year. A black magic cult seeks to conquer the world. Based on *Chandu, the Magician,* a radio series by Harry A. Earnshaw, Vera M. Oldham and R.R. Morgan.
(Video Yesteryear) VC

Revenge

(1972) Color, 89 min. Director: Sidney Hayers.
Joan Collins, James Booth, Ray Barrett, Kenneth Griffith. Family of a 10-year-old girl, victim of a brutal slaying, kidnaps the likeliest suspect when he is released by the police due to insufficient evidence and administers justice of its own.
(Embassy Home Entertainment) VC

Robot Monster

(1953) Color, 63 min. Director: Phil Tucker.
George Nader, Claudia Barrett, Selena Royle, Gregory Moffett. Near-legendary grade Z sci-fi monster flick featuring a man dressed in a gorilla suit and wearing a deep sea diver's helmet as the fearsome beast of the title. Genuinely awful. Originally filmed in 3-D
(Video Dimensions) VC

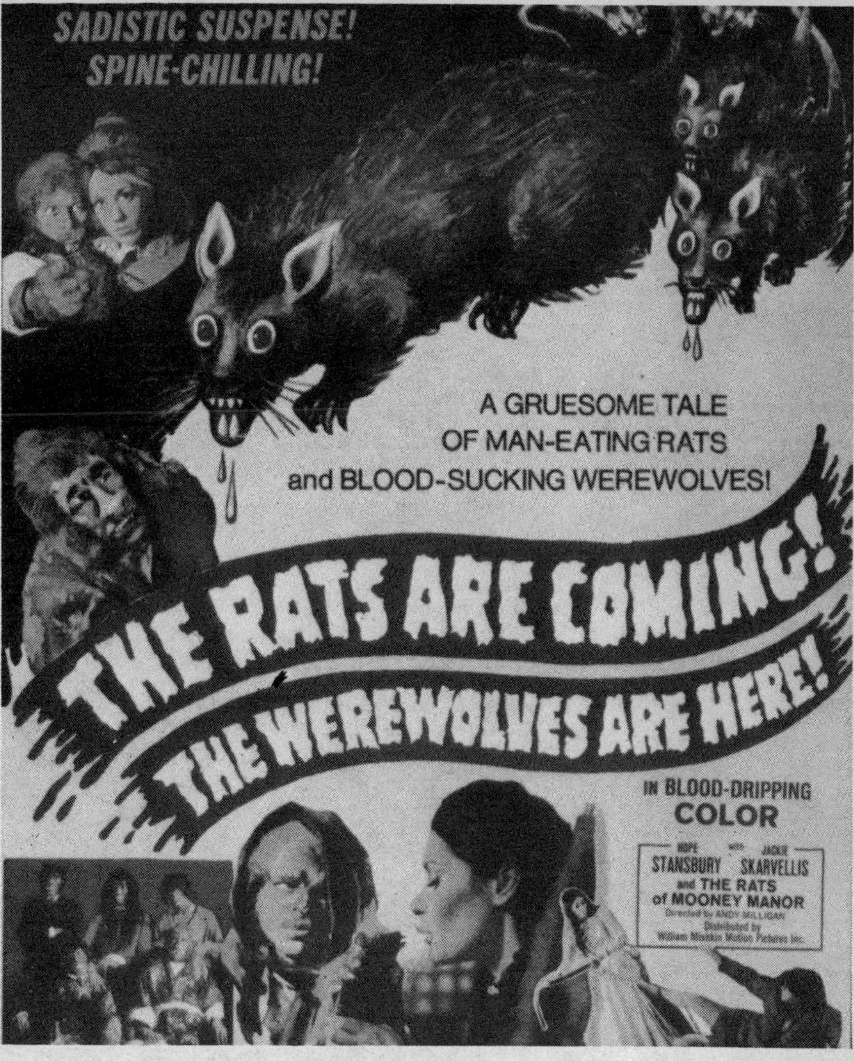

The Rats are Coming! The Werewolves are Here! (1972)

"You *know* the world's in trouble!"

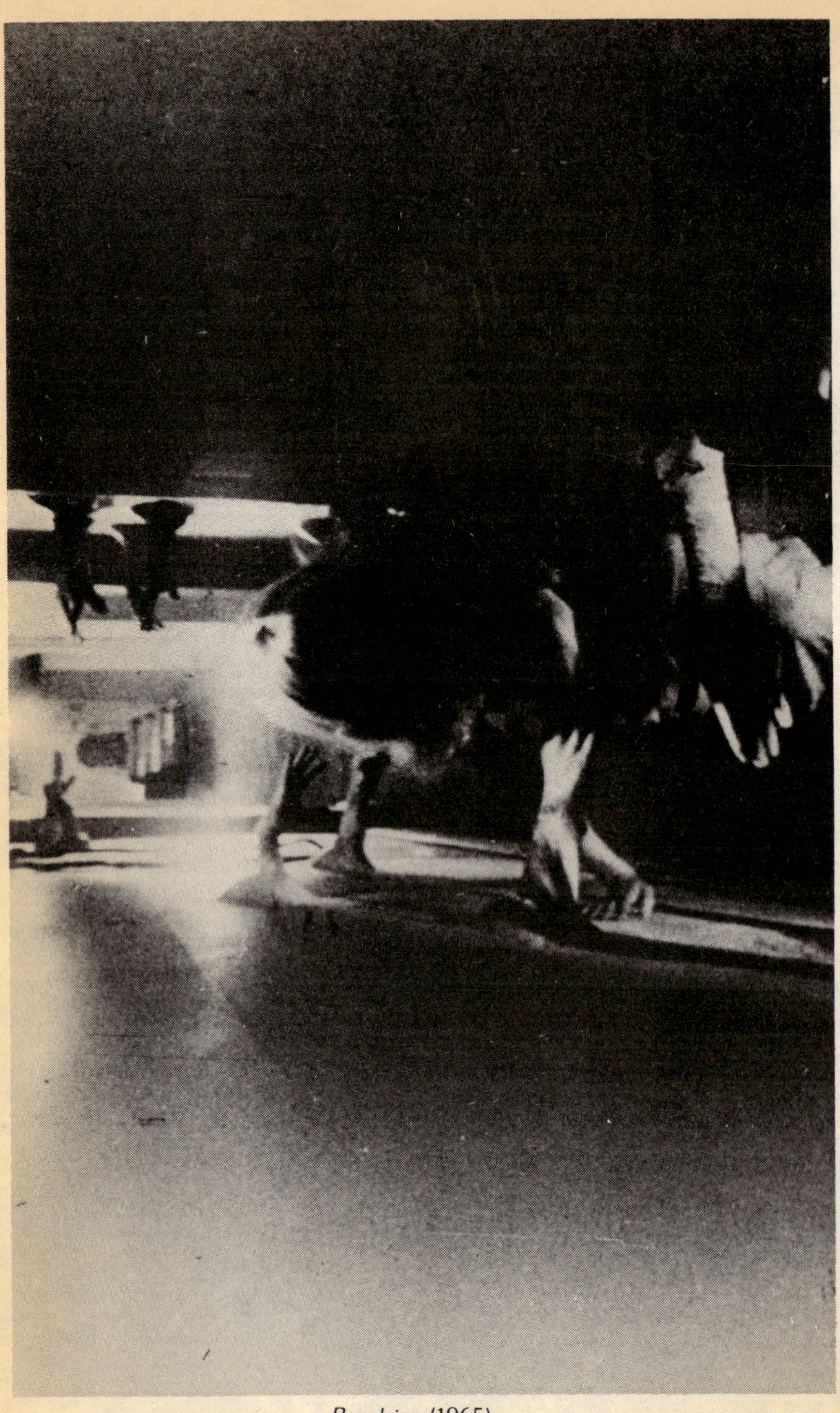

Repulsion (1965)

Rocketship X-M ✪✪

(1950) Color/B&W, 78 min. Director: Kurt Neumann.
Lloyd Bridges, Osa Massen, John Emery, Noah Beery, Jr., Hugh O'Brien. Earth's first manned rocket to the moon takes a wrong turn and lands on Mars instead, where the crew discovers evidence of an atomic holocaust and a race of mutants. A cult favorite, but not really very good. Music score by Ferde Grofe.
(Nostalgia Merchant) VC

Rollerball ✪½

(1975) Color, 123 min. Director: Norman Jewison.
James Caan, John Houseman, Moses Gunn, Maud Adams. It's the 21st century. Crime has virtually been eliminated so the masses have to get their violence fix from watching a futuristic variation on football called rollerball, which is played on roller skates or motorcycles, and involves deadly physical contact. Caan is a top rollerballer who begins to question it all. Some exciting sports sequences, but after two hours even they get repetitive and boring. Beyond that, the script is both pretentious and dull.
(CBS/Fox Video) VC

Rosemary's Baby ✪✪✪✪

(1968) Color, 136 min. Director: Roman Polanski.
Mia Farrow, John Cassavetes, Ruth Gordon, Sidney Blackmer, Ralph Bellamy, Maurice Evans. Housewife Farrow and actor-husband Cassavetes move into an old, but high rent New York City apartment building with an unsavory history and become involved with devil worshippers Gordon and Blackmer, who cook up a plot to get Farrow pregnant with the devil's child. Super slick contemporary horror film expertly directed by Polanski, who also adapted the script from Ira Levin's bestseller.
(Paramount Home Video, RCA VideoDisc) VC, CED, LV

Ruby ✪✪

(1977) Color, 85 min. Director: Curtis Harrington.
Piper Laurie, Stuart Whitman, Janet Baldwin, Fred Kohler. Laurie is a gun moll who absconds with her gangster boyfriend's loot—after he's dead, of course—and sets herself up as the owner of a drive-in. But then her lover returns from the grave to claim his revenge. Some offbeat humor, but otherwise nondescript.
(Video Communications) VC

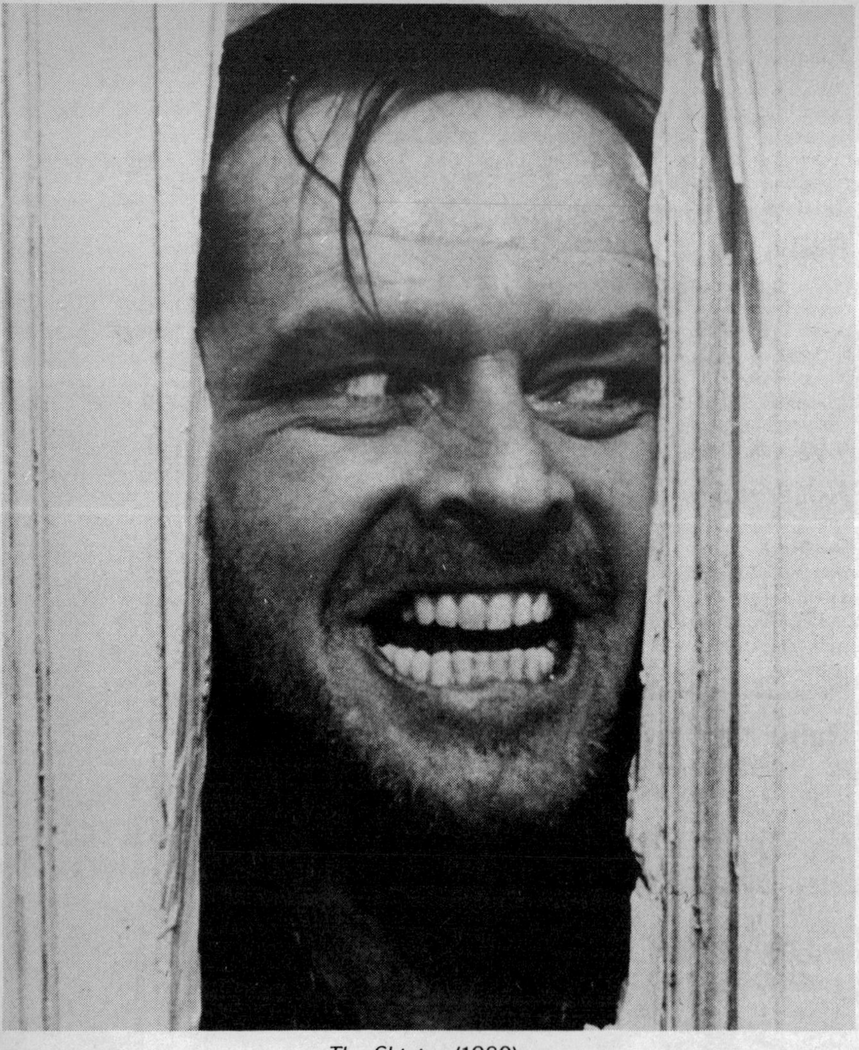

The Shining (1980)

". . .arguably Kubrick's best film to date."

S

Sasquatch ½

(1976) Color, 101 min. Director: Ed Ragozzin.
George Lauris, Jim Bradford, William Emmons. Ape-like creatures are discovered in the forests of British Columbia; scientists determine them to be the "missing link." Documentary-like flavor. A.k.a. *The Legend of Bigfoot.*
(Video Communications) VC

Saturn 3 ½

(1980) Color, 88 min. Director: Stanley Donen.
Kirk Douglas, Farrah Fawcett, Harvey Keitel. Douglas and Fawcett are a husband and wife team of outer space botanists who create an artificial Garden of Eden for research purposes—into which barge evil Keitel and a shiny killer robot. Pointless sci-fi which strives to emulate *Alien.*
(CBS/Fox Video) VC, LV

Savage Weekend ½

(1978) Color, 83 min. Director: David Paulsen.
Christopher Allport, James Doerr, Marilyn Hamlin, Kathleen Heaney, David Gale. The familiar masked killer of hundreds of previous horror films is loose again, this time using cars, fish hooks, chainsaws and benchsaws to dispatch his victims. Zero suspense but gobs of gore. A.k.a. *The Upstate Murders.*
(Paragon Video) VC

Scanners

(1981) Color, 102 min. Director: David Cronenberg.
Patrick MaGoohan, Stephen Lack, Jennifer O'Neill, Michael Ironside. An underground society of telepaths (scanners), whose "gifts" are the end-result of an experimental drug unleashed on their mothers during pregnancy by scientist MaGoohan, must conceal themselves from those who wish them harm because of their "separateness" as well as from those among their ranks who wish to use the group's powers as a weapon. Writer Cronenberg instills his provocative script with a number of interesting themes, but then director Cronenberg proceeds to obscure them with too many explosions into mindless violence. There are also frequent lapses in logic. O'Neill's character is a virtual non-entity and hero Lack delivers his lines like an amateur. MaGoohan and Dick Smith's special effects are very good, though.
(CBS/Fox Video) VC

Scared to Death

(1947) B&W, 70 min. Director: Walt Mattox.
Bela Lugosi, Joyce Compton, Douglas Fowley, George Zucco. A woman dies of fright when she is confronted with the death mask of the man she framed for a crime she committed. Thereafter, her corpse recounts the details of how all this came about. Weak.
(Nostalgia Merchant) VC

Scars of Dracula ½

(1970) Color, 94 min. Director: Roy Ward Baker.
Christopher Lee, Dennis Waterman, Jenny Hanley, Anouska Hempel. Hanley goes searching for a friend, who disappeared shortly after taking shelter for the night at Castle Dracula, and comes face to face with the old blood drinker himself. Typical entry in the Hammer Dracula series, though better than some. Nice period decor and costumes, but not very frightening, and Dracula himself is virtually reduced to a supporting role.
(Thorn/EMI Video) VC

Schizo ½

(1977) Color, 109 min. Director: Pete Walker.
David McGillivray, Lynn Rederick, John Layton. Splattery Jack-the-Ripper style whodunit in which the heroine and the knife-wielding psychopathic killer are revealed at fade-out to be one and the same person.
(Media Home Entertainment) VC

Schizoid ½

(1980) Color, 91 min. Director: David Paulsen.
Klaus Kinski, Marianna Hill, Craig Wasson, Donna Wilkes. An advice-to-the-lovelorn columnist receives a series of letters threatening her life and she begins to think they're from the same maniac who is currently running around the city scissoring people. Standard mad slasher movie, but Kinski always makes a great villain no matter how feeble his material. A.k.a. *Murder by Mail.*
(MCA Videocassette) VC

Schlock

(1973) Color, 78 min. Director: John Landis.
Eliza Garrett, Saul Kahan, John Landis. Schlock (short for Schlockthropus) is a prehistoric ape man who plays the piano, eats bananas and drinks milk very disgustingly. He falls in love with a curvaceous teenager named Mindy and carries her off to the top of her high school gym, at which time the National Guard shows up. Landis' directorial debut (he also plays Schlock) is full of off-the-wall humor in the *Animal House* vein.
(Wizard Video) VC

Scream Bloody Murder

(1972) Color, 85 min. Director: Robert J. Emery.
Fred Holbert, Leigh Mitchell, Robert Knox, Suzette Hamilton. A young boy grinds his father up with the family tractor, but mangles his own hand in the bargain. After being fitted with a steel claw, he is released from a mental institution, at which time he goes on a murder spree.
(Video Communications) VC

Screams of a Winter Night

(1979) Color, 92 min. Director: James L. Wilson.
Gill Glasgow, Mary Cox, Robin Bradley, Matt Borel, Patrick Byers. Anthology film in which kids camping at a remote mountain lake spin ghost stories to terrify one another. One by one, the stories come to life. One deals with a Bigfoot type monster that emerges from the lake, another is about a haunted apartment, and the last is about a female psychopath.
(Video Communications) VC

Scrooge ✪✪

(1935) B&W, 67 min. Director: Henry Edwards.
Sir Seymour Hicks, Donald Calthrop, Philip Frost, Eve Gray, Robert Cochrane, Maurice Evans. Early sound adaptation of Charles Dickens' *A Christmas Carol*, about a miser who changes his tune when he receives visits from the ghosts of Christmas past, present and future.
(Video Yesteryear) VC

Seance on a Wet Afternoon ✪✪✪

(1964) B&W, 115 min. Director: Bryan Forbes.
Kim Stanley, Richard Attenborough, Margaret Lacey. Fake spiritualist Stanley cooks up a plot with mousey husband Attenborough to kidnap a baby, then offer her services to the bereaved parents to find the missing child, all to enhance her reputation. But the plan goes awry and Stanley is forced to put her "powers" to the test for real. Superbly acted, intensely atmospheric mood piece that is absorbing throughout.
(Thunderbird Films, Cable Films) VC

Season of the Witch ✪✪

(1976) Color, 89 min. Director: George A. Romero.
Jan White, Ray Laine, Anne Muffly, Bill Thunhurst. A seemingly happily married housewife joins a neighborhood coven, has an affair with her teenage daughter's lover, and is chased in her dreams by a masked devil out to rape her. Waiting for her husband to return from a business trip, she hears noises at the door, and the dream begins for real. Subdued horror film from the director of the not so subdued *Night of the Living Dead*. A.k.a. *Jack's Wife*.
(Wizard Video) VC

Seeds of Evil ✪

(1981) Color, 81 min. Director: Jim Kay.
Joe Dallesandro, Katherine Houghton, Rita Gam, James Congdon. For those of you who developed a green thumb after being traumatized by *Day of the Triffids*. An evil gardener raises killer plants and helps cultivate a murderous human tree. Made in 1963 as *The Gardener* but retitled for its subsequent re-blooming.
(Unicorn Video) VC

Sergeant Pepper's Lonely Heart's Club Band ✪½

(1978) Color, 113 min. Director: Michael Schultz.
Peter Frampton, the Bee Gees, Steve Martin, George Burns, Aerosmith, Earth, Wind & Fire. Nitwit musical-fantasy based on the Beatles album of the same name that has only one thing going for it: all those great Beatle tunes. Unfortunately, the Beatles don't perform them.
(MCA Videocassette and Disc) VC, LV

Seven Brothers Meet Dracula, The ✪

(1974) Color, 89 min. Director: Roy Ward Baker.
Peter Cushing, John Forbes-Robertson, David Chiang, Julie Ege, Robin Stewart. Dracula uses a disciple's body to walk the earth once more, this time in Japan, where he puts the bite on some kung-fu masters and turns them into chop-socky vampires. Patchwork martial arts cum horror movie. Does neither very well. A.k.a. *Legend of the Seven Golden Vampires*.
(Electric Video) VC

Seven Percent Solution, The ★★

(1976) Color, 113 min. Director: Herbert Ross.

Nicol Williamson, Alan Arkin, Robert Duvall, Sir Laurence Olivier, Joel Grey, Vanessa Redgrave. Lead-footed, over-produced adaptation of Nicholas Meyer's enjoyable Sherlock Holmes pastiche of the same name in which Holmes (Williamson) is spirited off to Vienna by the faithful Watson (Duvall) to have the eminent Sigmund Freud (Arkin) cure him of his cocaine addiction. Lavishly mounted, but dull. Williamson, Duvall and Arkin—good actors all—are miscast.

(MCA Videocassette and Disc) VC, LV

Seventh Victim, The ★★★

(1943) B&W, 71 min. Director: Mark Robson.

Tom Conway, Kim Hunter, Hugh Beaumont. Searching for her missing sister, Hunter becomes involved with a cult of devil-worshippers to which her sister once belonged. This characteristically moody Val Lewton film offers up a lot of talk, but some genuine chills as well. There's also a shower scene involving a shadowy intruder that is so reminiscent of *Psycho's* shower scene that one cannot help but believe Hitchcock must have seen and been influenced by it. Nicely done.

(Nostalgia Merchant) VC

Seventh Voyage of Sinbad, The ★★★

(1958) Color, 87 min. Director: Nathan Juran.

Kerwin Mathews, Kathryn Grant, Torin Thatcher. Princess Grant is kidnapped by evil magician Thatcher, who reduces her to the size of a doll with his sorcery so that he may cart her around undetected. Sinbad (Mathews) sets out to rescue her and along the way makes pals with a cute little genie and does battle with a Cyclopian monster as well as various other villainous beasties. A spirited adventure-fantasy with marvelous special effects by master magician Ray Harryhausen and a suitably rousing score by Bernard Herrmann.

(Columbia Pictures Home Entertainment) VC

Severed Arm, The ★

(1973) Color, 92 min. Director: Thomas S. Alderman.

Deborah Walley, Paul Carr, Ray Dennis, Marvin Kaplan, David G. Cannon, John Crawford. An act of cannibalism (for survival) triggers this deranged tale of revenge. Lots of axe murders perpetrated by the title character. Grade Z.

(Video Gems) VC

Shadow of Chinatown ★

(1946) B&W, 65 min. Director: Robert F. Hill.

Bela Lugosi, Herman Brix, Joan Barclay, Luana Walters. A mad scientist invents a machine that can induce a hypnotic state over long distances and sends a wave of fear and panic through Chinatown. Adapted from the 1936 serial *Yellow Phantom.*

(Video Ten) VC

Shaggy Dog, The ★★½

(1959) B&W, 104 min. Director: Charles Barton.

Fred MacMurray, Jean Hagen, Tommy Kirk, Annette Funicello, Tim Considine. An antique ring with supernatural powers changes Kirk into a were-sheepdog. Amusing slapstick comedy from the Disney factory.

(Walt Disney Home Video, RCA VideoDisc) VC, CED

She Demons ★

(1958) B&W, 77 min. Director: Richard Cunha.

Irish McCalla, Tod Griffin, Victor Sen Yung, Gene Roth. Four people are marooned on a remote island where an escaped Nazi war criminal has set up shop and is conducting experiments in skin grafting. Naturally he screws up and his victims turn out as deformed monsters. Putrid.

(Nostalgia Merchant) VC

Sherlock Holmes and the Secret Weapon ½

(1942) B&W, 68 min. Director: Roy William Neill.
Basil Rathbone, Nigel Bruce, Lionel Atwill, Dennis Hoey, Mary Gordon, Kaaren Verne, Holmes Herbert. Holmes helps inventor of sophisticated bombsight weapon to escape Nazi agents and flee to England whereupon the inventor divides up the weapon into four parts, entrusting each to a scientist friend for protection. When the inventor is kidnapped by the Nazis right under Holmes' nose and the other scientists start turning up dead, the master sleuth must swing into action if he is to save the Allied cause. Nice atmosphere despite the updated treatment. Based on Conan Doyle's *The Dancing Men.*
(Electric Video) VC

Sherlock Holmes and the Voice of Terror

(1942) B&W, 65 min. Director: John Rawlins.
Basil Rathbone, Nigel Bruce, Evelyn Ankers, Reginald Denny, Thomas Gomez, Henry Daniell. After appearing in two successful period Holmes adventures for 20th Century Fox, Rathbone and Bruce moved over to Universal to continue the series, but in a more updated format. In this first adventure under the new banner, the pair takes on the Nazis. Mediocre.
(MGM/UA Home Video) VC

Shining, The

(1980) Color, 143 min. Director: Stanley Kubrick.
Jack Nicholson, Shelley Duvall, Danny Lloyd, Scatman Crothers, Joe Turkel. Alcoholic, self-hating Nicholson signs on as winter caretaker of a haunted Colorado mountain hotel and once the bad weather sets in, he starts going off the deep end, finally threatening the lives of his wife and son with an axe. Fans of the Stephen King novel on which it is based tend to hate this film because it's more of a meditation on some of the elements in King's story rather than a literal adaptation. But that's their problem. Accepted on its own terms, the film's a knock-out, a genuinely Jamesian ghost story decked out in modern dress—and arguably Kubrick's best film to date.
(Warner Home Video) VC

Shock, ½

(1946) B&W, 70 min. Director: Alfred Werker.
Vincent Price, Lynn Bari, Reed Hadley, Frank Latimore. A doctor attempts to destroy a patient's mind through the use of drugs and hypnotism because she saw him kill his wife. Sounds reasonable to me.
(Video Archive) VC

Shout, The

(1979) Color, 87 min. Director: Jerzy Skolimowski.
Alan Bates, Susannah York, John Hurt. Composer Hurt and wife York fall under the influence of mysterious stranger Bates, who claims to have been given supernatural powers by the aborigines, powers which include the ability to deliver a death-dealing shout. Obscure but interesting horror film which creates a subtle, but undeniable tension. Offbeat. Based on a story by Robert Graves.
(Columbia Pictures Home Entertainment) VC

Shriek in the Night, A

(1933) B&W, 67 min. Director: Albert Ray.
Lyle Talbot, Purnell Platt, Harvey Clark, Arthur Hoyt, Louise Beavers, Ginger Rogers. Early talkie thriller which puts the relatively young device of sound to melodramatic but good use. A murderer is at large in an exclusive apartment building. Every once in awhile a scream cuts into the relative quiet, signalling that there has been another victim.
(Thunderbird Films) VC

Silent Running ½

(1971) Color, 89 min. Director: Douglas Trumbull.
Bruce Dern, Cliff Potts, Ron Rifkin, Jesse Vint. Astronaut Dern and three cute robot companions are charged with tending an outer space greenhouse where food is being grown to feed a starving earth ravaged by nuclear war. Trumbull, who was part of the *2001* effects team, makes his directorial debut here, bringing the same level of technical sophistication to his film that he brought to Kubrick's. But he leaves out the ideas. Oh, yes, there is much pontificating about loneliness, but what does it all mean? The robots provide some comic high spots, but overall, the film just plods along. Co-scripted by Michael Cimino.
(MCA Videocassette) VC

Silent Scream

(1980) Color, 87 min. Director: Denny Harris.
Rebecca Balding, Cameron Mitchell, Avery Schreiber, Barbara Steele, Yvonne DeCarlo. Young lodgers in a rooming house run by DeCarlo are knocked off by a secret boarder, DeCarlo's psycho daughter (Steele), who has a thing for knives. Mitchell and Schreiber are the cops assigned to the case; their scenes together are unintentionally comic. Altogether too little tension and precious little logic, but lots of blood.
(Media Home Entertainment) VC

Simon ½

(1980) Color, 90 min. Director: Marshall Brickman.
Alan Arkin, Madeline Kahn, Judy Graubart, Austin Pendleton, Fred Gwynne. Scientists submerge Arkin in an isolation tank for 200 hours, during which time they convince him that he's an alien from outer space. They then turn him loose on society to see what happens. What happens is frequently hilarious, and just as frequently not.
(Warner Home Video) VC

Simon—King of the Witches ½

(1971) Color, 91 min. Director: Bruce Kessler.
Andrew Prine, Brenda Scott, Ultra Violet. Psychedelic horror flick about a warlock (Prine) and his predilection for human sacrifices involving nude young women. Undistinguished.
(Electric Video) VC

Sinbad and the Eye of the Tiger ½

(1977) Color, 113 min. Director: Sam Wanamaker.
Patrick Wayne, Taryn Power, Jane Seymour, Margaret Whiting, Patrick Troughton. Sinbad (Wayne) ventures to the ends of the earth in search of the secret that will release his prince from the spell of an evil sorceress and encounters a variety of monsters, including giant bees and walruses and skeletons. Ray Harryhausen's model animation effects are up to snuff but the script and acting are out to lunch. Weakest of Ray's Sinbad adventures.
(Columbia Pictures Home Entertainment) VC

Sinbad the Sailor

(1947) Color, 117 min. Director: Richard Wallace.
Douglas Fairbanks, Jr., Maureen O'Hara, Anthony Quinn, Walter Slezak, George Tobias, Jane Greer. Sinbad (Fairbanks) sails the seven seas in search of a fabulous treasure. Rollicking costume fantasy-adventure given lavish treatment.
(Nostalgia Merchant, King of Video) VC

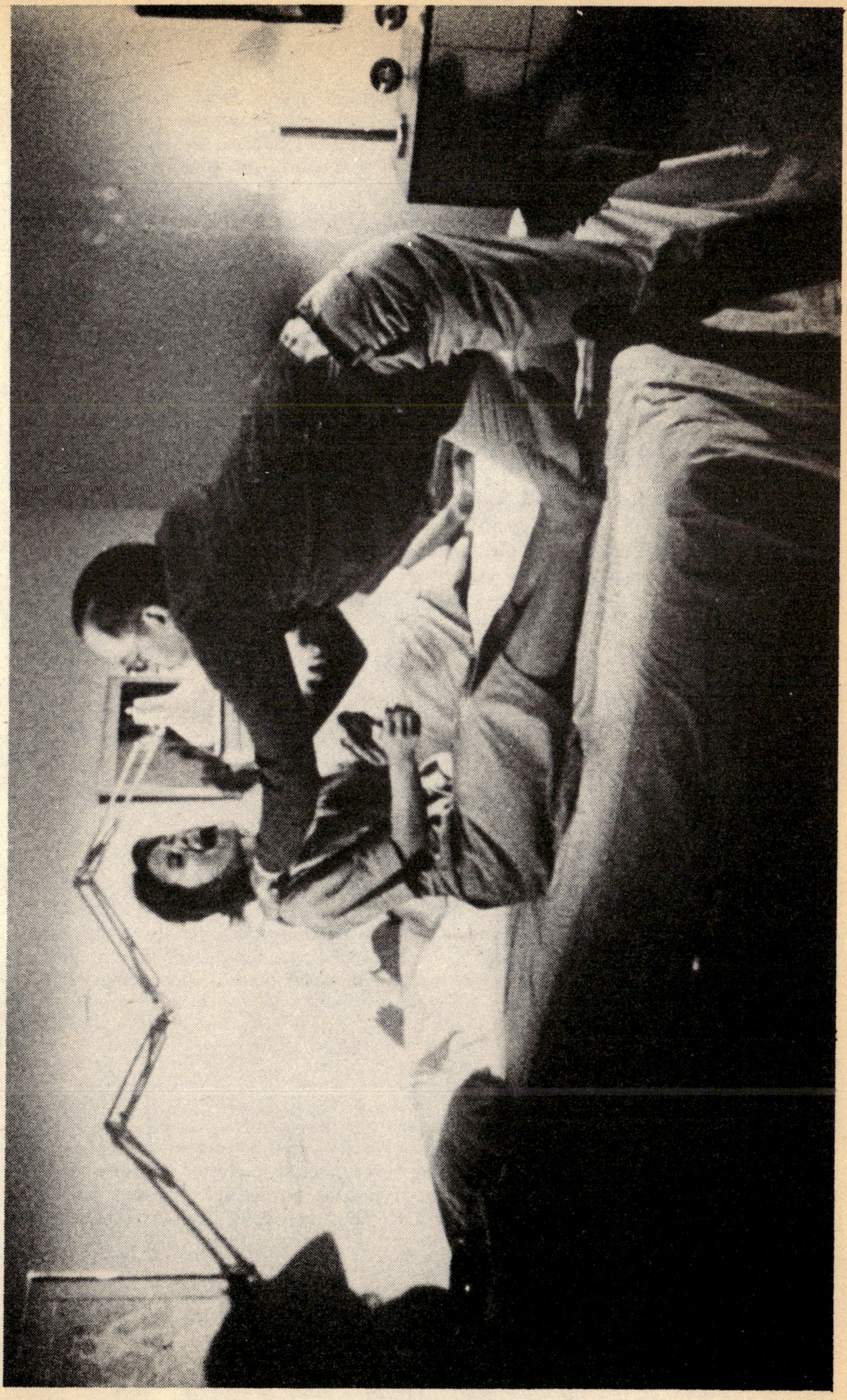

Sisters (1973)

Sisters ★★★

(1973) Color, 93 min. Director: Brian De Palma.
Margot Kidder, Jennifer Salt, Bill Finley, Charles Durning, Lisle Wilson. Kidder is one-half of a deadly Siamese twin sister act; she's a model, her sister's a deranged murderess. Finley is the creepy doctor who performed the operation that separated them. De Palma's first and best—probably because it was the first—Hitchcock pastiche is aided considerably by Bernard *(Psycho)* Herrmann's riveting score.
(Warner Home Video) VC

Slaughterhouse Five ★★★

(1972) Color, 104 min. Director: George Roy Hill.
Michael Sacks, Ron Liebman, Sharon Gans, Valerie Perrine. Billy Pilgrim (Sacks) becomes "unstuck in time," a phenomenon which propels him into the future and into the arms of a voluptuous Hollywood movie queen named Montana Wildhack (Perrine) as well as backward to WWII where he relives his experiences as a victim of the fire bombing of Dresden. Striking but not altogether coherent adaptation of the striking but not altogether coherent novel by Kurt Vonnegut. Oh, well. . .so it goes.
(MCA Videocassette) VC

Slaves of the Cannibal God ★

(1979) Color, 86 min. Director: Sergio Martino.
Ursula Andress, Stacy Keach, Claudio Cassinelli. Andress hires guide Keach to take her into the jungle in search of her missing husband and both are immediately taken captive by a vicious cult of cannibals. Chomp!
(Wizard Video) VC

Sleeper ★★½

(1973) Color, 88 min. Director: Woody Allen.
Woody Allen, Diane Keaton, John Beck, Mary Gregory. Musician Allen is thawed out TV-dinner-style after being in a state of suspended animation for 200 years and awakens to find himself the captive of a totalitarian regime. He becomes involved in a cloning project, is forced to disguise himself as a robot, and falls in love with revolutionary Keaton. This is one of Allen's most popular comedies, and yet, it's really only intermittently funny.
(CBS/Fox Video) VC, CED

Sleuth ★★★

(1972) Color, 138 min. Director: Joseph L. Mankiewicz.
Sir Laurence Olivier, Michael Caine. Mystery novelist Olivier, whose wife is having an affair with Caine, invites Caine to his estate for a heart-to-heart talk, but the discussion soon turns to murder. Stylish, two-character whodunit (or, rather whodun-what) designed to keep you guessing and guessing and guessing. Olivier hams it up to the hilt, and Caine matches him every step of the way. Good fun.
(CBS/Fox Video) VC

Slime People, The ★

(1963) B&W, 76 min. Director: Robert Hutton.
Robert Hutton, Les Tremayne, Robert Burton, Susan Hart. A temperature inversion over Los Angeles produces a race of mutants that grow from the city's refuse to prey on unsuspecting Angelenos. My favorite line, spoken by the callow youth to the ingenue in a moment of tenderness: "You know, being with you makes me forget all about the slime people." Now why couldn't I ever come up with lines like that to feed my dates?
(Video Gems) VC

Slithis 🎞½

(1978) Color, 90 min. Director: Stephen Traxler.
Hy Pyke, Win Condict, Alan Blanchard, Judy Motulsky. Radioactivity escaping from an energy plant mixes with mud to create an oozing, man-eating monster. You've heard of Swamp Thing? Well, this is Mud Thing.
(Media Home Entertainment) VC

Snuff 🎞

(1975) Color, 82 min.
This uncredited atrocity is a plotless gore-fest set in the jungles of South America and includes endless scenes of sadism, bondage, bloodshed and mutilation. As a splatter movie, it's really no worse than many, but its advertising campaign, which encourages audiences to believe that the killings are real, reaches a new low. Fortunately this claim has since been proven a hoax (fortunately!), and yet the film is still being hyped in the same manner on video. What a way to make a living!
(Wizard Video) VC

Something is Creeping in the Dark 🎞½

(1970) Color, 90 min. Director: Mario Colucci.
Farley Granger, Lucia Bose, Stan Cooper. A group of travelers is forced to seek shelter in an old country house when a storm blows up. Naturally the house is haunted and soon the evil forces within start claiming the uninvited guests one by one. Some effective moments. A.k.a. *Something is Crawling in the Dark.*
(Value Video) VC

Somewhere in Time 🎞🎞🎞

(1980) Color, 103 min. Director: Jeannot Szwarc.
Christopher Reeve, Jane Seymour, Christopher Plummer, Teresa Wright, George Voskovec. Contemporary playwright Reeve wills himself back to the year 1912 in search of lost love Seymour. Old-fashioned, *Portrait of Jenny*-style romantic fantasy. But it works. Adapted by Richard Matheson from his novel *Bid Time Return.*
(MCA Videocassette) VC

Son of Blob 🎞

(1972) Color, 81 min. Director: Larry Hagman.
Robert Walker, Jr., Richard Webb, Godfrey Cambridge, Carol Lynley, Shelley Burman, Burgess Meredith. Sequel to *The Blob* in which the killer mass of gelatinous glob that was disposed of in the Arctic at the end of the first film is thawed out and brought back to Los Angeles so that it can ooze terror once more. Essentially a comedy, but not a very funny one. A.k.a. *Beware the Blob.*
(Video Gems) VC

Son of Godzilla 🎞

(1967) Color, 86 min. Director: Jun Fukada.
Tadao Takashima, Akira Kubo, Akihito Hirata, Kenji Sahara. Godzilla sheds his monster image to don the role of loving parent, who must protect his clutzy son from villainous giant killer mantises and spiders. Disneyesque Japanese monster movie with lots of laughs, not all of them intentional. Bad.
(Budget Video) VC

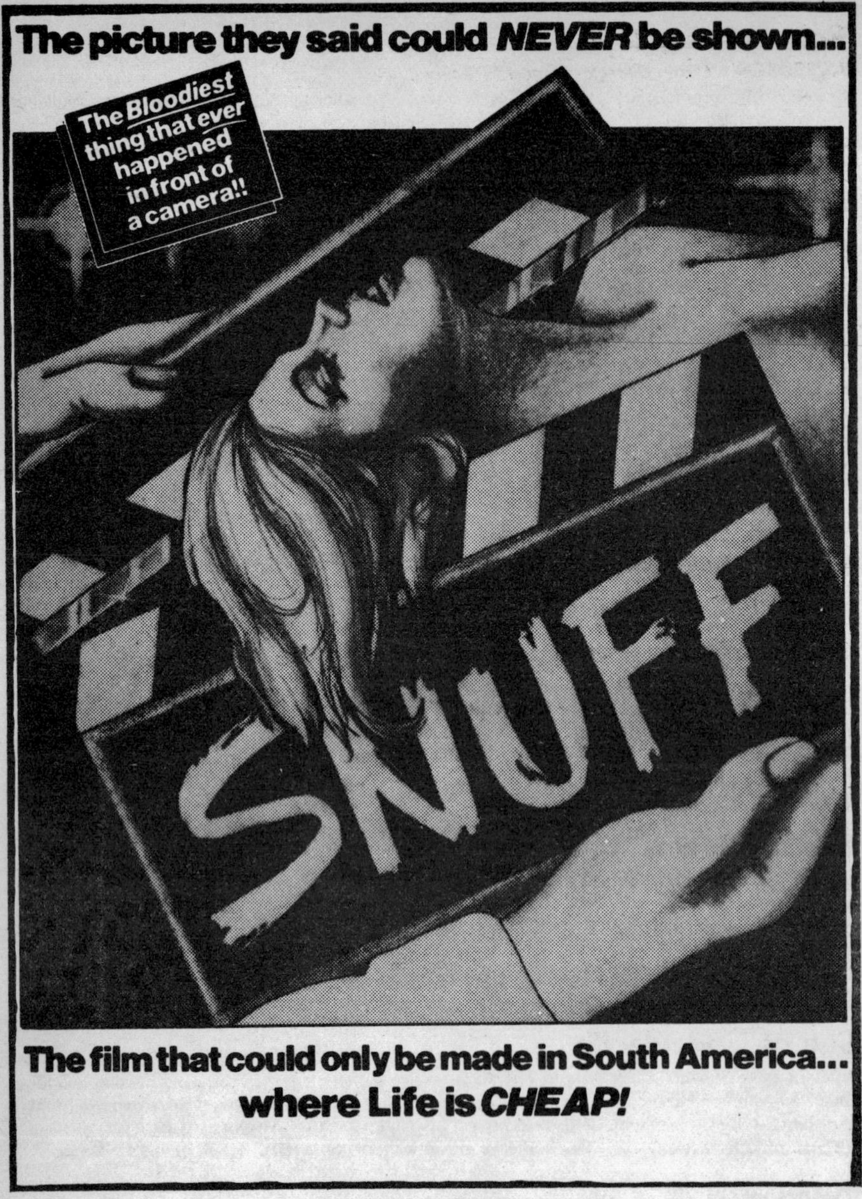

Snuff (1975)

"What a way to make a living!"

Son of Kong ☐ ½

(1933) B&W, 70 min. Director: Ernest B. Schoedsack.

Robert Armstrong, Helen Mack. Bloodied and broke but unbowed after his Empire State Building fiasco, entrepreneur Carl Denham (Armstrong) heads back to Skull Island and there discovers the offspring of the mighty Kong with whom he tries to make amends for having spirited daddy off to the big city. Kong's son is a blond by the way, which makes you wonder what really did transpire between the old boy and Fay Wray during those scenes when they weren't on screen. Anyway, this is a rather weak follow-up to the original that is played more for sentiment and/or laughs than adventure. Willis O'Brien's special effects are okay, but that old *Kong* magic is conspicuously absent.

(Nostalgia Merchant) VC

Son of Sinbad ☐ ½

(1955) Color, 88 min. Director: Ted Tetzlaff.

Dale Robertson, Sally Forest, Vincent Price, Lili St. Cyr, Mari Blanchard. Sinbad, Jr. (Robertson) is captured by the Caliph of Bagdad and commissioned to find the secret of Greek Fire in order to win his freedom. Lackluster fantasy-adventure.

(Video Communications) VC

Soylent Green ☐☐ ½

(1973) Color, 97 min. Director: Richard Fleischer.

Charlton Heston, Leigh Taylor-Young, Edward G. Robinson, Chuck Connors, Joseph Cotten. The setting is an overpopulated New York City in the year 2022. Police detective Heston is called in to investigate the murder of a top executive in the Soylent Company, a firm that manufactures synthetic food, and stumbles upon the sinister secret of the company's formula for success—recycled people. Muddled sci-fi with an interesting premise and a nice performance by Robinson, who died shortly after the film was completed. Based on Harry Harrison's *Make Room! Make Room!*

(MGM/UA Home Video) VC, CED

Sparrows ☐☐☐ ½

(1926) B&W, 75 min. Director: William Beaudine.

Mary Pickford, Roy Stewart, Gustav von Seyffertitz. Orphan Mary and her nine small wards are trapped on a baby farm run with an iron hand by the villainous von Seyffertitz. They decide to escape and must flee into the swamp, pursued by von Seyffertitz and his hounds, where they encounter crocodiles and other dangers. Terrific silent horror-melodrama with some truly hair-raising sequences in the swamp.

(Blackhawk) VC

Speckled Band, The ☐☐

(1931) B&W, 88 min. Director: Jack Raymond.

Raymond Massey, Lyn Harding, Athole Stewart, Nancy Price. Sherlock Holmes (Massey) is called in to unmask a diabolically clever killer who uses a poisonous snake to carry out his dirty work. Stiff, but entertaining early talkie Holmes mystery. Based on the short story *The Adventure of the Speckled Band* by Sir Arthur Conan Doyle.

(Thunderbird Films) VC

Spies ☐☐ ½

(1928) B&W, 90 min. Director: Fritz Lang.

Gerda Maurus, Rudolf Klein-Rogge, Willy Fritsch, Lupu Pick, Fritz Rasp. Master criminal Klein-Rogge uses the field of international banking as a front for his schemes to steal government secrets. His object: to topple the government, throw society into chaos, and assume leadership himself. Another of director Lang's eerie foreshadowings of Hitler's rise to power. Interesting, but very ponderous.

(Video Yesteryear, Blackhawk) VC

Spy Who Loved Me, The ☞☞ ½

(1977) Color, 125 min. Director: Lewis Gilbert.

Roger Moore, Barbara Bach, Curt Jurgens, Richard Kiel, Caroline Munro, Bernard Lee, Geoffrey Keene, Lois Maxwell. Spectacular James Bond adventure that bears absolutely no resemblance to the Ian Fleming novel on which it was based—the novel takes place in the Adirondack Mountains of northern New York State, while the film trots all over the globe. Anyway, this time out Bond is out to stop an evil shipping magnate (Jurgens) who is determined to destroy the world so that he can start up his own civilization—beneath the sea. Kiel is his bodyguard, a vicious killer with razor sharp steel teeth called "Jaws." Better than average in the series, but Moore is *so* lackluster as Bond!

(RCA VideoDisc) CED

Stanley ☞

(1972) Color, 96 min. Director: William Grefe.

Chris Robinson, Alex Rocco, Steve Alaimo, Susan Carroll. Seminole Indian and returned Vietnam vet Robinson uses his pet rattlesnake to drive poachers off his happy hunting ground. Creepy, but only if you dislike snakes.

(Video Communications) VC

Star Trek—The Motion Picture ☞½

(1979) Color, 132 min. Director: Robert Wise.

William Shatner, Leonard Nimoy, DeForest Kelley, Stephen Collins. Everything that made the original *Star Trek* TV series so entertaining—strong characterizations and a very real sense of fellowship among the series' leads—is conspicuously absent from this multi-million dollar turkey. If ever a movie were guilty of masturbating over its own special effects, this one is it. There's no plot to speak of, the familiar characters seem but empty shells of their former selves; there's nothing except eye-popping technology, a fact that eventually makes the film's running time seem interminable. Jerry Goldsmith's score is good though.

(Paramount Home Video, RCA VideoDisc) VC, CED, LV

Star Trek II: The Wrath of Khan ☞☞ ½

(1982) Color, 113 min. Director: Nicholas Meyer.

William Shatner, Leonard Nimoy, DeForest Kelley, James Doohan, Ricardo Montalban. This second theatrical feature based on the cult TV series stands head and shoulders above the leaden 1979 film by Robert Wise, but it still seems little more than a glorified TV show. In fact, *Trek II* is really a sequel of sorts to an episode of the old TV series called *Space Seed* in which Captain Kirk (Shatner) exiles the villainous Khan (Montalban) to a barren planet because of his misdeeds. In the feature, Khan returns to get even with his nemesis, now *Admiral* Kirk, who is undergoing a mid-life crisis. Entertaining, but not near as good as Meyer's debut sci-fi film, the superlative *Time After Time.*

(Paramount Home Video) VC

Star Wars ☞☞☞ ½

(1977) Color, 121 min. Director: George Lucas.

Mark Hamill, Carrie Fisher, Harrison Ford, Sir Alec Guinness, Peter Cushing. This spectacular space-fantasy lifts elements from such influences on popular culture as the western, the legend of King Arthur, and the space novels of Edgar Rice Burroughs and mixes them together to produce a new form of popular culture: the media phenomenon. Since its release the names Luke Skywalker, Han Solo, R2-D2, C-3PO have virtually become part of our language. The special effects are great, the action is non-stop, the acting as good as it needs to be. A slick, superficial entertainment that will eventually take its place as episode IV ("A New Hope") in director Lucas' planned nine-film saga.

(CBS/Fox Video) VC, LV, CED

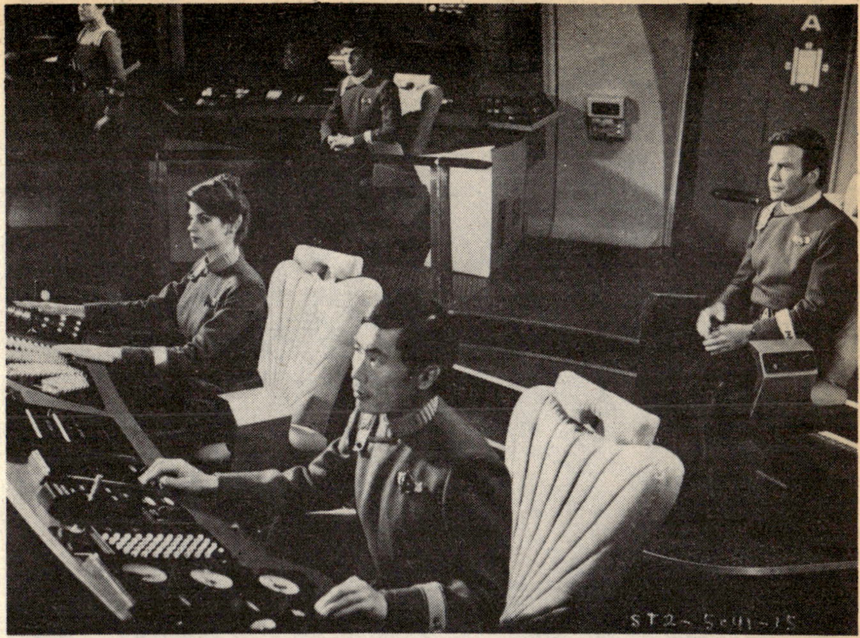

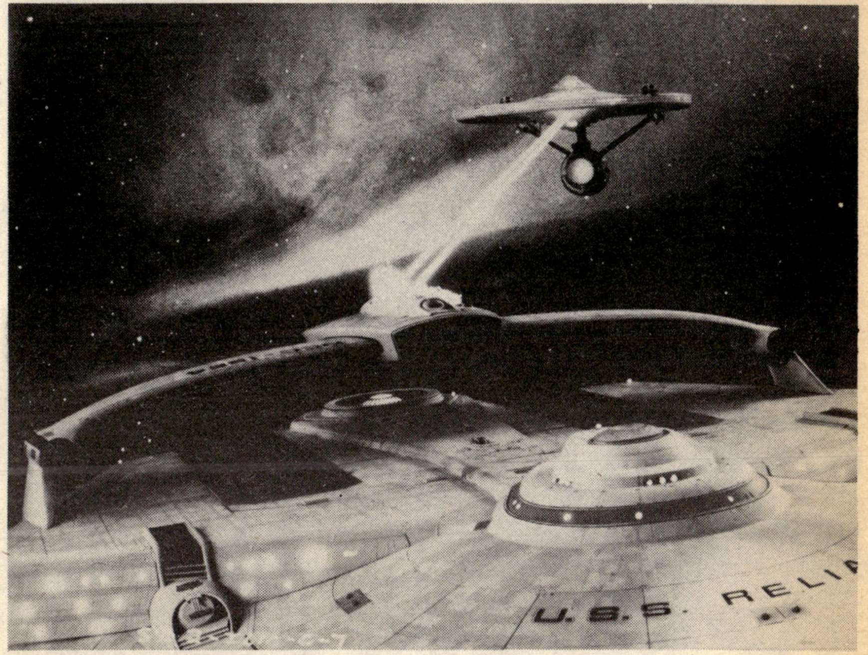

Star Trek II: The Wrath of Khan (1982)

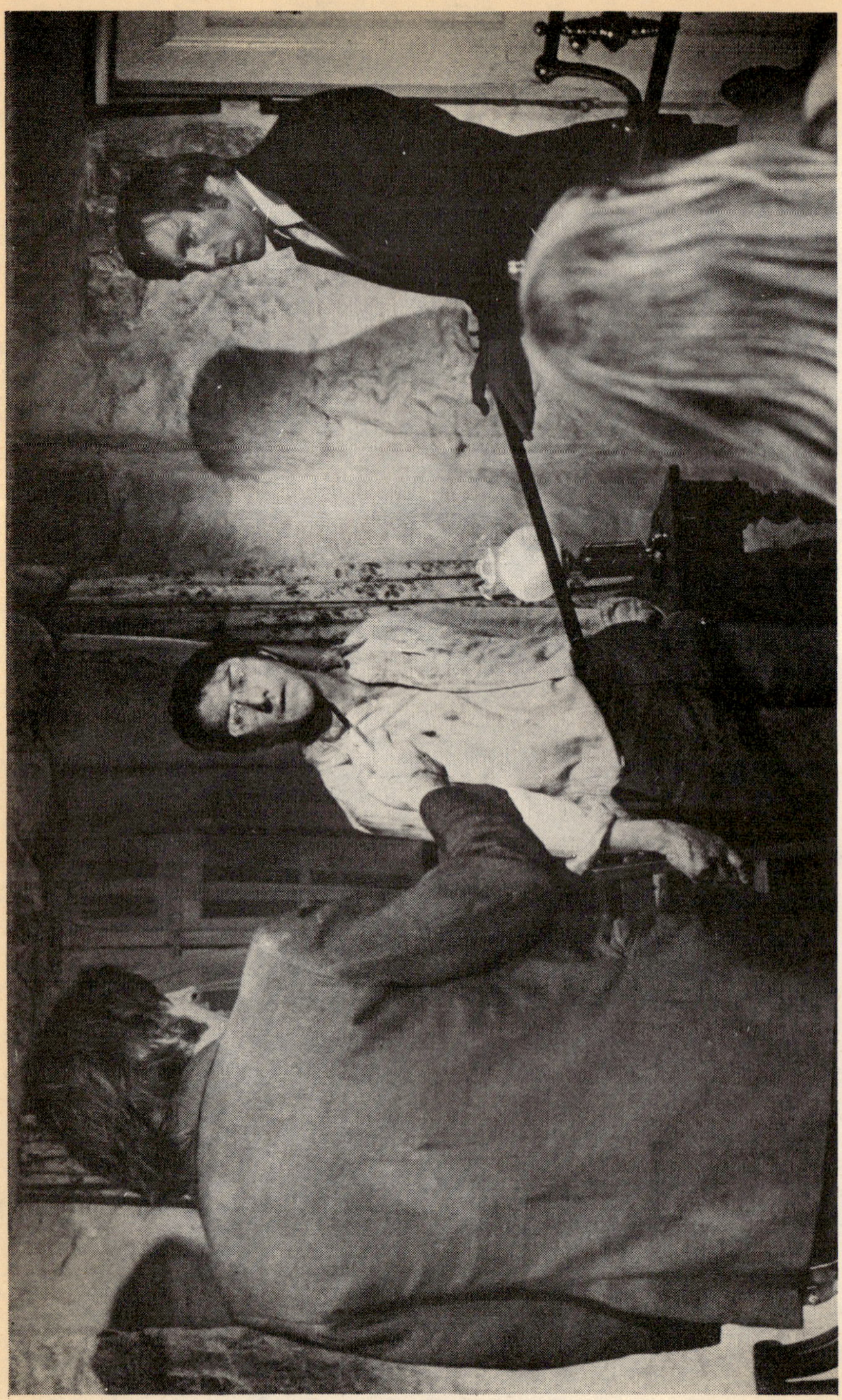

Straw Dogs (1972)

Stranger from Venus

(1954) B&W, 76 min. Director: Burt Balaban.
Patricia Neal, Helmut Dantine, Derek Bond. Essentially this is a remake of *The Day the Earth Stood Still* set in England. Dantine takes the Michael Rennie part as the benign but firm outer space visitor who comes to earth with a message of peace. . .or perish. Neal reprises her role as the helpful mom.
(Nostalgia Merchant) VC

Stranger is Watching, A ½

(1982) Color, 91 min. Director: Sean Cunningham.
Kate Mulgrew, Rip Torn. Crackpot Torn kidnaps TV reporter Mulgrew and the daughter of a prominent politician and conceals them in a special hideaway beneath Grand Central Station. Ludicrous thriller loosely drawn from Mary Higgins Clark's bestseller. Cunningham turns the finale into a replay of his *Friday the 13th*. A waste.
(MGM/UA Home Video) VC, CED

Straw Dogs

(1972) Color, 113 min. Director: Sam Peckinpah.
Dustin Hoffman, Susan George, David Warner, Peter Vaughan, T.P. McKenna. Mild-mannered American Hoffman settles down in Cornwall with kittenish wife George in order to write a book. The hostile villagers, who look upon him as an outsider, push him to the limits of his endurance until he is forced to turn to violence to protect both his honor and his home. Hoffman is alternately brilliant and miscast as the put-upon hero, but George is consistently real as the tease whose charms explode in her face. You can accept Peckinpah's message about man's inherent predatory nature, or reject it, but there's no denying that he hammers it home with skill and power.
(CBS/Fox Video) VC, CED

Student Bodies ½

(1981) Color, 80 min. Director: Mickey Rose.
Kristen Riter, Matt Goldsby, Richard Brando, Mimi Weddell. Parody of *Halloween, Friday the 13th* and others of their ilk in which crazed masked killer Brando, who is nicknamed The Breather on account of how he sounds behind his mask, wipes out a variety of school kids using such ingenious weapons as paper clips and chalk erasers. Frequently very funny put-down of mad slasher movies.
(Paramount Home Video) VC

Superman ½

(1978) Color, 138 min. Director: Richard Donner.
Christopher Reeve, Margot Kidder, Marlon Brando, Gene Hackman. Spectacular, definitive film version of the familiar comic strip, which, in its first hour, sets an epic tone, then shifts gears abruptly and strives for camp humor. This makes the film seem slightly schizoid—like two different films spliced together as one. But on their own terms, both parts work very effectively. Reeve has the thankless job of making the man of steel not only seem heroic but believable, and he succeeds at both. Top-notch entertainment.
(Warner Home Video, RCA VideoDisc) VC, CED

Superman II ½

(1980) Color, 127 min. Director: Richard Lester.
Christopher Reeve, Margot Kidder, Terence Stamp, Jack Halloran, Gene Hackman. Entertaining but weak follow-up in which the man of steel replays Samson when he makes it with his lady love and sacrifices his superhuman strength in the process—but only for a time. The film folds up completely during the last half hour, which is devoted to a self-indulgent exercise in wowie-type special effects, car crashes and stunts. Otherwise, it's okay.
(Warner Home Video) VC

Svengali ½

(1931) B&W, 76 min. Director: Archie Mayo.

John Barrymore, Marian Marsh, Donald Crisp, Carmel Myers, Bramwell Fletcher. Sinister impresario Barrymore falls for aspiring singer Marsh, binds her to him via hypnotism so that he can orchestrate not only her career but her whole life. Slow moving, stylized adaptation of George Du Maurier's *Trilby.* Barrymore's flamboyant performance pulls out all the stops.

(Classic Video Cinema Collector's Club) VC

Swamp Thing

(1981) Color, 92 min. Director: Wes Craven.

Adrienne Barbeau, Louis Jourdan, Ray Wise, David Hess. When biochemist Wise refuses to deliver his special formula for plant growth into the hands of enemy agents, the bad guys bomb his lab in the Louisiana bayou. The doc survives the blast but at the expense of his human form. He is transformed into Swamp Thing, a half-man/half-plant avenger. Based on the popular series of comic books written by Len Wein and drawn by Berni Wrightson.

(Embassy Home Entertainment) VC

Swarm, The

(1978) Color, 116 min. Director: Irwin Allen.

Michael Caine, Katherine Ross, Richard Widmark, Richard Chamberlain, Olivia de Havilland, Ben Johnson, Lee Grant, Henry Fonda. With an all-star cast like this, you just know this movie's gotta be a turkey, and you're right. Millions of killer bees fly up from South America to take over North America. Disaster movie maven Allen manages in almost two hours time to deliver not a single ounce of suspense nor one interesting special effect. An absolute disaster of a movie. Based on the novel by Arthur Herzog.

(Warner Home Video) VC

Swiss Family Robinson

(1960) Color, 126 min. Director: Ken Annakin.

John Mills, Dorothy McGuire, Sessue Hayakawa, James MacArthur. Disney version of the classic Johann Wyss novel about a shipwrecked European family and how its members stay alive on an island beset by wild animals and murderous pirates. Colorful and exciting fantasy-adventure.

(Walt Disney Home Video) VC

Sword and the Sorcerer, The ½

(1982) Color, 100 min. Director: Albert Pyun.

Lee Horsley, Kathleen Beller, Simon MacCorkindale, George Maharis, Richard Lynch, Richard Moll. Horsley's family is murdered by evil sorcerer Lynch, so when the lad grows up he naturally vows revenge and commits himself Conan-style to toppling the powerful magician from his throne. Empty-headed but fast moving adventure in the Robert E. Howard tradition with some very good special effects that belie the film's B-movie origins.

(MCA Videocassette) VC

Sybil

(1976) Color, 208 min. Director: Daniel Petrie.

Joanne Woodward, Sally Field, Brad Davis, Martine Bartlett. Field develops a case of multiple personality—16 personalities, in fact—as the result of her mother's (Bartlett) brutal mistreatment of her during childhood. Woodward is the doctor who patiently nurses her back to wholeness. Powerful drama based on a true story. Sally Field gives a smashing performance.

(MGM/UA Home Video) VC, CED

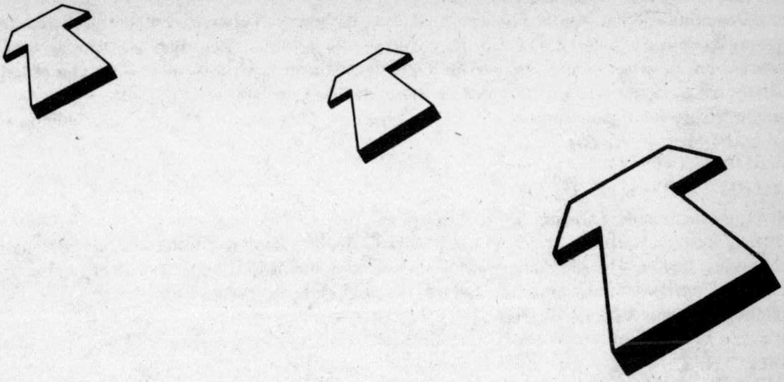

Tales of Terror ½

(1962) Color, 90 min. Director: Roger Corman.
Vincent Price, Basil Rathbone, Peter Lorre, Debra Paget. Trio of tales based on four Edgar Allen Poe short stories: *Morella, The Black Cat, The Facts in the Case of M. Valdemar,* and *The Cask of Amontillado.* Corman's treatment of each ranges from the overtly humorous to the genuinely ghoulish, with mixed results. But Peter Lorre *is* hilarious.
(Warner Home Video) VC

Targets

(1968) Color, 92 min. Director: Peter Bogdanovich.
Boris Karloff, Tim O'Kelly, Peter Bogdanovich. Old-time horror movie star Karloff decides to retire from the screen because the horrors of modern life have rendered his kind of movie monster obsolete. Meanwhile, Kelly, a Charles Whitman-like gun nut, goes bonkers and starts sniping at people as they drive by on the freeway. At the end, the pair meets at a drive-in where Karloff's latest film is premiering and where O'Kelly has pushed on for a final shoot out. Filmed before but released just after the Robert Kennedy/Martin Luther King, Jr. killings, this film (Bogdanovich's directorial debut) incurred the wrath of the NRA because of its implicit anti-gun (and therfore pro-gun control) message. It's strong stuff and remains Bogdanovich's best film to date.
(Paramount Home Video) VC

Target. . .Earth?

(1980) Color, 90 min. Director: Joost van Rees.
Victor Buono, Isaac Asimov, Carl Sagan. Pseudo-documentary in which a computer and a scientist (Buono) interminably discuss the meaning behind the meteorite explosion over Siberia in 1908, as well as other strange phenomena, concluding the fact that earth may be the target of alien beings from outer space. Sounds logical to me. Some special effects are thrown in to offset the boredom, and Asimov and Sagan are interviewed briefly to lend the film a certain amount of credibility.
(Video Communications) VC

Tarzan the Ape Man

(1932) B&W, 101 min. Director: W.S. Van Dyke.
Johnny Weissmuller, Maureen O'Sullivan, C. Aubrey Smith, Neil Hamilton. Olympic swimming champion Weissmuller's debut as Edgar Rice Burrough's legendary ape man is still impressive. O'Sullivan makes an appealing Jane—even if she does scream a bit too much—and the action sequences are not only very exciting, but for their time, very violent. A solid piece of action-adventure-fantasy filmmaking and one of the best Tarzan adventures in MGM's long-running series.
(MGM/UA Home Video) VC

Tarzan the Ape Man

(1981) Color, 112 min. Director: John Derek.
Bo Derek, Richard Harris, John Philip Law, Miles O'Keefe. Absolutely rotten vanity production by the talentless Dereks. Visually quite colorful—thanks to nature and a good film stock, but written, directed and acted with an astonishing lack of competence by all concerned.
(MGM/UA Home Video) VC, LV

Taste of Blood, A

(1967) Color, 120 min. Director: Herschell Gordon Lewis.
Bill Rogers, Elizabeth Wilkinson, Thomas Wood, Otto Schlesinger, Sheldon Seymour (H.G. Lewis). Businessman Rogers discovers he's a descendant of Count Dracula and embarks on a revenge spree. His victims: the ancestors of those who did his famous relative in. Talky gore film.
(Midnight Video) VC

Taste of Hell, A

(1973) Color. Director: ?
John Garwood, William Smith, Lisa Lorena. A hideously disfigured killer ("half corpse. . .all killer") leads a band of equally messed up guerillas on a doomed mission of revenge against an entire army. Obscure, low-budget horror cum war film.
(Astro Video) VC

Tattoo

(1981) Color, 103 min. Director: Bob Brooks.
Bruce Dern, Maud Adams, Leonard Frey. Dern turns in another of his patented performances as a crazy in this trashy, pointless melodrama about a deranged tattoo artist who wants to turn fashion model Adams' luscious bod into a canvas for his work. Adams is beautiful to look at, and Dern, as usual, is quite convincing as the psycho. But this film never really adds up to anything—except pure sleaze. The highly touted sex scenes between Dern and Adams, by the way, are a joke.
(CBS/Fox Video) VC, CED

Tell-Tale Heart, The

(1964) B&W, 81 min. Director: Ernest Morris.
Laurence Payne, Adrienne Corri, Dermot Walsh, Selma Vaz Dias. A murderer is haunted into confessing his deed by the constant beating of his victim's heart. Based on the story by Edgar Allen Poe. A.k.a. *Hidden Room of 1000 Horrors.*
(Thunderbird Films) VC

Terror

(1978) Color, 86 min. Director: Norman J. Warren.
Carolyn Courage, John Nolan, Sarah Keller, James Aubrey, Milton Reid. A witch burned at the stake 300 years ago lays a curse on her persecutors and their descendants, and the curse is later carried out by her ancestors.
(Video Communications) VC

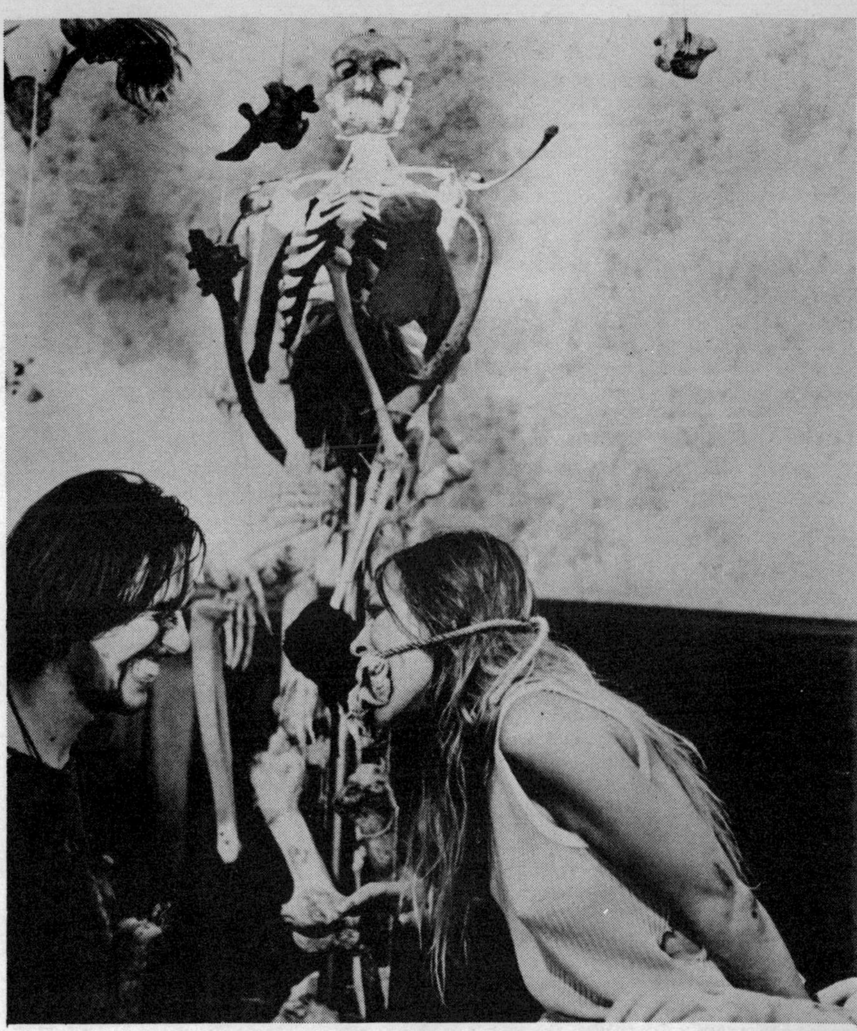

The Texas Chainsaw Massacre (1974)

". . .one of the scariest films ever made."

Terror, The ☐ ½

(1963) Color, 81 min. Director: Roger Corman.
Boris Karloff, Jack Nicholson, Sandra Knight, Richard Miller, Jonathan Haze. A French soldier (Nicholson) is led by a mysterious girl (Knight) to the castle of a mad baron (Karloff) who gets his kicks out of torturing people. A patchwork quilt shot by Corman in just a few short days using sets left over from his much more accomplished *The Raven*. Some additional scenes were also directed by Monte Hellman and Francis Ford Coppola. An incomprehensible mess.
(King of Video, Media Home Entertainment) VC

Terror By Night ☐☐ ½

(1946) B&W, 60 min. Director: Roy William Neill.
Basil Rathbone, Nigel Bruce, Alan Mowbray, Dennis Hoey. Fast-moving Sherlock Holmes mystery set aboard a moving train in which the master sleuth matches wits with the evil Colonel Sebastian Moran, who has disguised himself as one of the passengers. Good fun.
(Electric Video) VC

Terror of Tiny Town, The ☐☐

(1938) B&W, 63 min. Director: Sam Newfield.
Billy Curtis, Yvonne Moray, Little Billy, John Bambury. As the advertising for this film suggests: when the hero ambles into the saloon *under* the swinging doors, you know you're in for a rare treat. Rare is right, for this bizarre curio remains not only the first but the last all-midget western ever made.
(TV Cassette Corp. of America) VC

Texas Chainsaw Massacre, The ☐☐☐

(1974) Color, 86 min. Director: Tobe Hooper.
Marilyn Burns, Paul A. Partain, Edwin Neal, Jim Siedow, Gunnar Hansen. Young people on vacation run out of gas and seek help at a farmhouse inhabited by a family of crazed cannibal-killers, who proceed to stalk and kill them for their meat. Most viewers perceive this film as being gorier than it actually is, and this is Hooper's cleverest ploy: the title alone has you cringing before you even sit down to watch. Rather than constant explicitness, it's the pervading *atmosphere* of violence and depravity in this film which makes it seem so relentless in its terror. Undeniably one of the scariest films ever made.
(Wizard Video) VC

Theatre of Death ☐☐

(1966) Color, 91 min. Director: Samuel Gallu.
Christopher Lee, Julian Glover, Lisa Goldoni, Jenny Till. The Parisian police are confronted by a series of vampire-like slayings and the clues left behind lead them to Lee's Grand Guignol theatre where similar acts of violence are acted out each night for the pleasure of bloodthirsty patrons.
(Video Communications) VC

They Saved Hitler's Brain ☐

(1964) B&W, 74 min. Director: David Bradley.
John Holland, Walter Stocker, Scott Peters, Nestor Paiva, Carlos Rivas. Renegade Nazis living on a remote Caribbean island preserve the talking head of Adolf Hitler in a jug filled with formaldehyde with the aim of one day taking over the world. Der Fuhrer isn't the only jughead in this bomb. Bad, bad, bad. But funny. Photography by the great Stanley *(Magnificent Ambersons)* Cortez, who must have been at a low point in his career. A.k.a. *Madmen of Mandoras.*
(Video Communications) VC

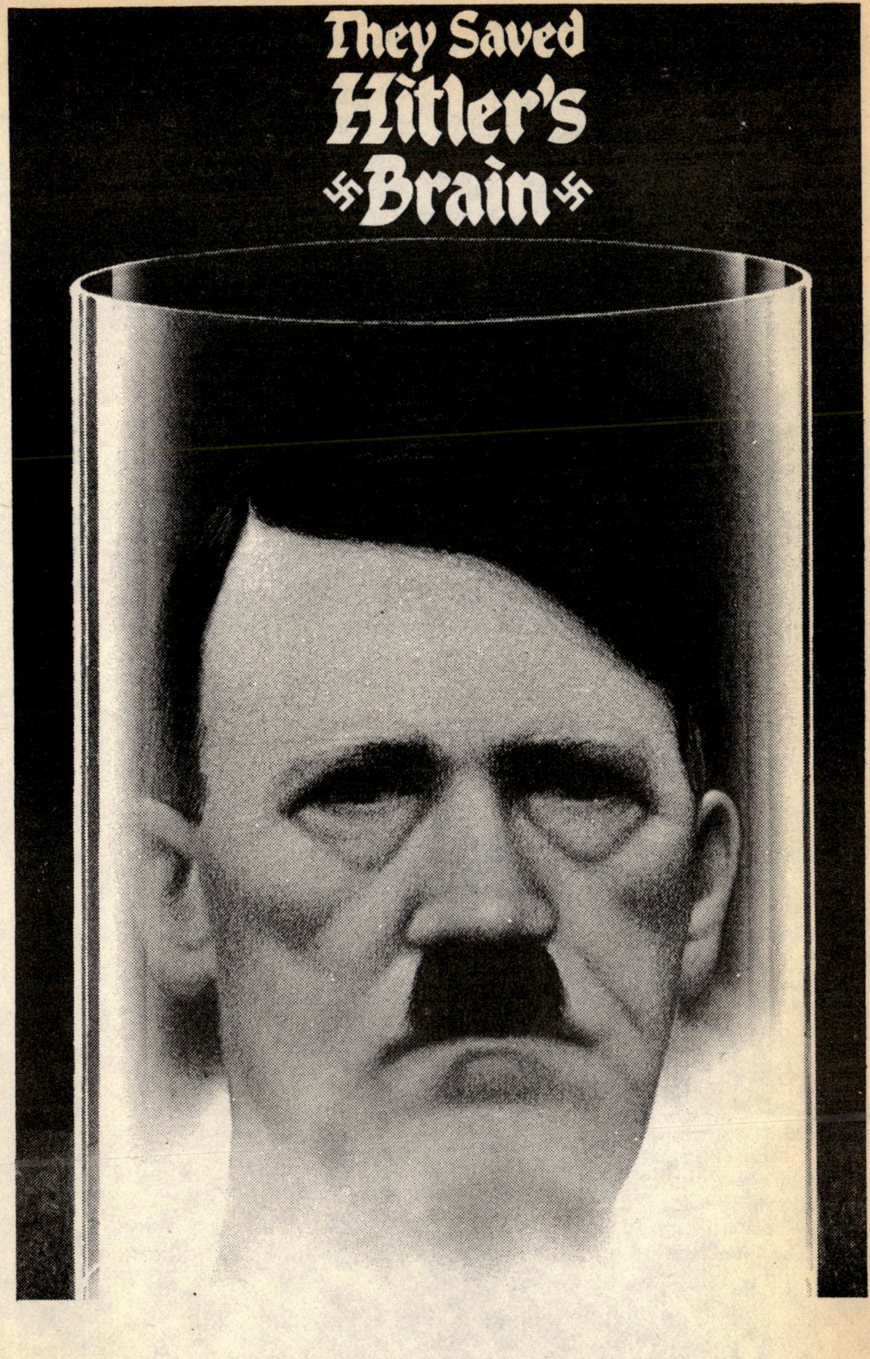

They Saved Hitler's Brain (1964)

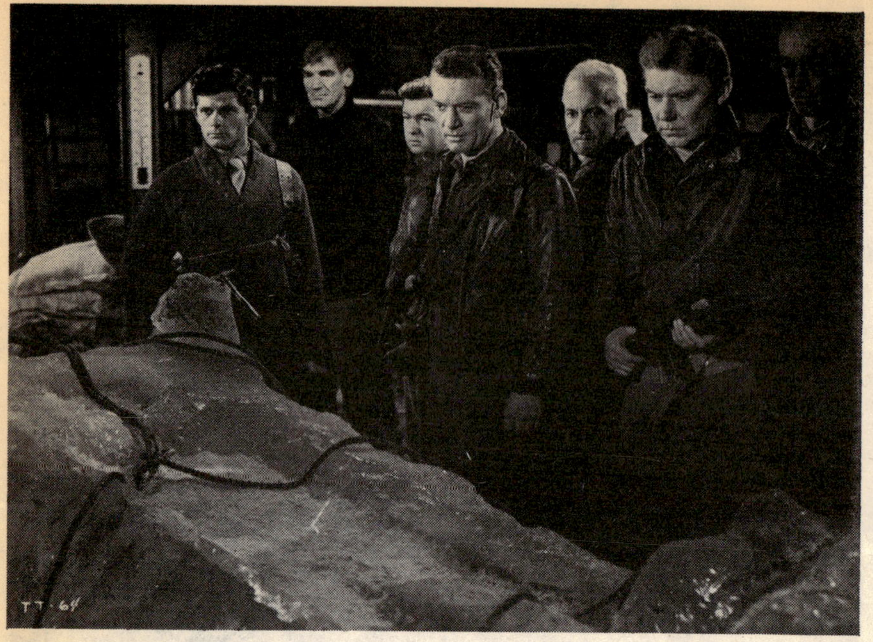

The Thing (1951)

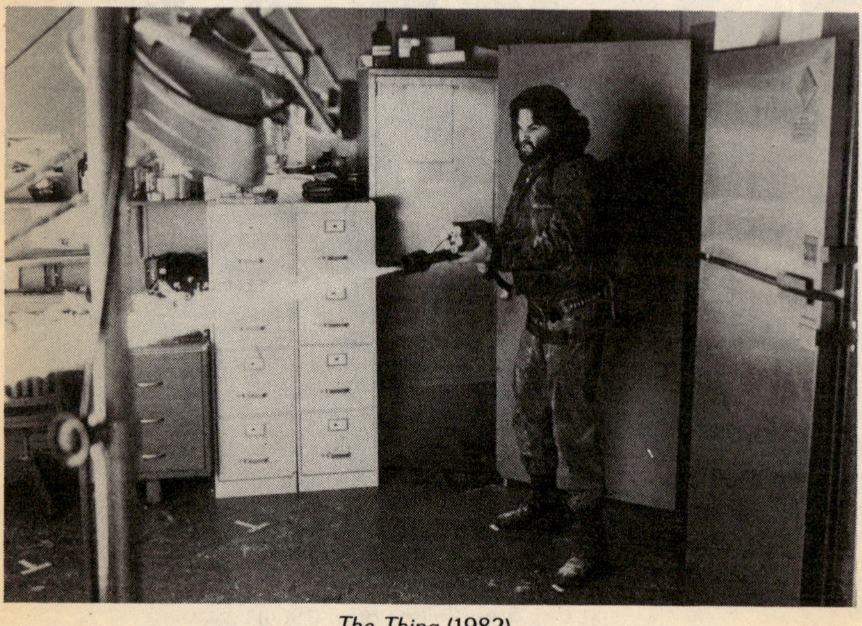

The Thing (1982)

Thief of Baghdad, The ★

(1978) Color, 104 min. Director: Clive Donner.

Peter Ustinov, Roddy McDowall, Kabir Bedi, Pavla Ustinov. Another version of the familiar Arabian Nights tale about the handsome prince (Bedir) who falls in love with the Caliph's daughter (Ms. Ustinov) and the lovable thief (McDowall) who helps him win a fortune and her hand. Tedious and unimaginative; originally made for TV, and it looks it. McDowall is totally miscast as the thief, and the usually impressive Peter Ustinov seems to be treating the whole affair like a bad joke. Which it is.

(Video Gems) VC

Thing, The ★★★★

(1951) B&W, 87 min. Director: Christian Nyby.

Kenneth Tobey, Margaret Sheridan, Dewey Martin, Robert Cornthwaite, Douglas Spencer, James Arness. One of the absolute best horror/science-fiction films ever made. Air Force officers and scientists at an Arctic research station discover the body of an alien creature buried in the polar ice, take it back to camp with them, and when it thaws out, the terror begins. Director Nyby and producer Howard Hawks elicit strong, believable performances from every member of the cast, which is one of the chief reasons why this movie continues to play so well and does not seem dated. Add to this the literate, witty script by Charles Lederer, Dimitri Tiomkin's nail-biting score and plenty of solid scares, and you come up with a classic. Based on the novella *Who Goes There?* by John W. Campbell, Jr.

(Nostalgia Merchant, King of Video, RCA VideoDisc) VC, CED

Thing, The ★★

(1982) Color, 106 min. Director: John Carpenter.

Kurt Russell, Richard A. Dysart. Carpenter's remake of the Howard Hawks classic has a lot of things going for it and they're all spelled Rob Bottin. Make-up wiz Bottin's astounding, splattery special effects of *Thing-ness* are the real stars of this picture—in fact, they're the only stars. Bill Lancaster's script harks back to the original John W. Campbell story upon which Hawks' film was also (loosely) based, but leaves out any sense of characterization. One simply doesn't care whether this Arctic team gets knocked off or not. But *oh, those effects!*

(MCA Videocassette and Disc) VC, LV

Things to Come ★★½

(1936) B&W, 92 min. Director: William Cameron Menzies.

Raymond Massey, Ralph Richardson, Sir Cedric Hardwicke. A devastating war breaks out, lasting from 1940 to 2036, by which time the earth has all but been destroyed and the stars remain the only habitable place for mankind to go. Stilted, preachy, but occasionally quite spectacular science-fiction film from the pen of H.G. Wells, who based his script on a number of his philosophical writings and short stories.

(Media Home Entertainment, Video Yesteryear, Budget Video) VC

Thirst ★★

(1979) Color, 89 min. Director: Rod Hardy.

David Hemmings, Henry Silva, Chantal Contouri. A young fashion designer is abducted by a secret society of modern day vampires who operate a large blood bank to fill the needs of its members. Hemmings is the scientific mastermind behind the international vampire cartel. Farfetched and unthrilling horror film made in Australia.

(Cult Video) VC

Thirsty Dead, The ★

(1974) Color, 96 min. Director: Terry Becker.

John Considine, Jennifer Billingsly, Tani Gutherie, Judith McConnell. Blood-drinking vampire corpses rise from the dead to form a cult ruled by a severed human head that has been kept alive for over 400 years by blood transfusions. Now *that's* thirsty! A.k.a. *Blood Cult of Shangri-La.*

(King of Video) VC

Three Ages, The

(1923) B&W, 60 min. Directors: Buster Keaton, Eddie Cline.
Buster Keaton, Wallace Beery, Margaret Leahy, Joe Roberts, Lilian Lawrence, Oliver Hardy. Comic genius Keaton's first feature film is a howler, an anachronistic look at historical periods ranging from the days of the caveman to imperial Rome to the present day (1923). Mel Brooks tried the same thing with *History of the World Part I,* but flopped miserably. Watch this one and weep, Mel. A comic gem from one of the cinema's greatest magicians.
(Video Dimensions) VC

Thunderball

(1965) Color, 129 min. Director: Terence Young.
Sean Connery, Claudine Auger, Adolfo Celi, Luciana Paluzzi, Rik Van Nutter, Martine Beswick, Bernard Lee. Villain Celi makes off with two atomic bombs, hides them underwater in the Bahamas, then threatens the allied powers with nuclear blackmail. Superagent James Bond goes to the rescue. Colorful fourth entry in the 007 series is eventually drowned by the weight of its own gimmickry. The underwater battle at the conclusion is just plain dull. Good John Barry score, though.
(RCA VideoDisc) CED

THX1138 ½

(1971) Color, 88 min. Director: George Lucas.
Robert Duvall, Donald Pleasence, Don Pedro Colley, Maggie McOmie, Ian Wolfe. Lucas' feature film debut is actually an expansion of an award-winning short he made while a student at USC. It deals with a computer-ruled future society policed by robots in which everything from sex to intellectual stimulation is monitored with an iron hand. Visually quite striking, but terribly confusing.
(Warner Home Video) VC

Time After Time ½

(1979) Color, 112 min. Director: Nicholas Meyer.
Malcolm McDowell, Mary Steenburgen, David Warner. Prior to writing his famous novel *The Time Machine,* H.G. Wells actually invents one, but before he can test it out for himself, Jack the Ripper (Warner) steals it to elude capture by Scotland Yard and is propelled forward in time to San Francisco circa 1979, where he finds contemporary society's wall-to-wall sex and violence very much to his taste. Wells follows him in the hope of bringing him to justice and saving utopia from his ravaging influence. Light, but thought-provoking fantasy expertly written and directed by Meyer with two very endearing performances by McDowell as Wells and Steenburgen as the 20th century girl with whom he falls in love.
(Warner Home Video) VC

Time Bandits ½

(1981) Color, 113 min. Director: Terry Gilliam.
Sean Connery, David Warner, Shelley Duvall, John Cleese, Michael Palin. Wide-eyed fantasy in which a little boy is whisked off into time by a group of dwarfs who are out to plunder the riches from various epochs in the world's history. Film alternates between being inventive and funny to foolish and tedious. It would have been twice as good if it had been half as long.
(Paramount Home Video, RCA VideoDisc) VC, CED, LV

Time Machine, The ½

(1960) Color, 103 min. Director: George Pal.
Rod Taylor, Yvette Mimieux, Alan Young, Sebastian Cabot, Whit Bissell. Faithful adaptation of H.G. Wells' novel about a London visionary who invents a machine which propels him far into the future—a post-holocaust world that is populated by two contrasting races: the peace-loving, sheep-like Eloi, and the cannibalistic Morlocks. Fine script by David Duncan acted by a superior cast. George Pal's finest hour.
(MGM/UA Home Video) VC, CED

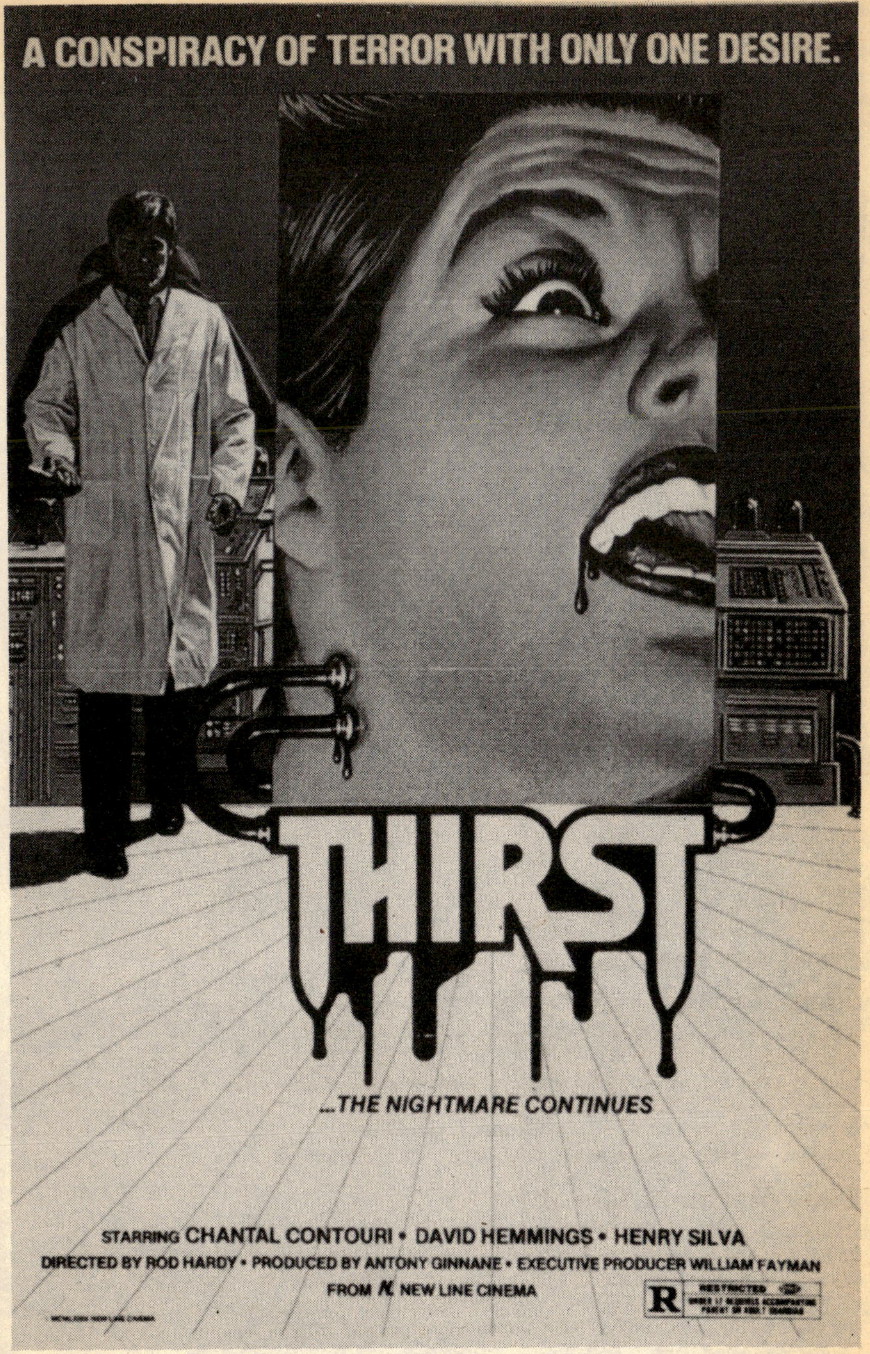
A CONSPIRACY OF TERROR WITH ONLY ONE DESIRE.
THIRST
...THE NIGHTMARE CONTINUES
STARRING CHANTAL CONTOURI • DAVID HEMMINGS • HENRY SILVA
DIRECTED BY ROD HARDY • PRODUCED BY ANTONY GINNANE • EXECUTIVE PRODUCER WILLIAM FAYMAN
FROM NEW LINE CINEMA
R RESTRICTED

Thirst (1979)

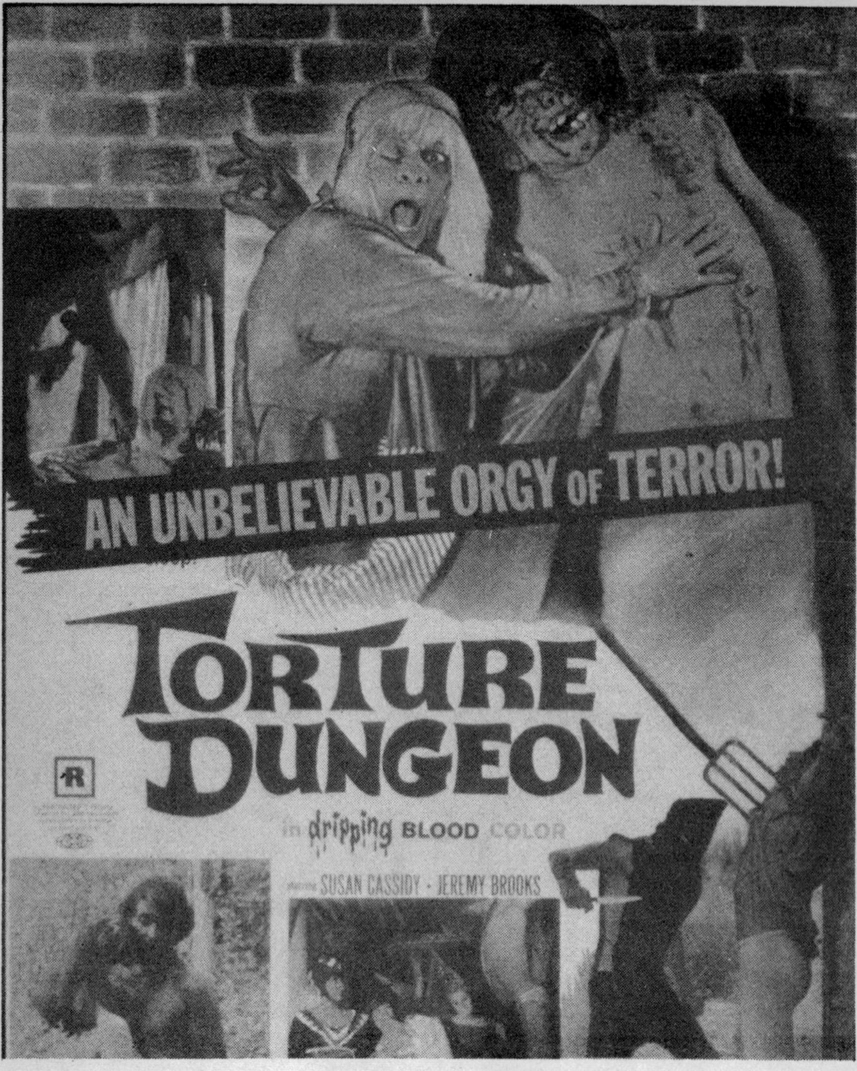

Torture Dungeon (1970)

". . .Grade Z gore film. . ."

Time Machine, The

(1978) Color, 94 min. Director: Henning Schellerup.
John Beck, Priscilla Barnes, John Hansen, Rosemary De Camp, Whit Bissell. Scientist Beck invents a machine that transports him into the future where a devastated earth remains populated by a weak race called the Eloi and a more malevolent race of Eloi-eating Morlocks. Don't confuse this with the great 1960 George Pal film based on the same H.G. Wells novel. This one is TERRIBLE!
(Video Communications) VC

Tommy

(1975) Color, 110 min. Director: Ken Russell.
Oliver Reed, Ann-Margret, Jack Nicholson, Roger Daltrey, Elton John, Robert Powell. Daltrey is struck deaf, dumb and blind when he sees his step-father accidentally kill his real father (Powell), who had been thought killed in the war. Later, he regains all three senses and is hailed as a messiah by a sea of lost souls in search of a quick miracle cure for their own woes. Telling commentary on 20th century man's amazing capacity for self-delusion, directed with eye-popping imagination by Russell, whose talent is not just wild, but awesome. Reed gives the performance of his career as Tommy's seedy but lovable step-pop, who is out to milk Tommy's fame for all it's worth.
(Columbia Pictures Home Entertainment, RCA VideoDisc) VC, CED

Toolbox Murders, The ½

(1977) Color, 95 min. Director: Dennis Donnelly.
Cameron Mitchell, Pamelyn Ferdin, Wesley Eure, Tim Donnelly, Aneta Corsaut. The police are called in to investigate a series of suburban murders in which the psycho killer is wiping out his victims with power drills, hammers, and nail-guns. Sleaze.
(Video Communications) vc

Topper ½

(1937) B&W, 96 min. Director: Norman Z. McLeod.
Cary Grant, Constance Bennett, Roland Young, Billie Burke. Grant and Bennett are a sophisticated couple who are killed in an accident and return as ghosts who turn the staid Topper's (Young) life totally upside down. Based on the novel *Topper* by Thorne Smith.
(Nostalgia Merchant) *VC*

Torture Dungeon

(1970) Color, 80 min. Director: Andy Milligan.
Jeremy Brooks, Susan Cassidy. Arguable plot deals with a nobleman who kills and dismembers all those who stand between him and the throne he covets. Grade Z gore film.
(Midnight Video) VC

Touch of Satan, A ½

(1974) Color, 90 min. Director: Don Henderson.
Michael Berry, Emby Mallay, Lee Amber, Yvonne Wilson. A young girl falls prey to a band of devil worshippers and is introduced to the *pleasures* of satanic rites. A.k.a. *A Touch of Melissa.*
(King of Video) VC

Tourist Trap

(1979) Color, 85 min. Director: David Schmoeller.
Chuck Connors, Joe Van Ness, Jocelyn Jones, Robin Sherwood. On a trip through the desert, a young couple runs into car trouble and is lured to an abandoned gas station which also doubles as a museum in which the mannequins on exhibit come dangerously alive. Some suspenseful moments.
(Media Home Entertainment) VC

Tower of Evil ½

(1972) Color, 89 min. Director: Jim O'Connolly.
Bryant Haliday, Jill Haworth, Anna Palk, Jack Watson, George Coulouris, Dennis Price. Archaeologists searching for a buried Phoenician treasure on a deserted island stumble upon a curse which soon starts taking its toll among their ranks. Predictable but scenic. A.k.a. *Horror on Snape Island.*
(Video Communications) VC

Trial, The

(1963) B&W, 118 min. Director: Orson Welles.
Orson Welles, Anthony Perkins, Jeanne Moreau. Government employee Perkins is arrested and relentlessly cross-examined by government officials, but the nature of his crime is never explained to him. Poor dubbing of some non-English-speaking players mars this otherwise striking (but obscure) film directed by Welles in his usual bravura style. Based on the novel by Franz Kafka.
(Budget Video, Cable Films) VC

Trilby ½

(1915) B&W, 60 min. Director: Maurice Tourneur.
Wilton Lackaye, Clara Kimball Young, Chester Barnett, Paul McAllister. Silent adaptation of Du Maurier's story about the sinister mesmerist and the singer he keeps in his power. Terribly dated, but Tourneur's remarkable pictorial style is well in evidence.
(Classic Video Cinema Collector's Club) VC

Triumph of Sherlock Holmes, The ½

(1935) B&W, 84 min. Director: Leslie S. Hiscott.
Arthur Wontner, Lyn Harding, Jane Carr, Leslie Perrins, Ian Fleming. Holmes (Wontner) is set to retire and devote his energies to bee keeping in Sussex when he is called in to investigate one last case, the murder of a Pinkerton detective by the still-at-large Professor Moriarty (Harding). Based on *The Valley of Fear* and parts of *The Final Problem* by Sir Arthur Conan Doyle.
(Budget Video, Cable Films) VC

Tron

(1982) Color, 96 min. Director: Steven Lisberger.
Jeff Bridges, Bruce Boxleitner, David Warner, Cindy Morgan, Barnard Hughes. Computer genius Bridges gets sucked inside a giant computer and must take part in a spectacular video game competition in order to save his life and win his freedom. This Walt Disney production eschews the studio's more familiar forms of animation to concentrate on an eye-popping display of the latest in computer graphics. And *that* is literally all there is to this movie. Pure bubble gum for the eyes.
(Walt Disney Home Video) VC

20,000 Leagues Under the Sea

(1954) Color, 118 min. Director: Richard Fleischer.
Kirk Douglas, James Mason, Paul Lukas, Peter Lorre. Douglas, Lukas and Lorre are cast adrift when the warship they are travelling on is torpedoed and sunk by what at first appears to be a sea monster, but is actually the world's first atomic powered submarine, piloted by the stern Captain Nemo (Mason). Nemo takes them aboard and introduces them to the wonders of the world beneath the sea. Fine adaptation of the Jules Verne classic, well acted with good special effects.
(Walt Disney Home Video, RCA VideoDisc) VC, CED

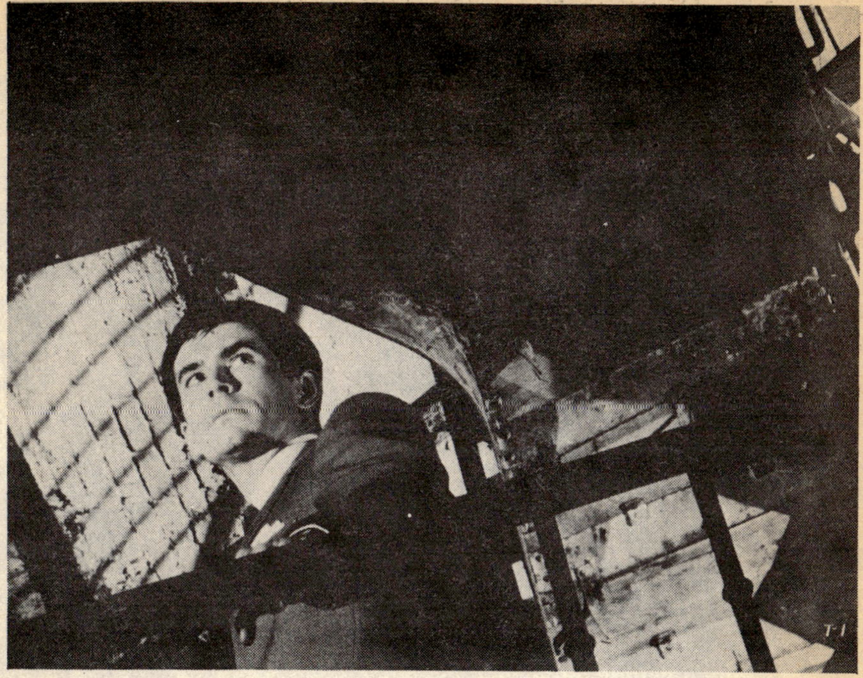

The Trial (1963)

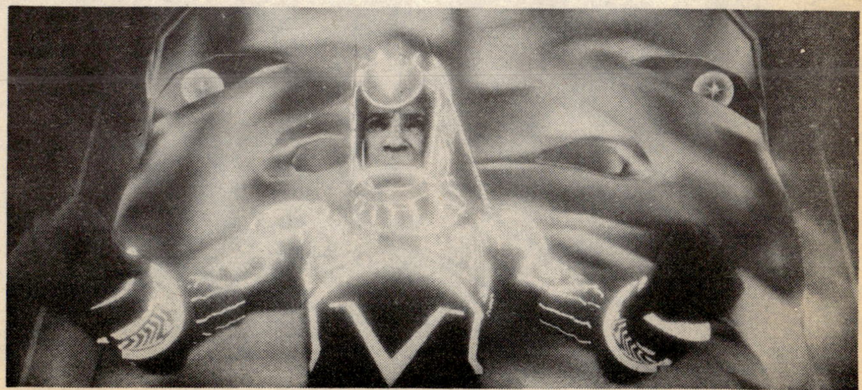

Tron (1982)

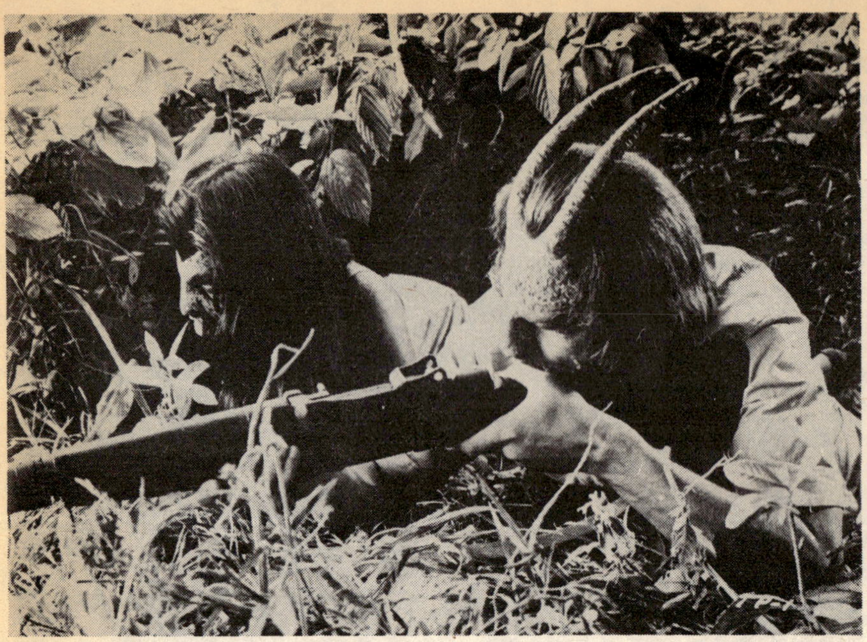

The Twilight People (1972)

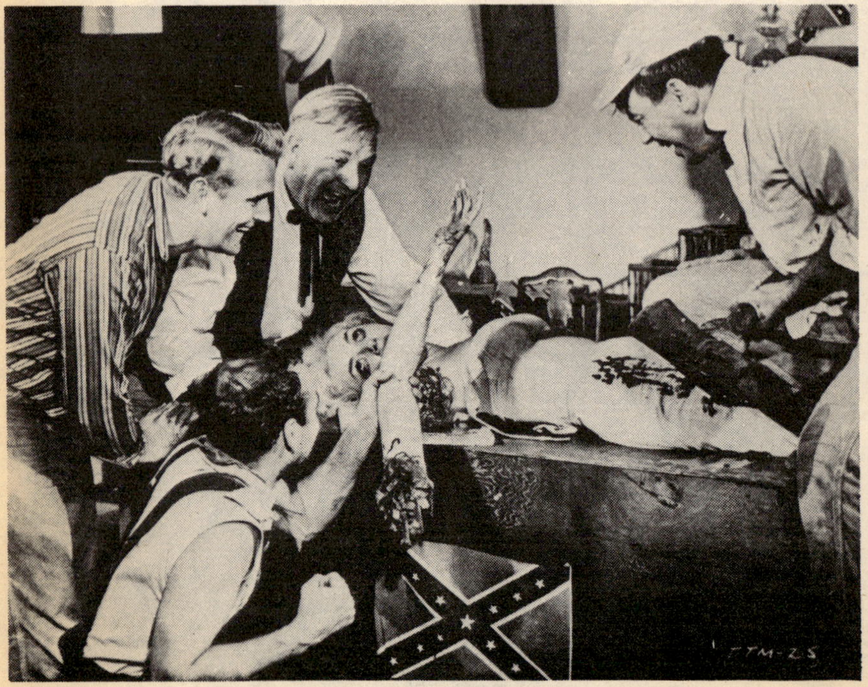

2000 Maniacs (1964)

Twilight People ✪

(1972) Color, 84 min. Director: Eddie Romero.
John Ashley, Pat Woodell, Pam Grier, Eddie Garcia, Jan Merlin. Return with us once more to *The Island of Dr. Moreau* (un-credited, of course) on which a mad scientist is busy experimenting in genetic engineering, turning animals into humans (or is it the other way around?) to create a super race. The humanimal make-ups are quite nice, but the script is ridiculous, and the direction worse. A.k.a. *Island of the Twilight People.*
(Wizard Video) VC

Twisted Brain ✪

(1974) Color, 90 min. Director: Larry N. Stouffer.
Pat Cardi, John Niland, Austin Stoker, Joy Hash, J. Greene. Guess where the filmmakers got this plot from: a mild-mannered high school student develops a formula in his lab, drinks it, and turns into a not-so-mild-mannered, in fact murderous, bowlegged monster. First he kills his biology teacher, then he kills his gym teacher, then. . .well, you get the idea. Too bad he didn't go after the scriptwriter. That sound you hear is Robert Louis Stevenson spinning in his grave. A.k.a. *Horror High.*
(Video Communications) VC

2000 Maniacs ✪

(1964) Color, 84 min. Director: Herschell Gordon Lewis.
Connie Mason, Thomas Wood, Jeffrey Allen. A Southern town magically reappears *Brigadoon*-style 100 years after its devastation by Yankee soldiers during the Civil War, and as a group of northern tourists pass through, the revenge-hungry townsfolk of the title take them captive, torture and murder them in a variety of graphically horrible ways. Colorfully photographed hack work.
(Wizard Video) VC

2001: A Space Odyssey ✪✪✪½

(1968) Color, 138 min. Director: Stanley Kubrick.
Gary Lockwood, Keir Dullea, William Sylvester, Douglas Rain as the voice of HAL. Kubrick and co-screenwriter Arthur C. Clarke trace the evolution of man from his humble origins as a lowly biped who is force-fed intelligence through extra-terrestrial intervention to his spectacular jump as a technological citizen of the stars. At this point, man enters his next evolutionary phase and is sent back to earth by those extra-terrestrials as a superman. Here's one science fiction film that is not only technically awesome, but mentally challenging as well—at least for its first two thirds. The metaphoric ending is little more than a light show and a muddle. But for most of its length, this is breathtaking cinema indeed.
(MGM/UA Home Video) VC, CED

Tunnel, The ✪✪

(1935) B&W, 94 min. Director: Maurice Elvey.
Richard Dix, Leslie Banks, Walter Huston, George Arliss, Madge Evans, Helen Vinson. Spectacular science fiction story about the construction of an undersea tunnel between England and the United States. Plenty of lavish sets, but not many thrills, and the cardboard characters are not very interesting either. The idea is great, but the end result is disappointing. A.k.a. *Transatlantic Tunnel.*
(Cable Films) VC

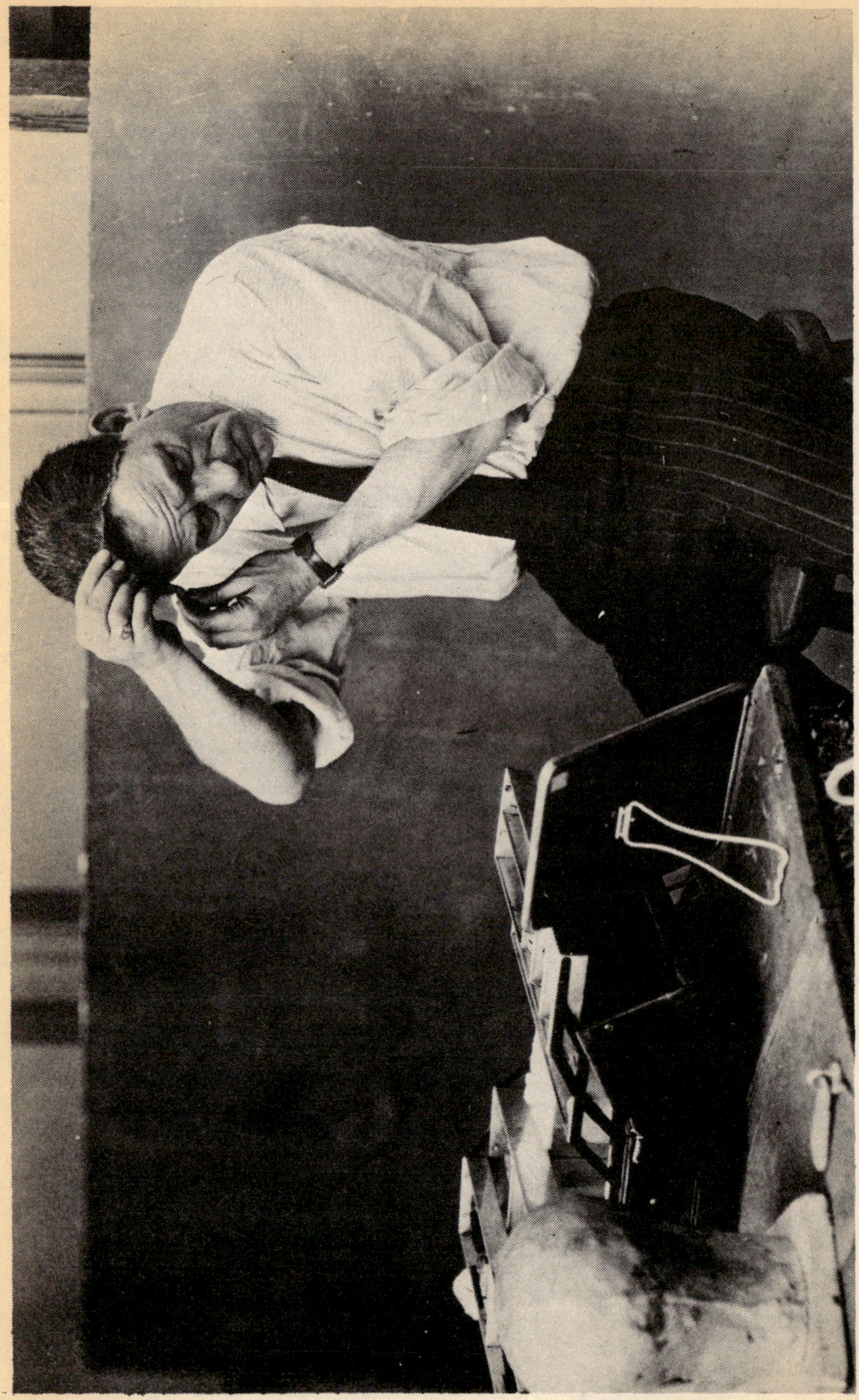

Lon Chaney, star of *The Unholy Three* (1930)

U

Uncanny, The

(1977) Color, 85 min. Director: Dennis Heroux.
Peter Cushing, Susan Penhaligon, Ray Milland, Joan Greenwood, Roland Culver, Samantha Eggar, Donald Pleasence. Trio of stories revolving around a horror movie star who's filming a feline-plagued version of Poe's *The Pit and the Pendulum* and an unscrupulous publisher (Milland) who can't quite swallow author Cushing's latest book, about the evil of cats. Top cast, well-made, but not very exciting.
(Nostalgia Merchant) VC

Unholy Three, The

(1930) B&W, 75 min. Director: Jack Conway.
Lon Chaney, Lila Lee, Elliott Nugent, Harry Earles, John Miljan. Remake of the 1925 Tod Browning silent which marked the great Chaney's only appearance in a talking picture. It's a bizarre crime drama in which Chaney plays a carnival ventriloquist who embarks on a life of crime abetted by the show's strongman and a midget. As a front, he disguises himself as a harmless old lady and plays most of the film in drag. Dated but memorable because of Chaney, who gives evidence that had he lived, he might have gone on to become the "man of a thousand voices" as well.
(Classic Video Cinema Collector's Club) VC

Unknown Powers ½

(1978) Color, 97 min. Director: (?)
Samantha Eggar, Jack Palance, Will Geer, Roscoe Lee Brown. Another of those pseudo-documentaries about paranormal phenomena which uses well-known personalities to guide us on our tour. Among other things, this one theorizes that the mass suicide by followers of the Reverend Jim Jones may have been a result of Jones' peculiar (and deadly) psychic gifts, powers which, the film says, we may all have. I sincerely hope not.
(Video Gems) VC

Unseen, The ½

(1981) Color, 88 min. Director: Peter Foleg.
Barbara Bach, Syney Lassick, Karen Lamm, Doug Barr, Three young women are forced to spend the night in a remote house inhabited by a weird family whose youngest member is kept locked in the cellar because he's badly deformed and virtually sub-human. You can no doubt guess what happens next. Nicely handled suspenseful thriller, well performed.
(VidAmerica) VC

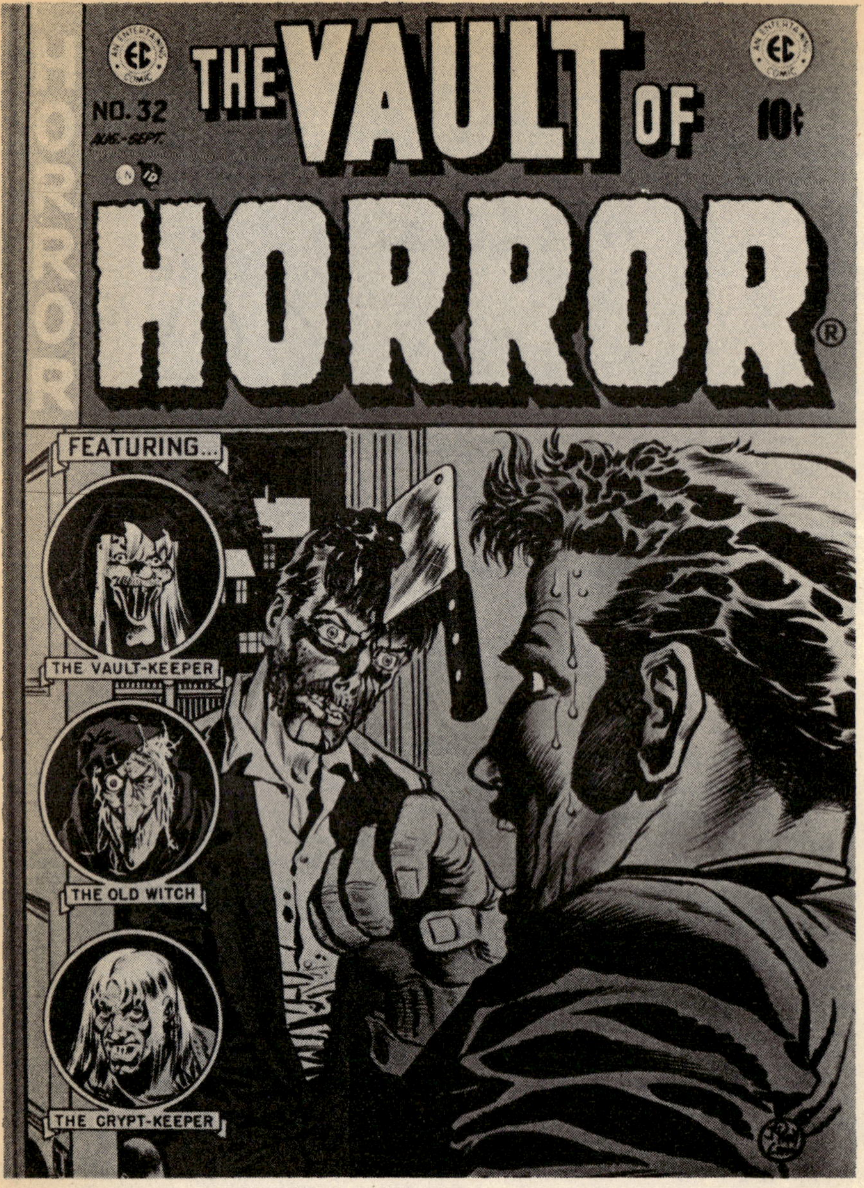

One of the issues of the 1950's comic series which inspired the film *Vault of Horror* (1973)

Vampyr

(1932) B&W, 66 min. Director: Carl Dreyer.
Julian West, Sybille Schmitz, Harriet Gerard, Albert Bras. Experimental, early talkie vampire tale based on the much-filmed Sheridan Le Fanu short story *Carmilla.* Slow moving and obscure, but boasts many memorable sequences, among which the most famous is West's imagined burial after he has been bitten by the female vampire, viewed entirely from his perspective inside the coffin. A.k.a. *The Strange Adventures of David Gray.*
(Thunderbird Films, Video Yesteryear) VC

Vault of Horror ½

(1973) Color, 86 min. Director: Roy Ward Baker.
Daniel Massey, Terry-Thomas, Glynis Johns, Anna Massey, Curt Jurgens, Michael Craig, Tom Baker. An anthology of five horror stories adapted from the pages of William M. Gaines' well-known series of E.C. horror comics of the same name from the early fifties. The wraparound story tells of five men trapped in an elevator, each of whom recounts a strange tale. When the door finally opens, it turns out that they're dead and in a cemetery. Fun.
(Nostalgia Merchant) VC

Village of the Damned ½

(1960) B&W, 78 min. Director: Wolf Rilla.
George Sanders, Barbara Shelley, Martin Stephens. Low-key science-fiction thriller in which the women of a small English town called Midwich are impregnated by alien seeds from space. Nine months later they give birth to malevolent blond haired babies with the power to kill with their thoughts. The first half of the film works best. Based on the novel *The Midwich Cuckoos* by John Wyndham.
(MGM/UA Home Video) VC

Visiting Hours

(1982) Color, 105 min. Director: Jean Claude Lord.
Michael Ironside, Lee Grant, William Shatner, Lenore Zann. Canadian made gore extravaganza in which a maniac rips his way through a crowded city hospital, slaughtering victims right and left—and all without the benefit of being a doctor himself.
(CBS/Fox Video) VC

Voyage to the Bottom of the Sea ★★

(1961) Color, 105 min. Director: Irwin Allen.

Walter Pidgeon, Joan Fontaine, Barbara Eden, Frankie Avalon, Peter Lorre, Robert Sterling, Henry Daniell. A meteor shower sets the Van Allen belt surrounding the earth aflame and a massive atomic submarine is sent to the polar ice cap to launch missiles and disperse the activity before the earth perishes. Personal conflicts arise on board which continuously threaten the mission. Nice special effects, but dull human adventure typical of the work of disaster specialist Allen. Later a very popular TV series.

(CBS/Fox Video) VC

Wait Until Dark

(1967) Color, 108 min. Director: Terence Young.

Audrey Hepburn, Alan Arkin, Richard Crenna, Jack Weston, Efrem Zimbalist, Jr. Blind housewife Hepburn is forced into a terrifying duel of wits to save herself from conmen Crenna and Weston and psycho Arkin who are out to retrieve a doll full of heroin. A first-class nail-biter based on the hit stage play by Frederick Knott, containing one scene that's guaranteed to lift you at least three feet off your chair.

(Warner Home Video) VC

War Game, The

(1965) B&W, 50 min. Director: Peter Watkins.

Harrowing "documentary" which cautions against the proliferation of nuclear arms by portraying the after-effects of nuclear war on Great Britain. Originally made for the BBC, but never aired because of its graphic presentation.

(Festival Films) VC

Warning Shadows ½

(1922) B&W, 70 min. Director: Arthur Robison.

Fritz Kortner, Fritz Rasp, Ruth Weyher. Experimental, expressionistic silent film made in Germany in which the mutual conflicts and inner hostilities of a group a dinner guests are acted out by their shadows. Intriguing, but not exactly fast-paced.

(Thunderbird Films) VC

War of the Worlds, The

(1953) Color, 85 min. Director: Byron Haskin.

Gene Barry, Ann Robinson, Les Tremayne, Henry Brandon. Terrific special effects highlight this classic George Pal production based on the H.G. Wells novel about the invasion of Earth by Martian death machines. Script and acting leave a lot to be desired, but the effects are the thing, and for them the film remains well worth seeing.

(Paramount Home Video, RCA VideoDisc) VC, CED, LV

Watcher in the Woods, The ½

(1980) Color, 108 min. Director: John Hough.

Bette Davis, Carroll Baker, David McCallum, Lynn-Holly Johnson, Ian Bannen. Adult-oriented ghost story from the Disney folks about a little girl who disappears from an English mansion on a stormy night, then returns as a ghost to haunt the place. Some effective, spooky moments, but the ending seems like patchwork.

(Walt Disney Home Video) VC

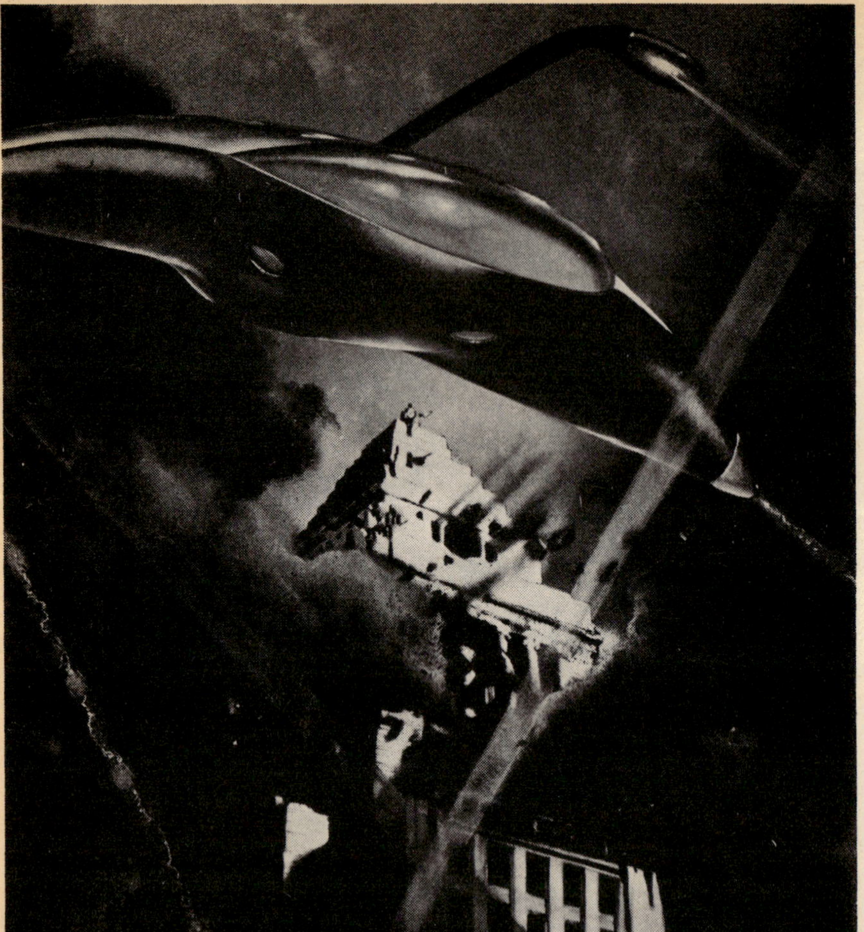

The War of the Worlds (1953)

". . .terrific special effects. . ."

Watership Down ★★★

(1978) Color, 97 min. Director: Martin Rosen.
Voices of John Hurt, Ralph Richardson, Michael Hordern, Harry Andrews, Denholm Elliott, Zero Mostel. Striking, animated film version of Richard Adams' best-seller about the exploits of a group of rabbits in search of a warren that's far from man and other dangers.
(Warner Home Video, RCA VideoDisc) VC, CED

Werewolves on Wheels ★

(1971) Color, 85 min. Director: Michael Levesque.
Stephen Oliver, Severn Darden, Billy Gray, D.J. Anderson, Barry McGuire. Sleazy riders get into a row with equally sleazy satanists, who get even by turning two of the bikers into werewolves—thus the title. Occasionally very funny, though I'm not sure it's supposed to be. Lots of slow motion violence, no doubt influenced by Sam Peckinpah's *The Wild Bunch* released two years before.
(Electric Video) VC

Westworld ★★★

(1973) Color, 88 min. Director: Michael Crichton.
Yul Brynner, Richard Benjamin, James Brolin. Pals Benjamin and Brolin vacation at an exclusive, futuristic amusement park run by androids, where they can act out their fantasies in various "worlds" modelled after the old west, the middle ages, or ancient Rome, challenging robot gunfighters to duels or jousting with robot knights. The trouble begins when a technical malfunction causes the androids to go beserk and the fun-loving pals have to start fighting for their lives against android gunslingers who are no longer playing a game but are actually out to kill them. Ingenious science-fiction thriller that is both scary and exciting. Lots of fun.
(MGM/UA Home Video) VC

Whatever Happened to Aunt Alice? ★★½

(1969) Color, 101 min. Director: Lee H. Katzin.
Geraldine Page, Ruth Gordon, Rosemary Forsyth. Page hires her housekeepers on the basis of the size of their savings accounts, murders them for the loot, then buries them in her garden. Gordon, a relative of one of the vanished victims, grows suspicious and decides to investigate on her own by posing as a housekeeper in search of employment. Not very suspenseful, but the leads have a great time. One of Gordon's few recent performances in which she doesn't chew up the scenery with her eccentric old lady bit.
(CBS/Fox Video) VC

What's Up, Tiger Lily? ★★★

(1966) Color, 80 min. Director: Woody Allen.
Woody Allen, Tatsuya Mihashi, Mie Hana. Allen made his directorial debut (loosely speaking) with this farcical thriller consisting of images drawn from an unreleased Japanese spy movie and a totally at odds script and soundtrack written and created by him. In it, Japanese thugs speak with Brooklyn accents and hurl epithets at each other like: "Saracen dog, Spanish fly!" Not consistent, but when it's funny, it's funny!
(Thunderbird Films) VC

When a Stranger Calls ★½

(1979) Color, 97 min. Director: Fred Walton.

Charles Durning, Carol Kane, Colleen Dewhurst, Tony Beckley. The first 20 minutes of this film are scary as hell. A babysitter (Kane) starts getting threatening phone calls from psycho Beckley; when she has the police trace them, she finds they're coming from inside the house. The police arrive in time to save her, but not the children. The film then skips forward some years. Beckley is released from prison and is bent on taking his revenge on Kane by going after her own kids this time. Ludicrous horror-thriller full of implausibilities.

(Columbia Pictures Home Entertainment) VC

When Worlds Collide ★★

(1951) Color, 81 min. Director: Rudolph Mate.

Richard Derr, Barbara Rush, Peter Hanson, John Hoyt. Earth is on a collision course with another planet and floods and other global disasters ensue. Scientists team up to build and launch a spaceship manned by a select group of men and women whose mission it will be to colonize the stars and perpetuate the human race. Dull George Pal production.

(Paramount Home Video) VC, LV

Werewolf vs. Vampire Woman, The ★

(1972) Color, 86 min. Director: Leon Klimovsky.

Paul Naschy, Patty Shepard, Gaby Fuchs, Andres Resino, Julio Pena, Barbara Capell. Naschy is werewolf Waldemar who teams up with a pair of young researchers to destroy the evil Countess Bathory (Shepard) whom they have accidentally resurrected. Sequel to Naschy's *Mark of the Wolfman.*

(King of Video) VC

White Zombie ★

(1932) B&W, 73 min. Director: Victor Halperin.

Bela Lugosi, Madge Bellamy, John Haron, Brandon Hurst. Lugosi runs a sugar mill operated by zombies over whom he exerts total control. He falls for Bellamy and decides to turn her into a zombie too. There are some genuinely eerie scenes in this film—especially those set in the sugar mill—but not enough to counteract the otherwise melodramatic plot and archaic treatment of it.

(Nostalgia Merchant, TV Cassette Corp of America) VC

Wicker Man, The ★★½

(1975) Color, 102 min. Director: Robin Hardy.

Edward Woodward, Britt Ekland, Diane Cilento, Christopher Lee, Ingrid Pitt. While investigating the case of a missing girl on a remote Scottish isle, policeman Woodward becomes entangled in a weird pagan ritual that culminates with the burning of the Wicker Man and the sacrifice of a virgin to appease the gods so they'll renew the island's blighted crops. Despite an interesting screenplay by Anthony *(Sleuth)* Schaffer and good performances by all concerned, the film never quite manages to grab hold. And some scenes are quite unintentionally funny.

(Media Home Entertainment) VC

Windows ★½

(1980) Color, 93 min. Director: Gordon Willis.

Talia Shire, Joseph Cortese, Elizabeth Ashley. Lesbian Ashley has a yen for Shire, and so she hires a man to terrorize her, hoping that this will have the effect of driving Shire into her arms for solace. But Shire turns the tables on her and falls for the policeman assigned to her case instead. The plot twists don't end here, though perhaps they should have. A pitiful directorial debut by ace cinematographer Gordon *The Godfather* Willis. Shire is really terrible.

(VidAmerica) VC

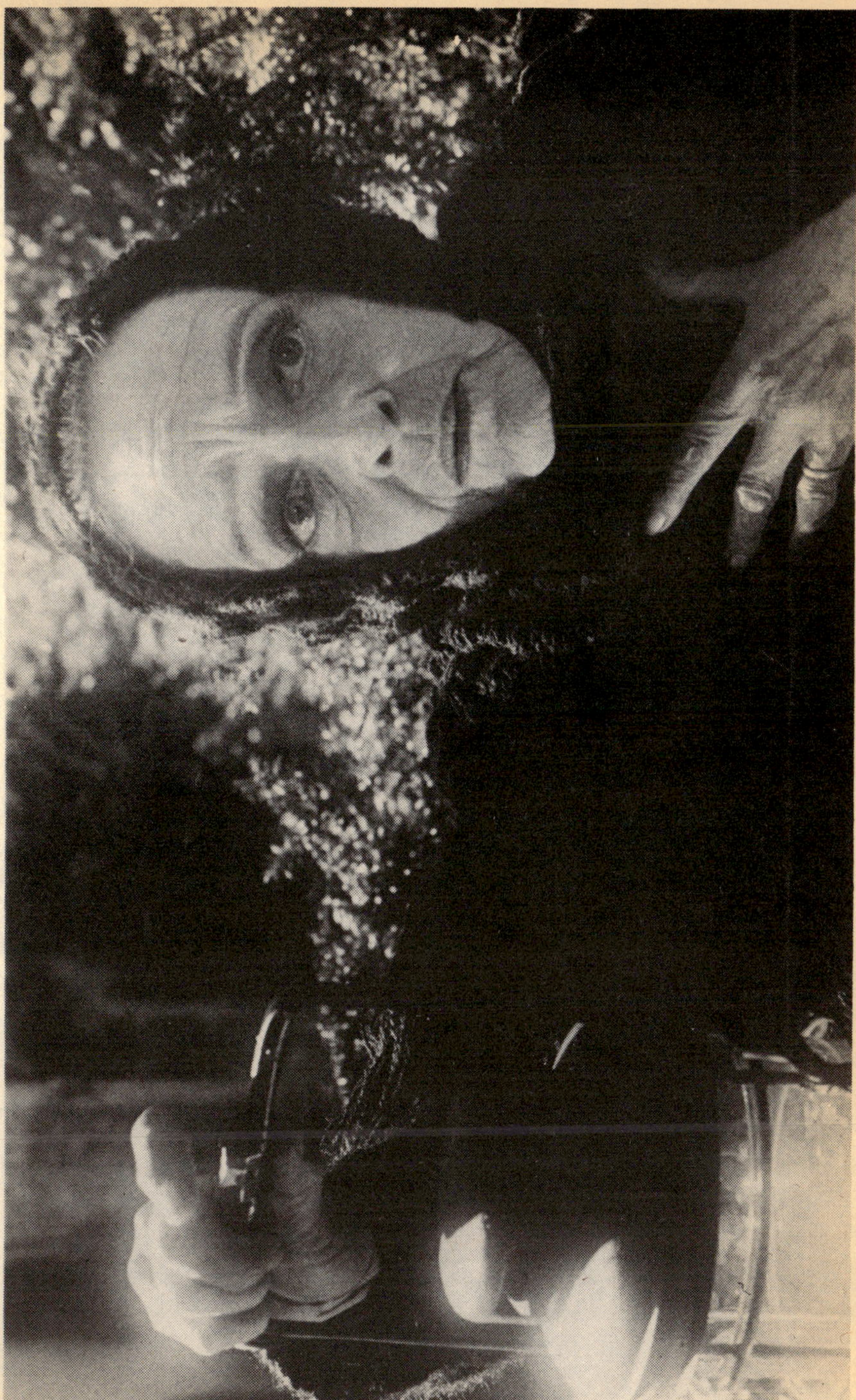

The Watcher in the Woods (1980)

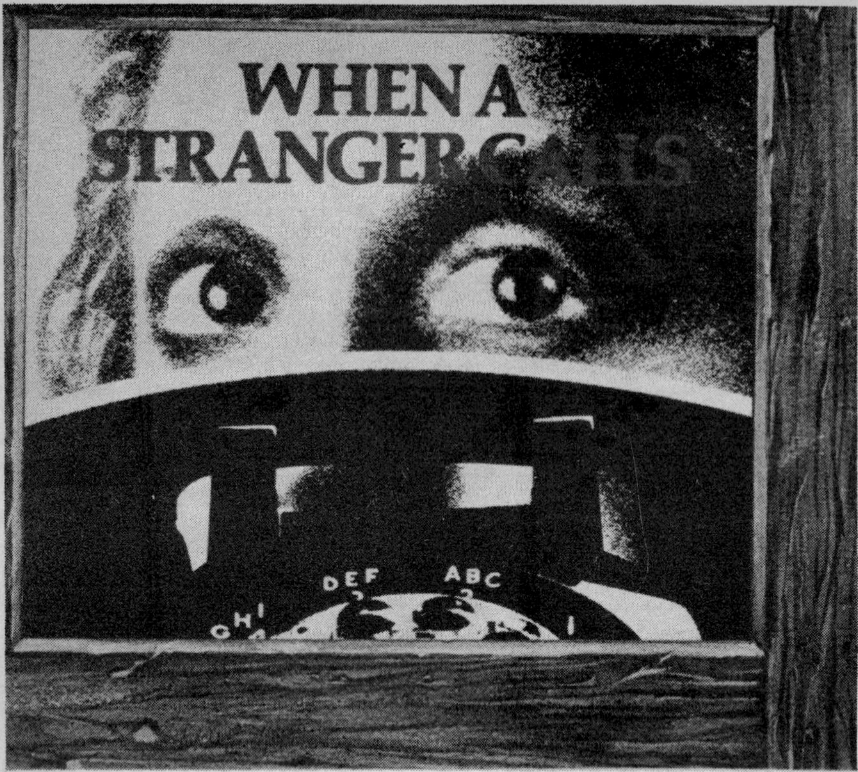

When a Stranger Calls (1979)

"The first 20 minutes. . .are scary as hell."

Winter Kills ★

(1980) Color, 97 min. Director: William Richert.
Jeff Bridges, John Huston, Anthony Perkins. Bridges delves into the fifteen-year-old case of an assassinated American president and begins uncovering one conspiracy after another. A totally incomprehensible mish-mash derived from Richard Condon's speculative novel about the murder of John F. Kennedy.
(CBS/Fox Video) VC

Witchcraft Through the Ages ★★

(1922) B&W, 90 min. Director: Benjamin Christensen.
Maren Pedersen, Astrid Holm, Elith Pio, Oscar Stribolt. The title of this film betrays its documentary-like aspirations. Director Christensen examines the history of witchcraft from the middle ages to modern times, evocatively illustrating such practices as the making of potions, Black Sabbaths and other such activities. The remainder of the film consists of an analysis of witchcraft today (1922), tying such practice in the post-Freudian age to a "natural" inclination in the female of the species towards hysterical behavior. Some nudity and gore got the film banned for a number of years.
(Thunderbird Films) VC

Witchmaker, The ★

(1969) Color, 97 min. Director: William O. Brown.
Anthony Eisley, Thordis Brandt, Alvy Moore, John Lodge, Diane Webber, Larry Vincent. Young girls are lured to a crocodile-infested Louisiana bayou by satanists, who murder and mutilate them for their blood, which is thought to have rejuvenating powers. Bloody but tepid.
(Cinema Concepts) VC

Wiz, The ★★½

(1978) Color, 133 min. Director: Sidney Lumet.
Diana Ross, Nipsy Russell, Michael Jackson, Ted Ross. Energetic, tuneful, but overlong and massively overproduced adaptation of the all-black-cast Broadway hit musical, which, in turn, was based on L. Frank Baum's *The Wizard of Oz* and the Judy Garland film made from it. Ross is Dorothy, a spinsterish New York City school marm, who is transported to Oz by means of a storm; there she meets her three companions who accompany her along that yellow brick road.
(MCA Videocassette and Disc) VC, LV

Wizard of Gore, The ★

(1970) Color, 96 min. Director: Herschell Gordon Lewis.
Ray Sager, Judy Cler, Wayne Ratay. Mad magician Montag the Magnificent (how's *that* for alliteration!) re-enacts the mutilation tricks he performs on stage when he starts slicing and dicing young girls for real. A splatter classic!
(Midnight Video) VC

Wizard of Oz, The ★★★½

(1939) B&W/Color, 101 min. Director: Victor Fleming.
Judy Garland, Ray Bolger, Bert Lahr, Jack Haley, Billie Burke, Margaret Hamilton. This classic musical fantasy ranks among the most popular films ever made. Garland is the Kansas farm girl who, with her dog Toto, is transported to the magical land of Oz where she meets the tin man (Haley), the scarecrow (Bolger) and the cowardly lion (Lahr), and does battle with the wicked witch of the west (Hamilton). Movie magic.
(MGM/UA Home Video) VC, CED

Wolfen ½

(1981) Color, 114 min. Director: Michael Wadleigh.
Albert Finney, Edward James Olmos, Diane Venora, Gregory Hines. A race of supernatural creatures that have evolved from wolves preys on derelicts and others who trespass onto its bombed-out South Bronx turf. Finney is the police detective who discovers their existence and in the end pacifies them despite the fact that they have eaten a number of his friends. Some mumbo-jumbo about the white man's mistreatment and misunderstanding of the American Indian and how that relates to the plight of the wolfen is thrown in to give the film a measure of social significance, but it's all rather fuzzy and slows the plot down to a crawl. The wolves are scary, though, and there is some bright repartee between Finney and Hines. Based on Whitley Strieber's virtually unreadable novel.
(Warner Home Video) VC

Wolfwoman ½

(1976) Color, 100 min. Director: Rino Di Silvestro.
Anne Borel, Frederick Stafford, Rossini, Dagmar Lassander, Osvaldo Ruggieri. A young woman's dream about an ancestor of hers who was a wolfwoman prompts her to transform into a werewolf as well. Feminist variation on an old theme. But that's the only new twist. A.k.a. *Legend of the Wolfwoman.*
(Video Communications) VC

Women in the Moon

(1929) B&W, 115 min. Director: Fritz Lang.
Klaus Pohl, Willy Fritsch, Gustav von Wangenheim, Gerda Maurus. Lang collaborated with rocket scientist Willy Ley to make this story of mankind's first expedition into space as scientifically accurate as possible, and the first part of the film, which details the building and testing of the rocket, is impressive indeed. The voyage itself, however, is rather a letdown, as is the human story. Trite as much of it may be, this film remains a landmark in science-fiction cinema by virtue of its subject matter. A.k.a. *Girl in the Moon.*
(Video Ten) VC

World of the Vampires

(1960) B&W, 75 min. Director: Alfonso Corona Blake.
Mauricio Garces, Silvia Fournier, Erna Martha Bauman, Joe Baviera. Mexican horror movie specialist Abel Salazar produced this perfectly awful story of an evil count who unleashes a plague of vampires on the house of the family whose ancestors condemned him as a witch. Just dreadful.
(Budget Video) VC

Wrestling Women vs. The Aztec Mummy, The

(1964) B&W, 75 min. Director: Rene Cardona.
Lorena Velazquez, Armando Silvestre, Maria Eugenia San Martin. An evil magician known as The Black Dragon is out to steal a fabulous treasure buried inside an Aztec pyramid, but two lady wrestlers are determined to stop him. To do so, they must overcome the reanimated corpse of an Aztec mummy as well as two Oriental *hitgirls.* Can you *believe* that plot? Well, to be honest, you're not supposed to, for this is intended to be a horror movie designed along the lines of a comic strip. Still, it's absurd, contrived and awful.
(Budget Video) VC

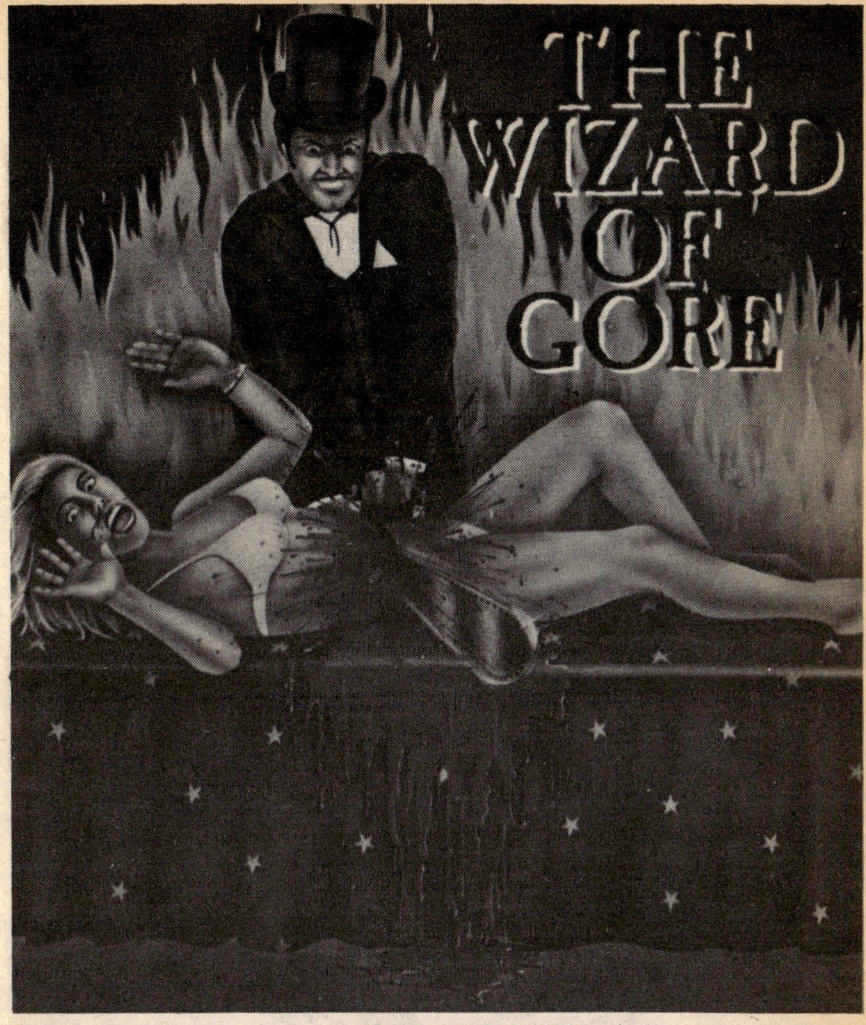

The Wizard of Gore (1970)

"A splatter classic!"

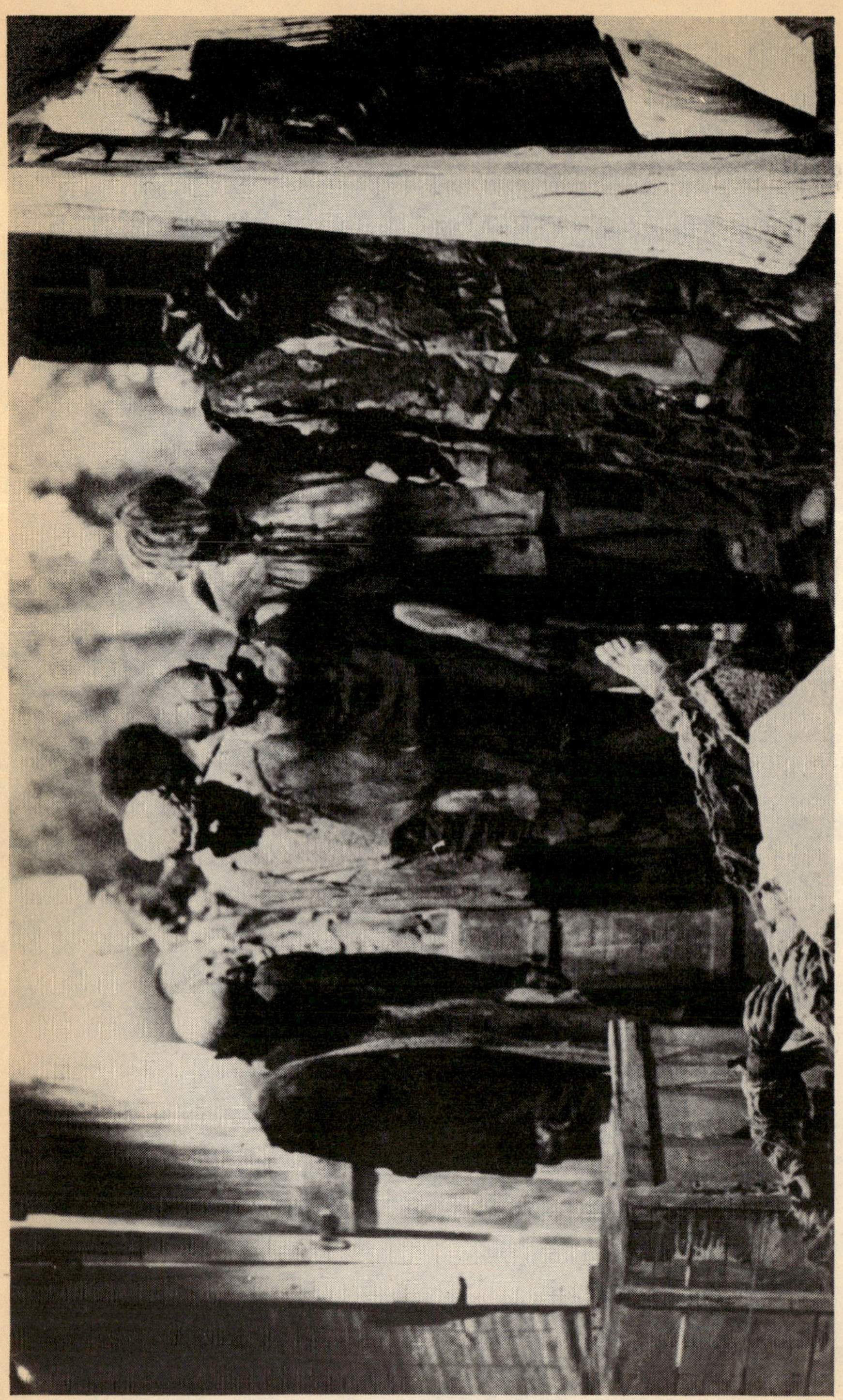

Zombie (1980)

XYZ

Xanadu ½

(1980) Color, 93 min. Director: Robert Greenwald.
Olivia Newton-John, Gene Kelly, Michael Beck. Kira (Newton-John), a golden-haired, singing muse, comes down to earth to help free-lance artist Beck and nightclub owner Kelly realize their dream of opening a glittering roller-disco. There are a few notable songs and no notable dance numbers in this very boring musical fantasy.
(MCA Videocassette and Disc) VC, LV

You Only Live Twice

(1967) Color, 116 min. Director: Lewis Gilbert.
Sean Connery, Donald Pleasence, Tetsuro Tampa, Karin Dor. Agent 007 (Connery) goes to Japan to track down his arch enemy Blofeld (Pleasence), who is shooting down American and Russian spacecraft with rockets launched from a secret lair inside a dormant volcano. Dull James Bond science-fiction adventure; even Connery looks bored. And Pleasence is totally miscast as Blofeld; why, he doesn't even *sound* like him!
(CBS/Fox Video, RCA VideoDisc) VC, LV

Young Frankenstein ½

(1974) B&W, 106 min. Director: Mel Brooks.
Gene Wilder, Peter Boyle, Marty Feldman, Madeline Kahn, Terri Garr, Cloris Leachman. A parody of Universal's *Frankenstein* films of the thirties with Wilder as a descendent of the original Baron, who resurrects his ancestor's monster (Boyle) and turns him into a song and dance man. The film's photography and set design beautifully recapture the flavor of the original films, and there are some genuinely funny moments, but Brooks' tendency to overdo everything—especially the bathroom humor and sex jokes—wears very thin after a while.
(CBS/Fox Video) VC, LV, CED

Zombie ½

(1980) Color, 93 min. Director: Lucio Fulci.
Ian McCulloch, Tisa Farrow, Richard Johnson. While investigating the case of a missing scientist who disappeared off his yacht in New York Harbor, reporter McCulloch is led to a remote island called Matool where he finds a mad doctor conducting bizarre experiments in secret, his island compound under the protection of a race of killer zombies. Gore-filled rip-off of George A. Romero's *Dawn of the Dead* by Italy's reigning king of spaghetti splatter.
(Wizard Video) VC

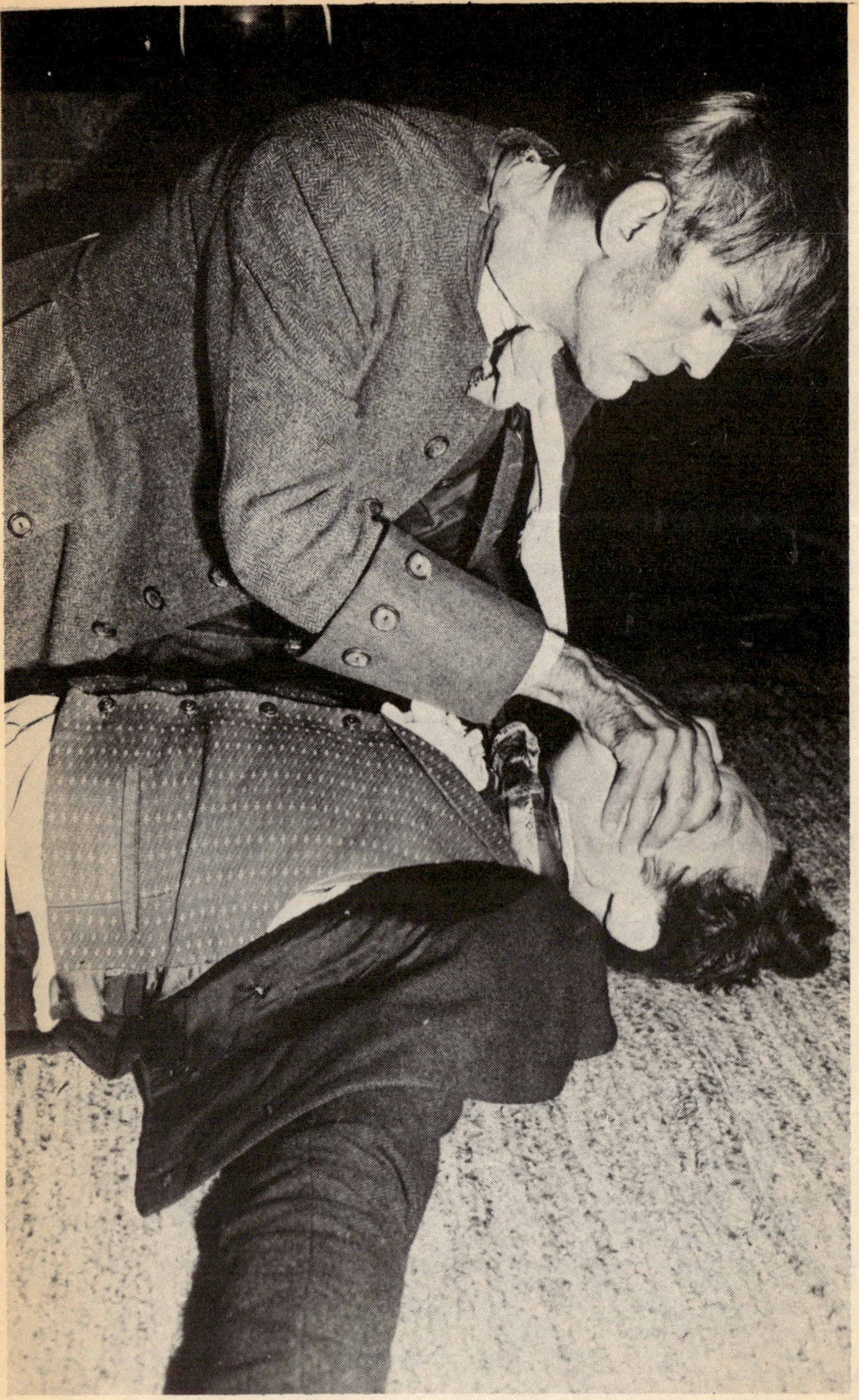

The Body Snatcher (1945)

Table of Contents: Appendices

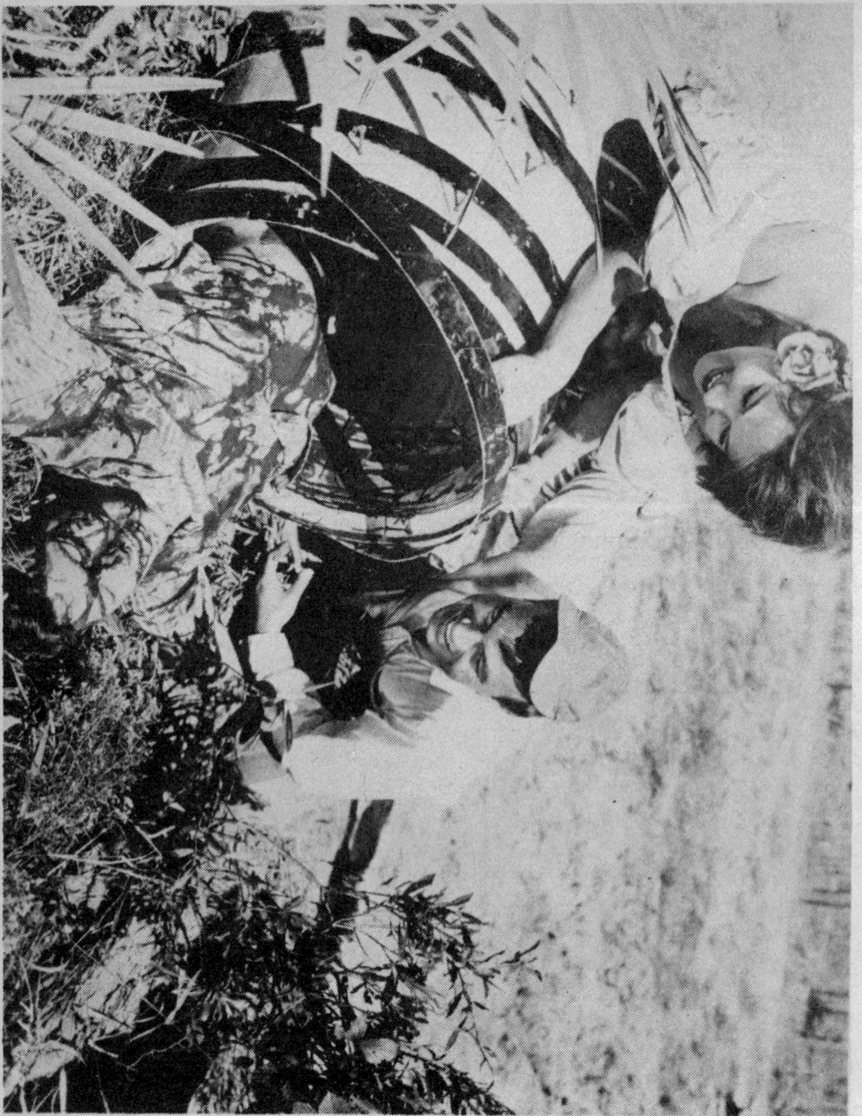

Two Thousand Maniacs (1964)

APPENDIX I: Additional Titles

The following titles are presently in release but obscure enough that apparently no one has seen them. I know I haven't. Nor was I able to find out anything about them during my research for this book. So that the next edition of *Video Screams* may include more in-depth descriptions of these films, I invite the companies that issue them—or anyone else with knowledge of these films for that matter—to supply me with more complete information about them. You may write to me in care of the publisher.

Axe (AstroVideo) VC (horror)
Beyond and Back (Video Communications) VC (documentary)
Beyond Death's Door (Video Communications) VC (documentary)
Day It Came to Earth, The (Paragon Video) VC (science fiction)
Demented (Media Home Entertainment) VC (horror)
Devil's Daughter, The (Video Yesteryear) VC (horror)
Dunder Klumpen (Video Gems) VC (animated fantasy)
Hospital Massacre (Embassy Home Entertainment) VC (horror)
Humongous (Embassy Home Entertainment) VC (horror)
Kidnapped Coed (AstroVideo) VC (horror)
Mardis Gras Massacre (Midnight Video) VC (horror)
Microwave Massacre (Midnight Video) VC (horror/satire)
Next Victim (Demonique Video) VC (horror)
Northville Cemetery Massacre, The (Paragon Video) VC (horror)
Once Upon the Brothers Grimm (Video Communications) VC (animated fantasy)
Perversion (Budget Video) VC (horror)
Pinocchio (Video Gems) VC (animated fantasy)
Savage Fury (Thunderbird Films) VC (horror)
Sinister Urge (Budget Video) VC (fantasy)
Sisters of Death (Video Communications) VC (horror)
Spaced Out (Thorn/EMI Video) VC (science fiction comedy)
Vortex (Value Video) VC (science fiction)
Whose Child Am I? (Electric Video) VC (science fiction/horror)
Zapped (Embassy Home Entertainment) VC (fantasy)

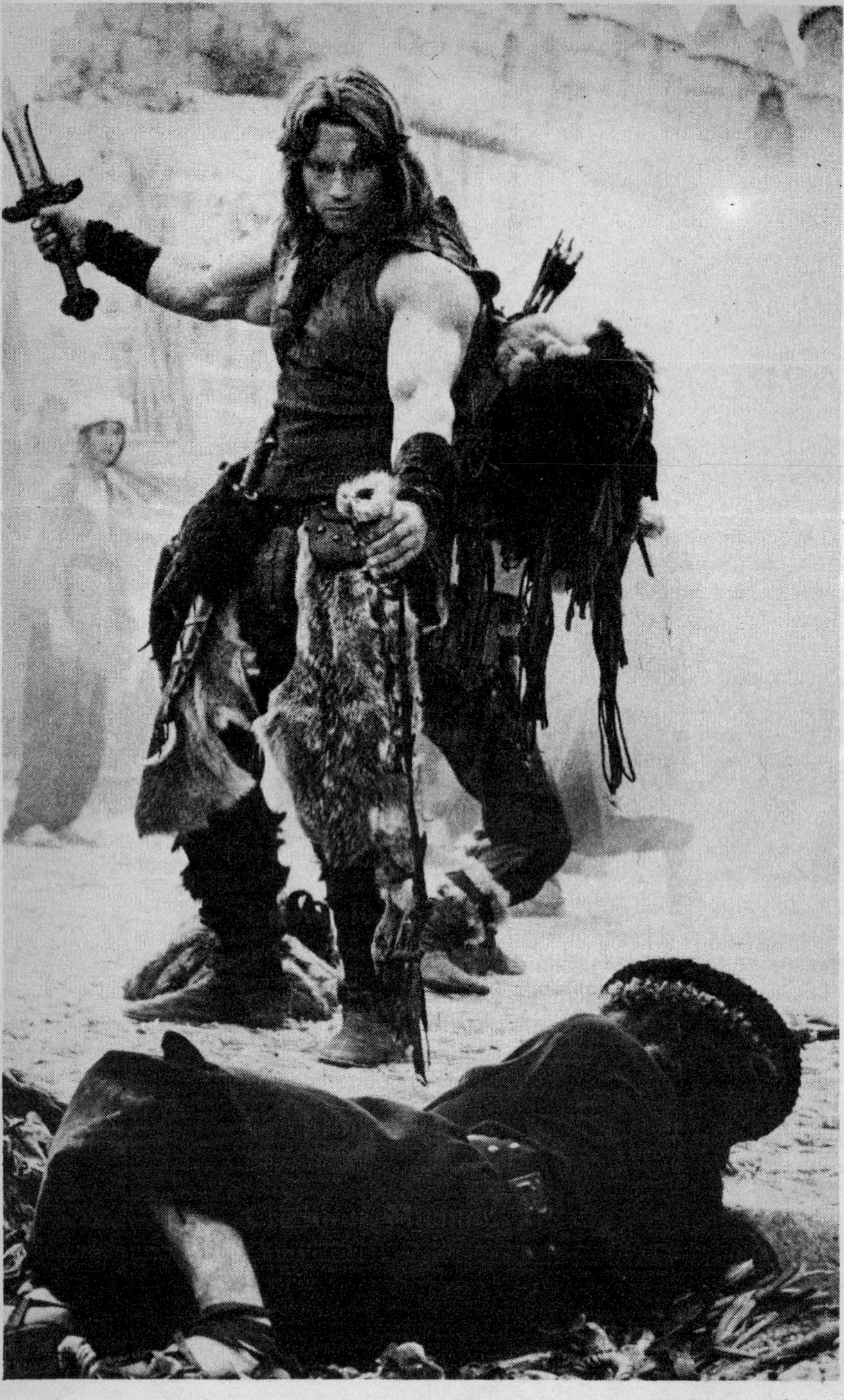

Conan the Barbarian (1982)

APPENDIX II: Video Sources

The following is a list of companies whose titles appear in this book. I have made every effort to supply the reader with the proper name and address of these companies so that they may be contacted directly about titles of particular interest. This has not been an easy task for video is such a rapidly evolving industry that it sometimes resembles the old shell game.

For example, during the course of this book's evolution, Magnetic Video changed its name to 20th Century Fox Video. Andre Blay, former head of Magnetic Video, left to form his own company, Blay Video, which was purchased shortly thereafter by Embassy Pictures and rechristened Embassy Home Entertainment. In the meantime, CBS/MGM Home Video split up. MGM merged with United Artists to form MGM/UA Home Video and CBS merged with 20th Century Fox Video which summarily underwent its second name change to become CBS/Fox Video—are you following all of this?

Well, as of this writing, all of the dust has apparently settled and all the various mergers, name and address changes appear to be over. This situation could change overnight, however, and if it does, any subsequent name and address changes will be reflected in future editions of *Video Screams*. But for the moment, this list of video sources and where to write to them is as accurate and up to date as I could possible make it.

One final note. All of the films listed in *Video Screams* are available in formats for use on the U.S. and Canada NTSC television standard. These videocassettes and discs *cannot* be played on foreign television systems. However, some companies do make their films available in foreign standards as well. PAL is the standard for the United Kingdom and elsewhere, SECAM for France and other countries. Companies which do so are denoted by a P (PAL) or an S (SECAM) next to their names. Foreign readers of *Video Screams* should contact them about which of their films are available on these standards.

And, of course, when contacting any of the following sources about their films, don't forget to mention you read about them in *Video Screams*. Good luck and happy hunting.

AstroVideo, Inc.
90 Golden Gate Avenue
San Francisco, CA 94102
1-415-673-4320

Blackhawk Films
1235 W. 5th Street
Box 3990
Davenport, Iowa 52808
1-319-323-9736

Budget Video (P)
4590 Santa Monica Blvd.
Los Angeles, CA 90029
1-213-660-0187

Cable Films (P) (S)
Country Club Station
Box 7171
Kansas City, MO 64113
1-913-362-2804

Cinema Concepts, Inc.
1805 Berlin Turnpike
Newington, CT 06109
1-203-667-1251

Classic Video Cinema Collector's Club, Inc.
17240 Goldwin
Southfield, MI 48075

Columbia Pictures Home Entertainment
Columbia Plaza South
Burbank, CA 91505
1-213-954-6000

CBS/Fox Video
23434 Industrial Park CT.
Farmington Hills, MI 48024
1-313-476-2250

Demonique Video
Webb Towers #201
1015 West 34th St.
Los Angeles, CA 90007

Direct Video (P)
1800 N. Highland Avenue
Suite 709
Hollywood, CA 90028
1-213-902-0326

Discount Video Tapes, Inc.
1117 N. Hollywood Way
Box 7122
Burbank, CA 91510
1-213-843-3366

Electric Video, Inc. (P)
1116 Edgewater Avenue
Ridgefield, N.J. 07657
1-201-943-7860

Embassy Home Entertainment
424 North Center Street
Northville, MI 48167
1-313-348-8122

Family Home Entertainment (P)
7920 Alabama Avenue
Canoga Park, CA 91304
1-213-888-3040

Festival Films
4445 Aldrich Avenue South
Minneapolis, MN 55409
1-612-870-4744

Harmony Vision
1697 Broadway
Suite 1410
New York, NY 10019
1-213-556-0680

Homevision
8124 Central Park Avenue N.
Skokie, IL 60076
1-312-674-6270

King of Video
2480 Industrial Road
Las Vegas, NV 89102
1-702-362-2520

MCA Videocassette, Inc.
70 Universal City Plaza
Universal City, CA 91608
1-213-508-4306

MCA VideoDisc, Inc.
100 Universal City Plaza
Universal City, CA 91608
1-800-228-5444

Media Home Entertainment (P) (S)
116 North Robertson Blvd.
Suite 701
Los Angeles, CA 90048
1-213-855-1611

MGM/UA Home Video
1700 Broadway
New York, NY 10019
1-212-975-3121

Midnight Video (P) (S)
8750 Holloway Drive
Los Angeles, CA 90069
1-213-652-6552

Nostalgia Merchant
6255 Sunset Blvd.
Suite 1019
Hollywood, CA 90028
1-213-464-1406

NTA Home Entertainment
Dept. 106
12636 Beatrice Street
P.O. Box 66930
Los Angeles, CA 90066-0930
1-800-228-6505

Paragon Video Productions
3820 Vanessa Drive
Las Vegas, NV 89103

Paramount Home Video
5451 Marathon St.
Hollywood, CA 90038
1-213-468-5000

Planet Video
1650 Broadway
Suite 1400
New York, NY 10019

RCA SelectaVision (VideoDisc)
30 Rockefeller Plaza
New York, NY 10020
1-212-621-6000

Sun Video
P.O. Box 27583
Los Angeles, CA 90027

Thorn/EMI Video
800 Third Avenue
New York, NY 10022
1-212-759-7964
1-212-256-1034

Thunderbird Films
3500 Verdugo Road
Box 65157
Los Angeles, CA 90065

TV Cassette Corp. of America
Canaan, New Hampshire 03741

Unicorn Video
P.O. Box 1084
Reseda, CA 91335

Value Video
1015 Gayley Avenue
Suite 1055
Los Angeles, CA 90024
1-213-837-8756

Vestron Video
911 Hope St.
Box 4000
Stamford, CT 06907
1-203-358-0000

VidAmerica, Inc.
235 E. 55th Street
New York, NY 10022
1-212-355-1600

Video Archive, Inc.
64 Lawrence Avenue
Highland Park, N.J. 08904

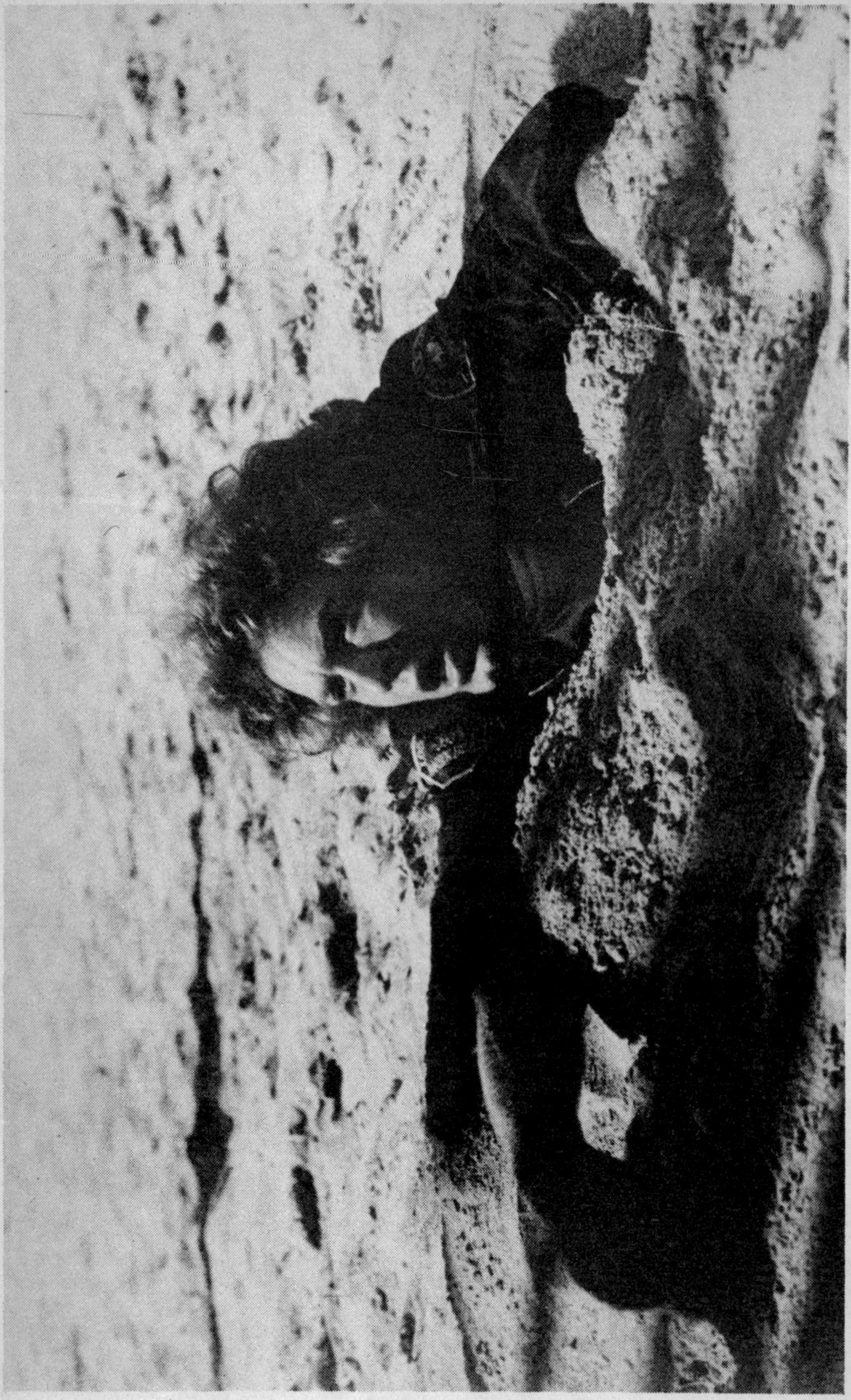

Blood Beach (1980)

Video Communications, Inc.
6555 E. Skelly Drive
Tulsa, OK 74145
1-918-622-6460

Video Dimensions
110 E. 23rd Street
New York, NY 10010
1-212-533-5999

Video Gems
731 N. La Brea Avenue
Los Angeles, CA 90038
1-212-938-2385

Video TEN, Inc.
121 La Veta Drive N.E.
Albuquerque, NM 87108
1-505-266-8619

Video Yesteryear (P)
Box C
Sandy Hook, CT 06482
1-203-426-2574

Walt Disney Home Video
500 South Buena Vista Street
Burbank, CA 91521
1-213-840-1875

Warner Home Video
75 Rockefeller Plaza
New York, NY 10019
1-212-484-8000

Wizard/Cult Video (P)
8160 Amor Road
Los Angeles, CA 90069
1-213-274-9193

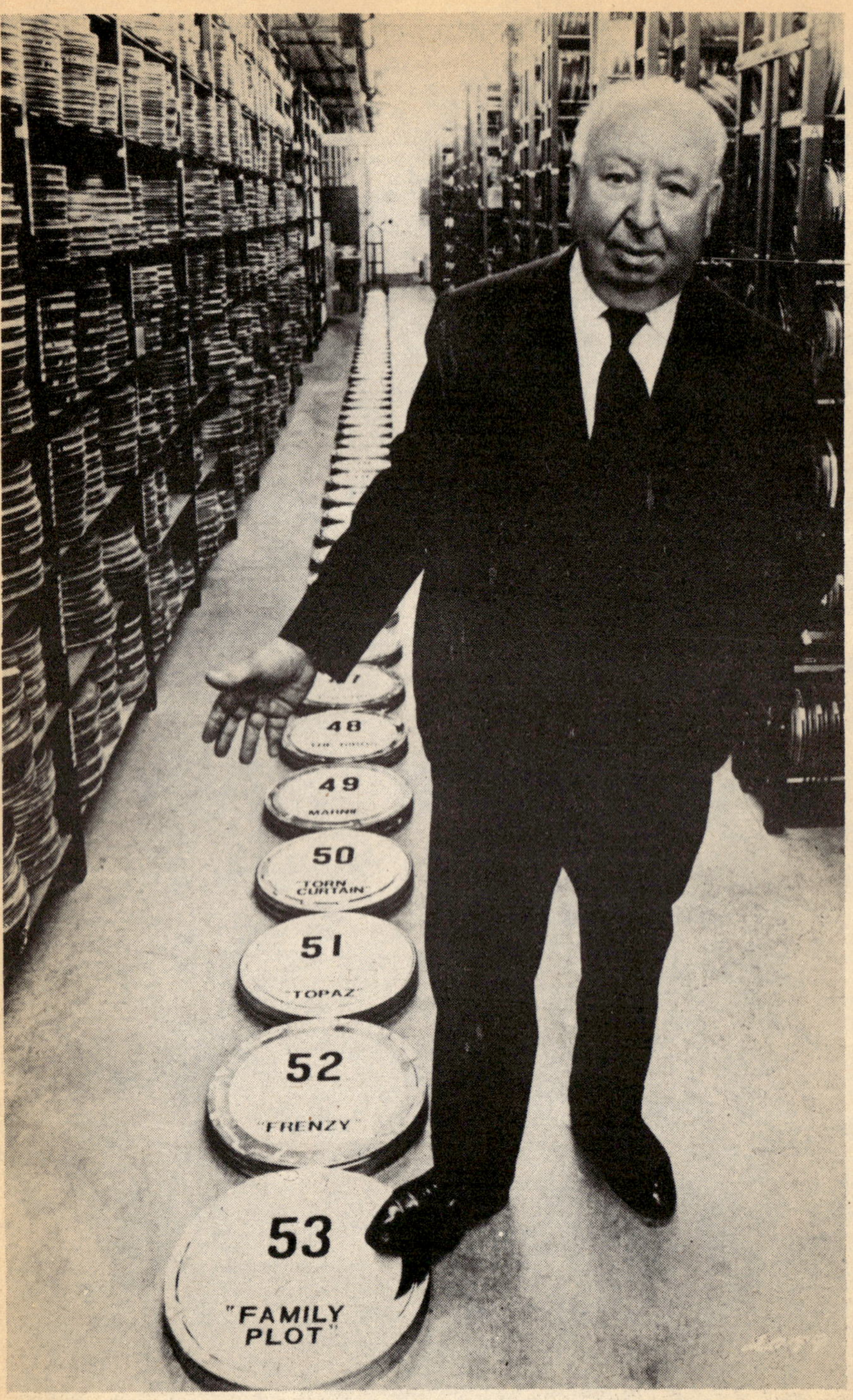

Alfred Hitchcock

Appendix III: Directors and Their Films

Adamson, Al
Blood of Dracula's Castle

Adlum, Ed
Invasion of the Blood Farmers

Alderman, Thomas S.
Severed Arm, The

Allen, Irwin
Swarm, The
Voyage to the Bottom of the Sea

Allen, Woody
Everything You Always Wanted to Know About Sex
Love and Death
Sleeper
What's Up, Tiger Lily?

Allston, Emmett
New Year's Evil

Alonso, Carlos Aured
Horror Rises from the Tomb

Altman, Robert
Popeye

Anderson, Lindsay
If

Anderson, Michael
Logan's Run
Orca

Annakin, Ken
Swiss Family Robinson

Annaud, Jean-Jacques
Quest for Fire

Annett, Paul
Beast Must Die, The

Argento, Dario
Bird with the Crystal Plumage, The
Hatchet Murders (Deep Red)

Arkush, Allan
Death Sport
Heartbeeps

Arnold, Jack
Creature from the Black Lagoon, The
Incredible Shrinking Man, The
It Came from Outer Space

Attenborough, Richard
Magic

Austin, Ray
House of the Living Dead

Badham, John
Dracula

Baker, Graham
Final Conflict, The

Baker, Roy Ward
And Now the Screaming Starts
Asylum
Scars of Dracula
Seven Brothers Meet Dracula, The
Vault of Horror

Bakshi, Ralph
Lord of the Rings, The

Balaban, Burt
Stranger from Venus

Balch, Antony
Horror Hospital

Baledon, Raphael
Curse of the Crying Woman

Band, Albert
Dracula's Dog
I Bury the Living

Band, Charles
Parasite, The

Bartel, Paul
Death Race 2000

Barton, Charles
Abbott & Costello Meet Frankenstein
Shaggy Dog, The

Batchelor, Joy
Animal Farm

Beaudine, William
Ape Man, The
Ghosts on the Loose
Sparrows

Beatles, The
Magical Mystery Tour, The

Beatty, Warren
Heaven Can Wait

Beaumont, Gabrielle
Godsend, The

Becker, Terry
Thirsty Dead, The

Beebe, Ford
Buck Rogers Conquers the Universe
Flash Gordon: Mars Attacks the World
Planet Outlaws

Benedek, Laslo
Night Visitor, The

Bentley, Thomas
Living Dead, The
Murder at the Baskervilles

Benveniste, Michael
Flesh Gordon

Bianchi, Edward
Fan, The

Biberman, Herbert J.
Master Race

Blackburn, Robert
Lemora, Lady Dracula

Blake, Alfonso Corona
World of the Vampires, The

Bloom, Jeffrey
Blood Beach

Bogdanovich, Peter
Targets

Boorman, John
Excalibur
Exorcist II—The Heretic

Bowers, George
Hearse, The

Bradley, David
They Saved Hitler's Brain

Brickman, Marshall
Simon

Brooks, Bob
Tattoo

Brown, William O.
Witchmaker, The

Browning, Tod
Dracula

Brownrigg, S.F.
Don't Look in the Basement
Keep My Grave Open

Bunuel, Juan
Leonor

Camus, Marcel
Black Orpheus

Capra, Frank
It's a Wonderful Life
Lost Horizon

Carayiannis, Costa
Land of the Minotaur

Cardona, Rene
Wrestling Woman vs. the Aztec Mummy, The

Cardos, John "Bud"
Dark, The
Day Time Ended, The
Kingdom of the Spiders

Carpenter, John
Assault on Precinct 13
Dark Star
Escape from New York
Fog, The
Halloween
Thing, The

Carreras, Michael
Maniac, The

Cassarino, Thomas
Hideous Sun Demon

Cates, Gilbert
Oh, God—Book II

Cavalcanti, Alberto
Dead of Night

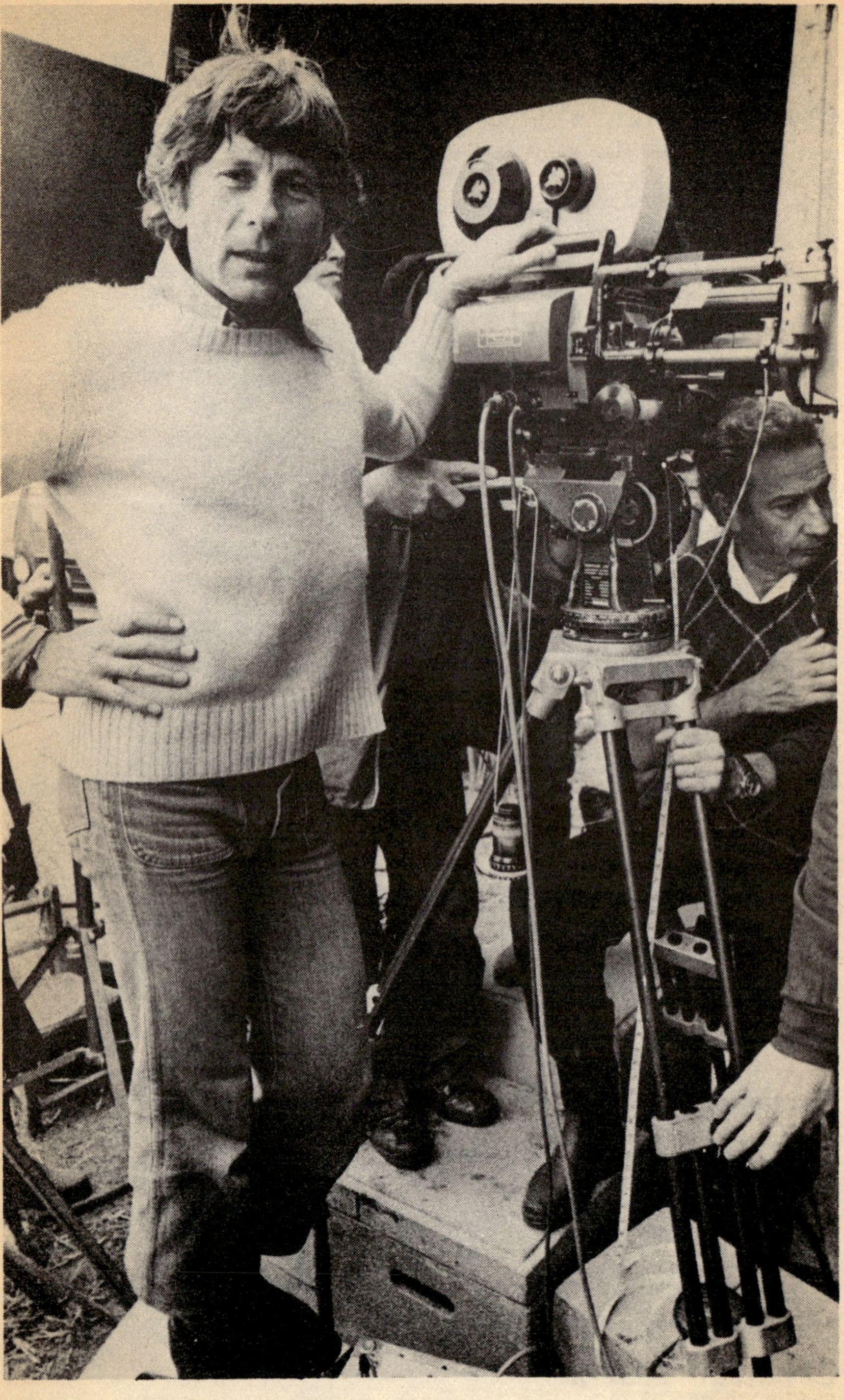

Roman Polanski

Chaffey, Don
Persecution
Pete's Dragon

Christensen, Benjamin
Witchcraft Through the Ages

Clair, Rene
Crazy Ray, The

Clark, Bob
Children Shouldn't Play with Dead Things
Murder by Decree

Clark, Greydon
Return, The

Clarke, Robert
Hideous Sun Demon

Clemens, Brian
Captain Kronos: Vampire Hunter

Clift, Denison
Phantom Ship

Cline, Eddie
Three Ages, The

Clouzot, Henri-Georges
Diabolique
Raven, The

Cocteau, Jean
Beauty and the Beast
Blood of a Poet
Orpheus

Colla, Richard A.
Battlestar Galactica

Colucci, Mario
Something is Creeping in the Dark

Conrad, Mikel
Flying Saucer

Conway, Jack
Unholy Three, The

Conway, James L.
Fall of the House of Usher, The
In Search of Noah's Ark

Coppola, Francis Ford
Dementia 13

Corman, Roger
Creature from the Haunted Sea, The
Fall of the House of Usher, The
Little Shop of Horrors
Pit and the Pendulum, The
Tales of Terror
Terror, The

Coscarelli, Don
Phantasm

Cozzi, Luigi
Alien Contamination

Crabtree, Arthur
Fiend Without a Face

Crain, William
Dr. Black and Mr. Hyde

Crane, Kenneth
Monster from Green Hell, The

Craven, Wes
Hills Have Eyes, The
Swamp Thing

Crichton, Charles
Dead of Night

Crichton, Michael
Coma
Looker
Westworld

Cronenberg, David
Rabid
Scanners

Crowley, Lawrence
Big Foot—Man or Beast?

Cruze, James
Great Gabbo, The

Cunha, Dick
Frankenstein's Daughter
Giant from the Unknown
Missile to the Moon
She Demons

Cunningham, Sean S.
Friday the 13th
Stranger is Watching, A

Curtiz, Michael
Adventures of Robin Hood, The

Daalder, Renee
Massacre at Central High

Dante, Joe
Howling, The

Danton, Ray
Crypt of the Living Dead

Day, Robert
Haunted Strangler, The

Dearden, Basil
Dead of Night
Man Who Haunted Himself, The

DeBello, John
Attack of the Killer Tomatoes

De Gaetano, Michael
Haunted, The

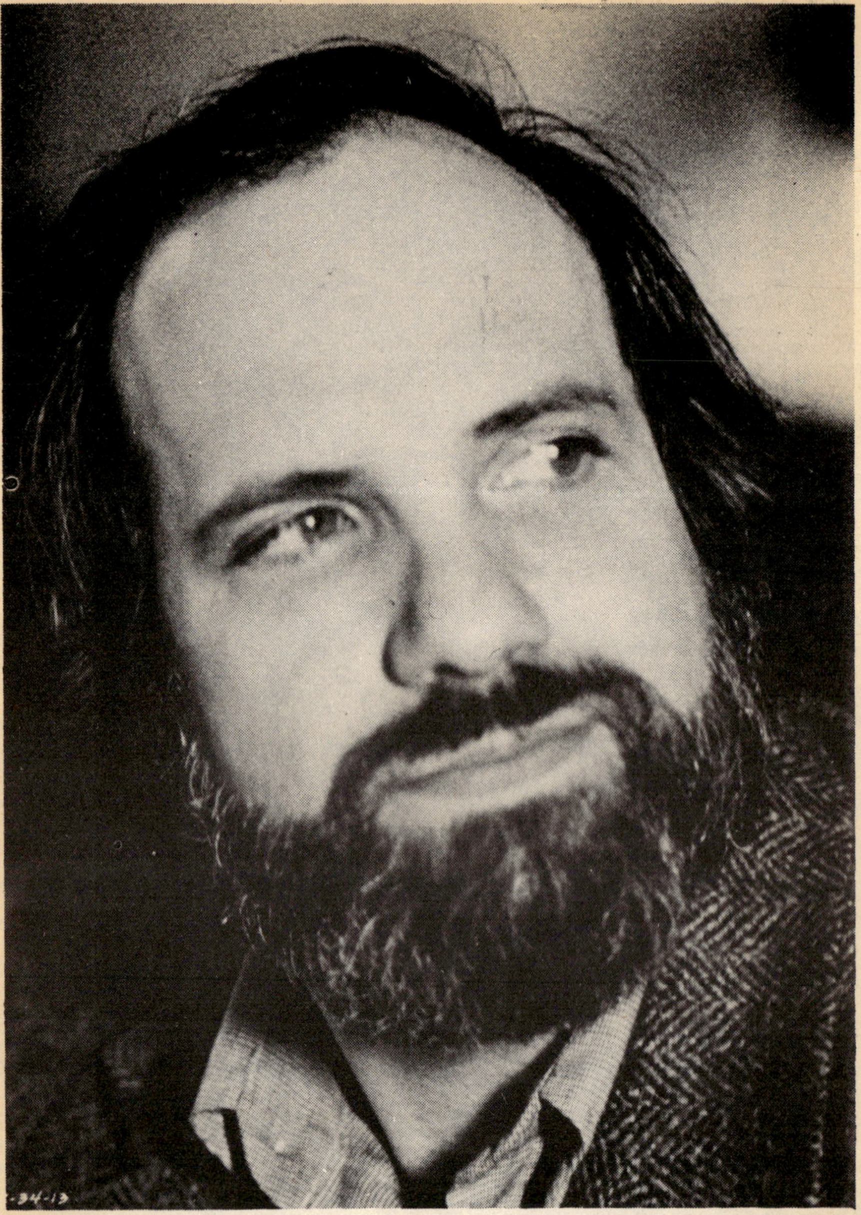

Brian De Palma

De Palma, Brian
Blow Out
Carrie
Dressed to Kill
Fury, The
Sisters

Derek, John
Tarzan the Ape Man

De Simone, Tony
Hell Night

Dieterle, William
Hunchback of Notre Dame, The

Di Silvestro, Rino
Wolfwoman

Donen, Stanley
Bedazzled
Little Prince, The
Saturn 3

Donnelly, Dennis
Toolbox Murders, The

Donner, Clive
Thief of Baghdad, The

Donner, Richard
Omen, The
Superman

Donohue, Jack
Babes in Toyland

Dragoti, Stan
Love at First Bite

Dreyer, Carl
Day of Wrath
Vampyr

Dwan, Allan
Gorilla, The

Eastwood, Clint
Firefox
High Plains Drifter
Play Misty for Me

Edwards, Blake
Pink Panther Strikes Again

Edwards, Henry
Scrooge

Edwards, Vince
Mission Galactica/Cylon Attack

Ellison, Joseph
Don't Go in the House

Elvey, Maurice
Evil Mind, The
Tunnel, The

Emery, Robert J.
Scream Bloody Murder

Endfield, Cy
Mysterious Island

Esper, Dwain
Maniac, The

Farris, John
Dear Dead Delilah

Ferrara, Abel
Driller Killer, The

Fisher, Terence
Hound of the Baskervilles, The

Fithian, Douglas
Hunted, The

Fleischer, Dave
Gulliver's Travels

Fleischer, Richard
Fantastic Voyage
Soylent Green
20,000 Leagues Under the Sea

Fleming, Victor
Wizard of Oz, The

Flocker, James T.
Ghosts That Still Walk

Foleg, Peter
Unseen, The

Forbes, Bryan
Seance on a Wet Afternoon

Fosselius, Ernie
Hardware Wars and Other Film Farces

Fowler Jr., Gene
I Married a Monster from Outer Space

Francis, Freddie
Creeping Flesh, The
Ghoul, The
Legend of the Werewolf

Franco, Jesus
Castle of Fu Manchu, The
Jack the Ripper
Kiss Me Monster

Franju, Georges
Judex

Frankenheimer, John
Prophecy

Franklin, Richard
Patrick

Frawley, James
Big Bus, The
Muppet Movie, The

Freleng, Friz
Looney, Looney, Looney Bugs Bunny Movie, The

Friedenberg, Richard
Bermuda Triangle, The

Friedkin, William
Exorcist, The

Fuest, Robert
Devil's Rain, The
Final Programme, The

Fukada, Jun
Son of Godzilla

Fulci, Lucio
Zombie

Gale, George
Mysteries from Beyond Earth

Gallu, Samuel
Theatre of Death

Gariazzo, Mario
Eerie Midnight Horror Show, The

Geronimi, Clyde
Alice in Wonderland

Gilbert, Lewis
Spy Who Loved Me, The
You Only Live Twice

Gilliam, Terry
Monty Python and the Holy Grail
Time Bandits

Girdler, William
Day of the Animals
Manitou, The

Glen, John
For Your Eyes Only

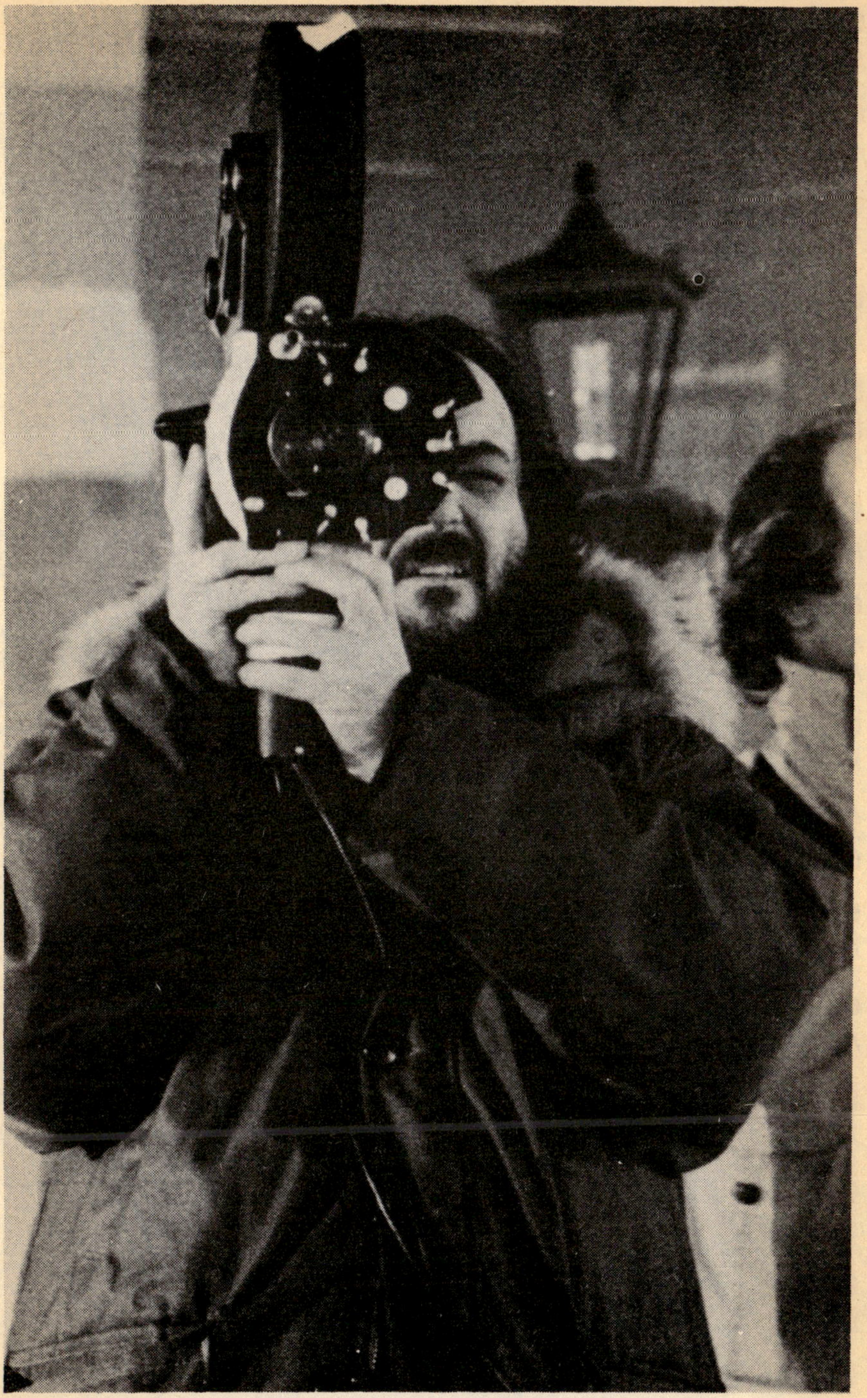

Stanley Kubrick

Gochis, Constantine S.
Redeemer, The

Godard, Jean-Luc
Alphaville

Gold, Jack
Medusa Touch, The

Goodell, J. Gregory
Human Experiments

Goodkind, Saul A.
Buck Rogers Conquers the Universe
Planet Outlaws

Goossens, Ray
Pinocchio in Outer Space

Gordon, Bert I.
Mad Bomber, The
Magic Sword, The

Goslar, Jurgen
Albino

Gottlieb, Carl
Caveman

Gottlieb, F.J.
Hansel and Gretel

Greene, David
Madame Sin

Greenwald, Robert
Xanadu

Grefe, William
Stanley

Griffith, Charles B.
Dr. Heckyl and Mr. Hype

Griffith, D.W.
Avenging Conscience, The
One Million B.C.

Grunewald, Allan
Nightmare Castle

Guest, Val
Day the Earth Caught Fire, The

Guillermin, John
King Kong

Gunn, Gilbert
Cosmic Monsters

Haggard, Piers
Fiendish Plot of Fu Manchu, The

Hagman, Larry
Son of Blob

Halas, John
Animal Farm

Hall, Alexander
Here Comes Mr. Jordan

Halperin, Victor
White Zombie

Hamer, Robert
Dead of Night

Hamilton, Guy
Diamonds are Forever
Goldfinger

Hammer, Robert
Don't Answer the Phone!

Hardy, Robin
Wicker Man, The

Hardy, Ron
Thirst

Harper, Rick
Hardware Wars and Other Film Farces

Harrington, Curtis
Killing Kind, The
Ruby

Harris, Denny
Silent Scream

Harrison, Paul
House of the Seven Corpses, The

Haskin, Byron
From the Earth to the Moon
War of the Worlds

Hayers, Sidney
Assault
Galactica III: Conquest of the Earth
Revenge

Hayes, John
End of the World

Heffron, Richard
Futureworld

Hellman, Oliver
Beyond the Door

Henderson, Don
Touch of Satan, A

Henry, Buck
Heaven Can Wait

Hensen, Jim
Great Muppet Caper, The

Heroux, Dennis
Uncanny, The

Hessler, Gordon
Golden Voyage of Sinbad, The

Hewitt, David L.
Lucifer Complex, The

Hewitt, Jean
Blood of Dracula's Castle

Hickox, Douglas
Clash of the Titans

Hill, George Roy
Slaughterhouse Five

Hill, Robert
Flash Gordon: Mars Attacks the World
Shadow of Chinatown

Hilliard, Richard
Psychomania

Hilton, Arthur
Cat Women of the Moon

Hiscott, Leslie S.
Triumph of Sherlock Holmes, The

Hitchcock, Alfred
Birds, The
Frenzy
Lodger, The
Psycho

Hodges, Mike
Flash Gordon

Honda, Inoshiro
Ghidrah, the Three-Headed Monster
Gorath
Mysterians, The

Hooker, Ted
Crucible of Terror

Hooper, Tobe
Funhouse, The
Poltergeist
Texas Chainsaw Massacre, The

Hough, John
Escape to Witch Mountain
Watcher in the Woods, The

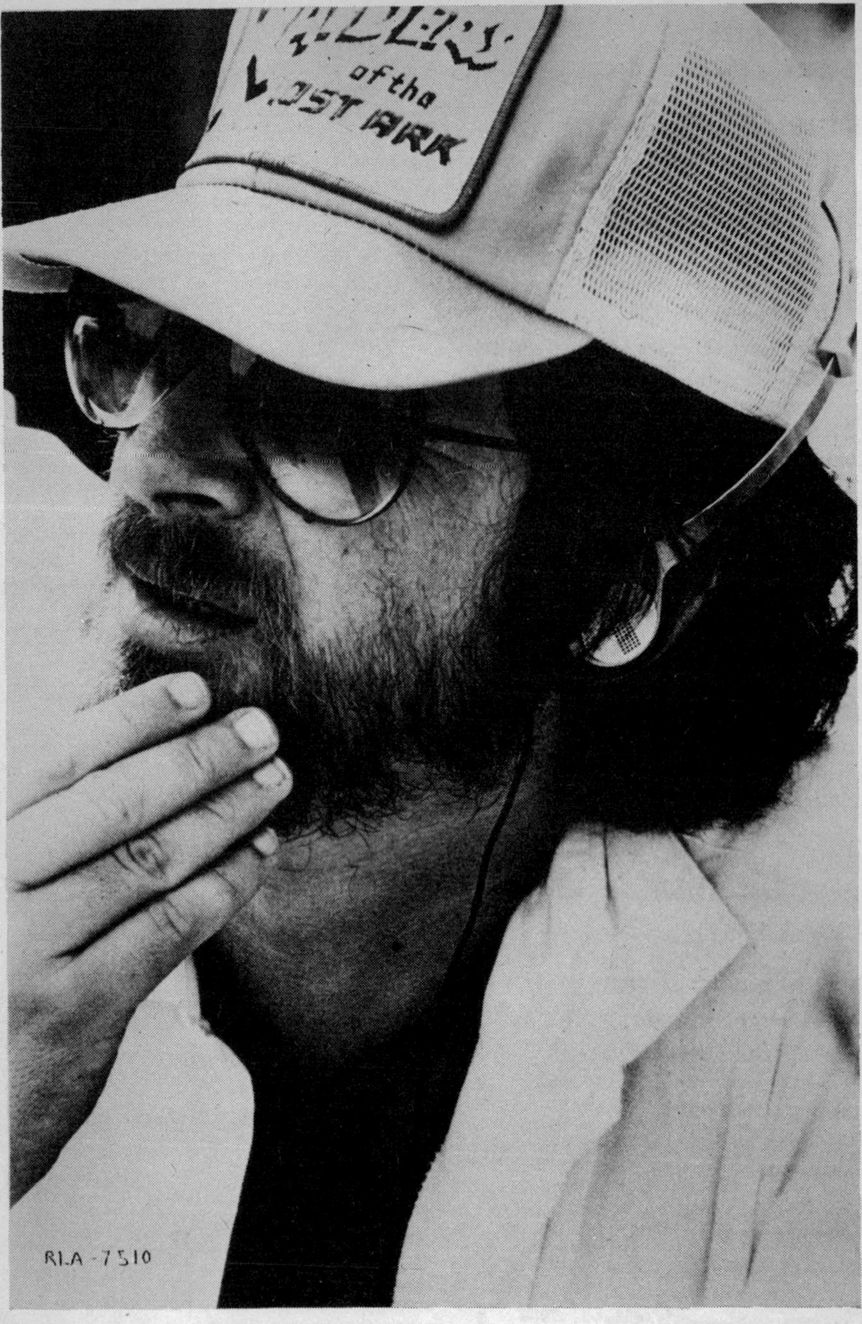

Steven Spielberg

Julian, Rupert
Phantom of the Opera, The

Juno, Victor
Last House on Dead End Street

Juran, Nathan
Seventh Voyage of Sinbad, The

Kay, Jim
Seeds of Evil

Katzin, Lee H.
Whatever Happened to Aunt Alice?

Keaton, Buster
Three Ages, The

Kershner, Irvin
Eyes of Laura Mars, The

Kessler, Bruce
Simon—King of the Witches

Kirtman, Leonard
Carnival of Blood

Klimovsky, Leon
People Who Own the Dark, The
Werewolf vs. Vampire Woman, The

Kramer, Stanley
On the Beach

Kubrick, Stanley
Clockwork Orange, A
Shining, The
2001: A Space Odyssey

Kyriazi, Paul
Death Machines

Laloux, Rene
Fantastic Planet

Landis, John
American Werewolf in London, An
Schlock

Landsburg, Alan
In Search of Ancient Astronauts

Lang, Fritz
Dr. Mabuse: The Fatal Passion
M
Metropolis
Spies
Woman in the Moon

Larraz, Joseph
House That Vanished, The

Lawrence, Quentin
Crawling Eye, The

Leacock, Philip
Baffled

Leder, Paul
I Dismember Mama

Leni, Paul
Cat and the Canary, The

Lester, Richard
Superman II

Levesque, Michael
Werewolves on Wheels

Levey, William A.
Blackenstein

Levitow, Abe
Phantom Tollbooth, The

Lewis, Herschell Gordon
Blood Feast
Color Me Blood Red
Gore, Gore Girls, The
Gruesome Twosome, The
Taste of Blood, A
2000 Maniacs
Wizard of Gore, The

Lewis Joseph H.
Invisible Ghost, The

Lisberger, Steven
Tron

Logan, Joshua
Camelot

Lommel, Ulli
Boogey Man, The

Loncraine, Richard
Haunting of Julia, The

Lord, Jean Claude
Visiting Hours

Lourie, Eugene
Gorgo

Lucas, George
Making of Star Wars, The/S.P.F.X. The Empire Strikes Back
Star Wars
THX1138

Lumet, Sidney
Fail Safe
Wiz, The

Luske, Hamilton
Alice In Wonderland

Lustig, William
Maniac

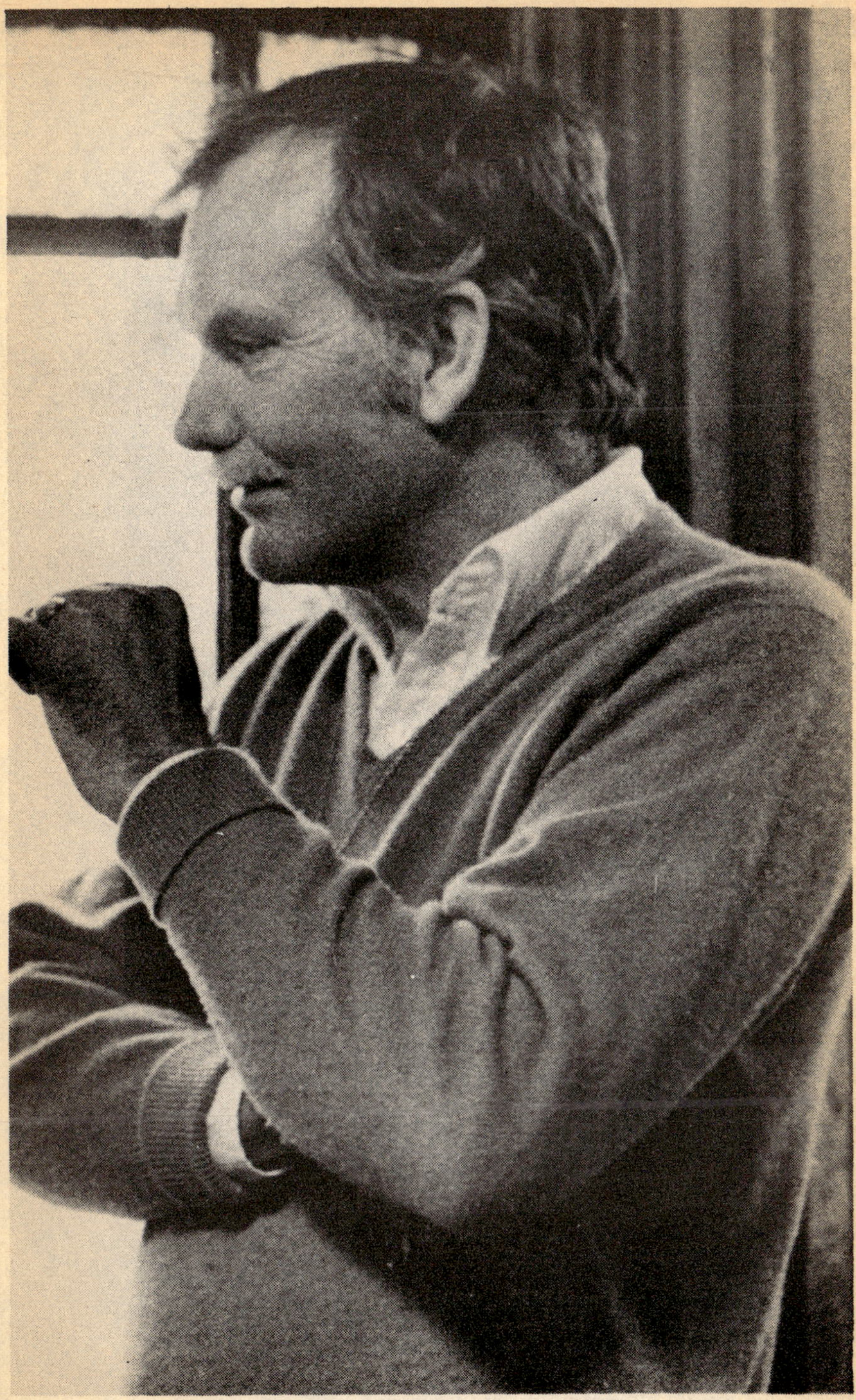

Sam Peckinpah

Lynch, David
Elephant Man, The
Eraserhead

Lynch, Paul
Prom Night

MacDonald, David
Devil Girl from Mars

MacGregor, Sean
Devil Times Five

MacKendrick, Alexander
Man in the White Suit, The

Madden, Lee
Night Creature

Mankiewicz, Joseph L.
Sleuth

Marshak, Philip
Dracula Sucks

Martin, Eugenio
Horror Express

Martin, Frank
Dr. Butcher, M.D.

Martin, Richard
Legend of the Loch Ness, The

Martino, Sergio
Slaves of the Cannibal God

Massaccessi, Aristide
Death Smiles on a Murderer

Matalon, Eddie
Cathy's Curse

Mate, Rudolph
When Worlds Collide

Mattox, Walt
Scared to Death

Matzig, Kurt
First Spaceship on Venus

Maylam, Tony
Burning, The

Mayo, Archie
Svengali

McLeod, Norman Z.
Topper

Medak, Peter
Changeling, The

Menzies, William Cameron
Invaders from Mars
Things to Come

Metzger, Radley
Cat and the Canary, The

Meyer, Nicholas
Star Trek II: The Wrath of Khan
Time After Time

Meyer, Russ
Beyond the Valley of the Dolls

Mihalka, George
My Bloody Valentine

Mikels, Ted V.
Astro-Zombies

Milius, John
Conan the Barbarian

Milligan, Andy
Bloodthirsty Butchers
Man with Two Heads, The
Rats are Coming, the Werewolves are Here, The
Torture Dungeon

Miner, Steve
Friday the 13th—Part II

Minnelli, Vincente
Brigadoon

Molinaro, Eduardo
Dracula and Son

Monson, Carl
Blood Legacy

Moore, Robert
Murder by Death

Monahan, David
Phantom Tollbooth, The

Morris, Ernest
Tell-Tale Heart, The

Morse, Terry
Fog Island

Morrissey, Paul
Andy Warhol's Dracula
Andy Warhol's Frankenstein

Moxey, John
Horror Hotel
Night Stalker, The

Murnau, F.W.
Faust
Nosferatu

Neame, Ronald
Meteor

Needham, Hal
Megaforce

Neill, Roy William
Dressed to Kill
Sherlock Holmes and the Secret Weapon
Terror by Night

Nelson, A.J.
Creeping Terror, The

Nelson, Gary
Black Hole, The
Freaky Friday

Nelson, Ralph
Charly

Neufeld, Sam
Mad Monster, The

Neufield Jr., Sam
Galactica III: Conquest of Earth

Neumann, Kurt
Kronos
Rocketship X-M

Newell, Mike
Awakening, The

Newfield, Sam
Terror of Tiny Town, The

Newland, Marv
Hardware Wars and Other Film Farces

Nichols, Charles
Charlotte's Web

Nigh, William
Mysterious Mr. Wong

Nyby, Christian
Thing, The

O'Connolly, Jim
Tower of Evil

Okabe, Kazuhiko
Panda and the Magic Serpent

Oliver, Robert H.
Frankenstein's Castle of Freaks

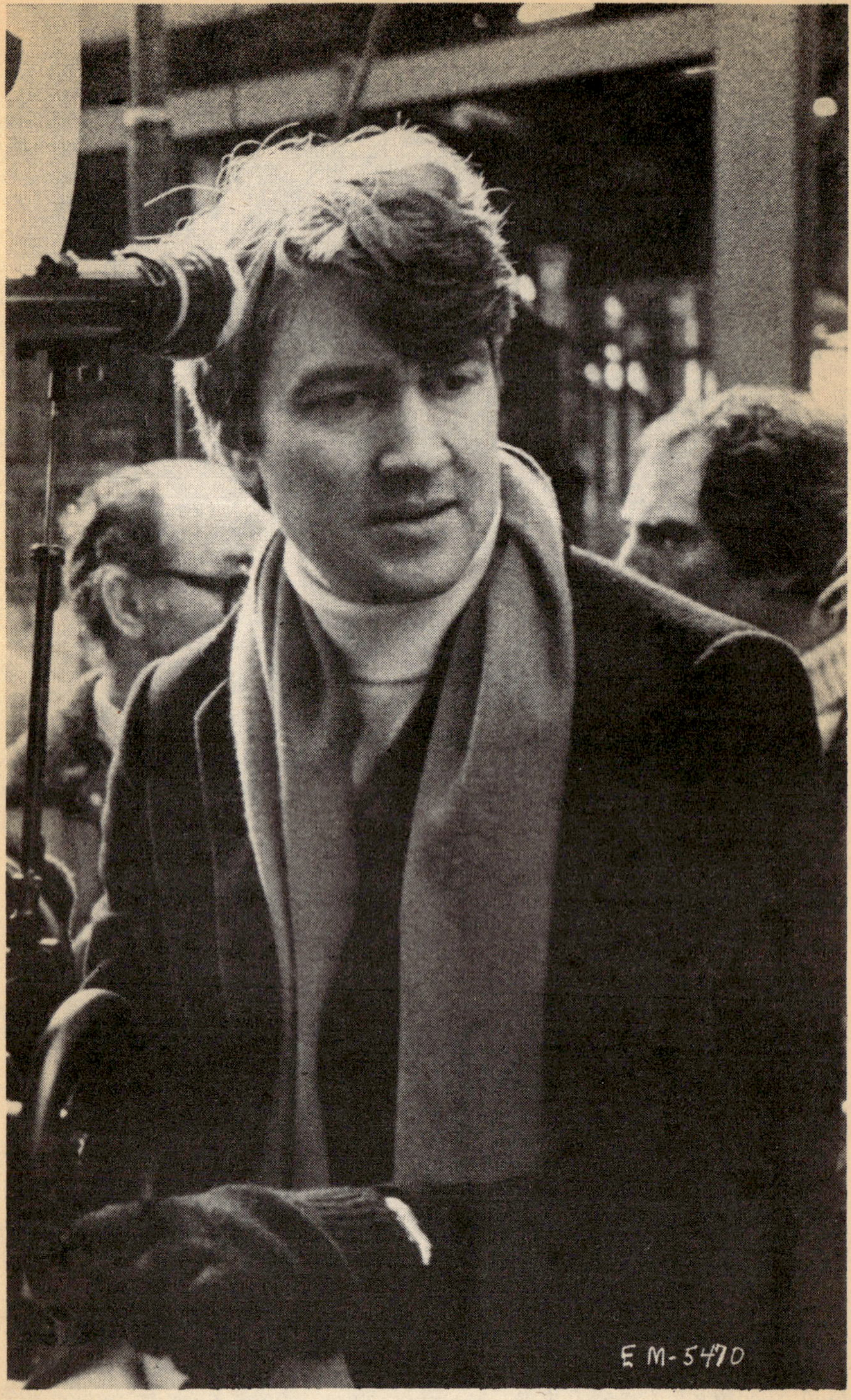

David Lynch

Olson, Rolf
Journey into the Beyond

Pal, George
Time Machine, The

Paris, Dominic
Dracula's Last Rites

Parker, John
Daughter of Horror

Paulsen, David
Savage Weekend
Schizoid

Peckinpah, Sam
Straw Dogs

Peeters, Barbara
Humanoids from the Deep

Petrie, Daniel
Sybil

Peyser, John
Centerfold Girls

Pichel, Irving
Destination Moon
Most Dangerous Game, The

Polanski, Roman
Repulsion
Rosemary's Baby

Post, Ted
Baby, The

Pyun, Albert
Sword and the Sorcerer, The

Quine, Richard
Bell, Book and Candle

Rae, Michael
Laserblast

Ragozzin, Ed
Sasquatch

Rankin Jr., Arthur
Hobbit, The

Ratoff, Gregory
Black Magic

Rawlins, John
Sherlock Holmes and the Voice of Terror

Ray, Albert
Shriek in the Night, A

Raymond, Jack
Speckled Band, The

Rebane, Bill
Invasion from Inner Earth

Reed, Herb
Graduation Day

Reiner, Carl
Oh, God!

Reinl, Dr. Harald
Chariots of the Gods?

Reisz, Karel
Morgan

Richards, Dick
Death Valley

Richert, William
Winter Kills

Riesner, Dean
Bill and Coo

Rilla, Wolf
Village of the Damned

Ritchie, Michael
Island, The

Roach, Hal and Hal Jr.
One Million B.C.

Robbins, Matthew
Dragonslayer

Robertson, John S.
Dr. Jekyll and Mr. Hyde

Robison, Arthur
Warning Shadows

Robson, Mark
Bedlam
Earthquake
Isle of the Dead
Seventh Victim, The

Roeg, Nicolas
Don't Look Now
Man Who Fell to Earth, The

Romero, Eddie
Beast of the Yellow Night, The
Beyond Atlantis
Twilight People, The

Romero, George A.
Creepshow
Night of the Living Dead
Season of the Witch (Jack's Wife)

Rose, Mickey
Student Bodies

Rosen, Martin
Watership Down

Rosenberg, Stuart
Amityville Horror, The

Rosenthal, Rick
Halloween II

Ross, Herbert
Seven Percent Solution, The

Russell, Ken
Altered States
Devils, The
Lisztomania
Tommy

Sachs, William
Force Beyond, The
Galaxina

Sanforth, Clifford
Murder by Television

Sangster, Jimmy
Fear in the Night
Horror of Frankenstein
Lust for a Vampire

Sargent, Joseph
Goldengirl

Scardmaglia, Elio
Murder Clinic, The

Scavolini, Romano
Nightmare

Schaffner, Franklin J.
Boys from Brazil, The
Planet of the Apes

Schellerup, Henning
Legend of Sleepy Hollow, The
Time Machine, The

Schmoeller, David
Tourist Trap

Schoedsack, Ernest B.
King Kong
Mighty Joe Young
Most Dangerous Game, The
Son of Kong

Schrader, Paul
Cat People

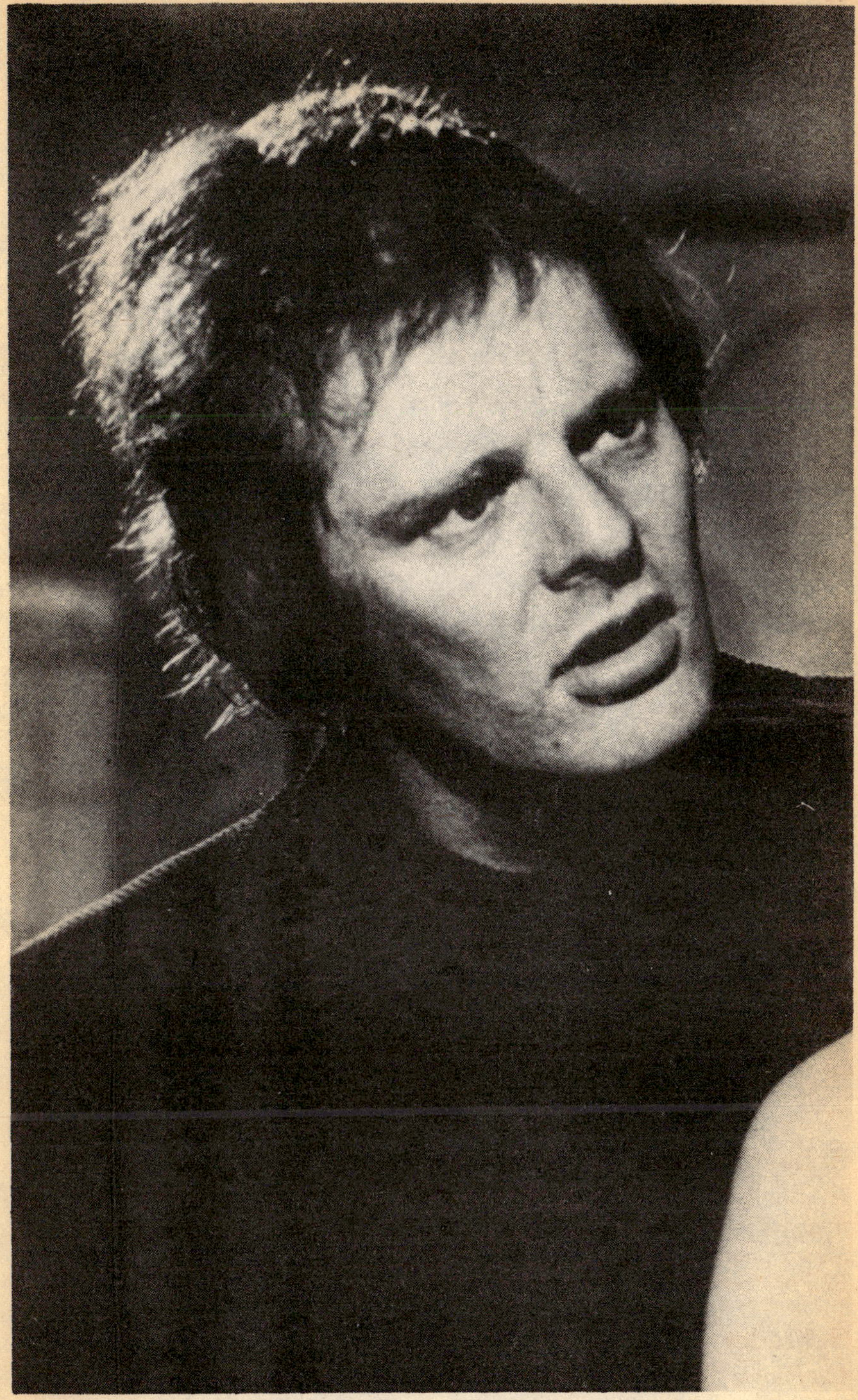

Paul Morrissey

Schultz, Michael
Sergeant Pepper's Lonely Hearts Club Band

Schumacher, Joel
Incredible Shrinking Woman, The

Scott, Ridley
Alien
Blade Runner

Segall, Stuart
Drive-In Massacre

Sekely, Steve
Day of the Triffids

Selander, Lesley
Flight to Mars

Sharp, Don
Psychomania

Sharpsteen, Ben
Dumbo

Siegel, Don
Invasion of the Body Snatchers, The

Silverman, Lewis
Amazing Transplant, The

Skolimowski, Jerzy
Shout, The

Sole, Alfred
Alice, Sweet Alice

Solvay, Paul
Devil's Wedding Night, The

Spielberg, Steven
Close Encounters of the 3rd Kind
Duel
Great Movie Stunts/Making of Raiders of the Lost Ark
Jaws
1941

Stephani, Frederick
Flash Gordon: Rocketship

Stern, Steven Hilliard
Devil and Max Devlin, The

Stevenson, Robert
Absent-Minded Professor, The
Bedknobs and Broomsticks
Blackbeard's Ghost
Darby O'Gill and the Little People
Herbie Rides Again
King Solomon's Mines
Love Bug, The
Mary Poppins

Stone, Oliver
Hand, The

Stouffer, Larry N.
Twisted Brain

Strayer, Frank
Monster Walks, The

Strock, Herbert L.
Crawling Hand, The

Stromberg, William
Crater Lake Monster, The

Summers, Walter
Human Monster, The

Suso, Henry
Death Sport

Swackheimer, E.W.
Amazing Spiderman, The

Sykes, Peter
Legend of Spider Forest, The

Szwarc, Jeannot
Bug
Jaws II
Somewhere in Time

Truffaut, Francois
Green Room The

Tucker, Phil
Robot Monster

Urueta, Chano
Brainiac, The
Living Head, The

Vadim, Roger
Barbarella

Van Dyke, W.S.
Tarzan the Ape Man

Van Rees, Joost
Target. . .Earth?

Von Fritsch, Gunther
Curse of the Cat People, The

Voskanian, Robert
Child, The

Wadleigh, Michael
Wolfen

Walker, Pete
Flesh and Blood Show, The
Schizo

Wallace, Richard
Sinbad the Sailor

Walton, Fred
When a Stranger Calls

Wanamaker, Sam
Sinbad and the Eye of the Tiger

Warren, Norman J.
Terror

Warshofsky, Fred
Outer Space Connection, The

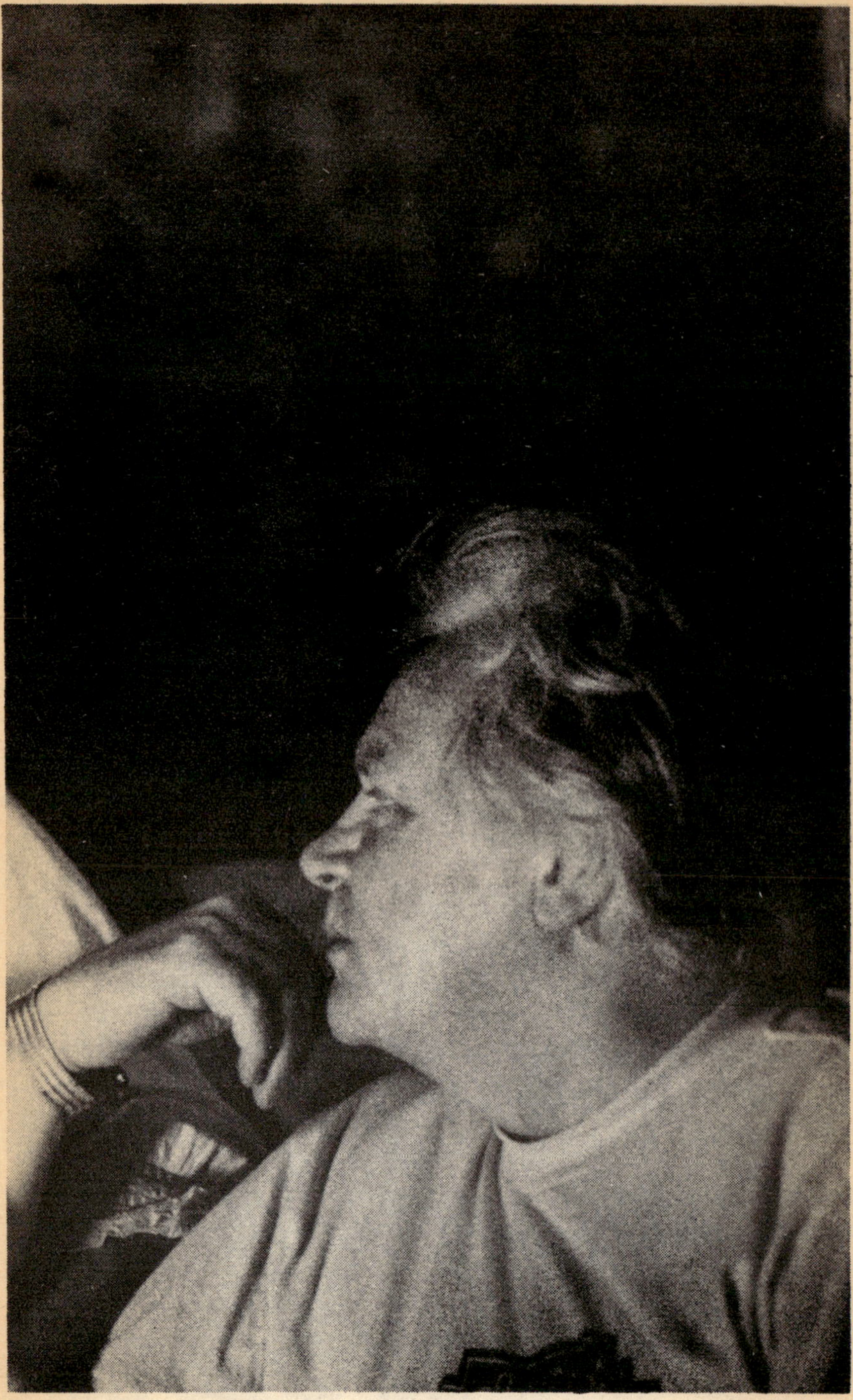

Ken Russell

Waters, John
Desperate Living
Female Trouble
Mondo Trasho
Multiple Maniacs
Pink Flamingos

Watkins, Peter
Gladiators, The
War Game, The

Weir, Peter
Cars That Eat People, The
Last Wave, The
Picnic at Hanging Rock

Welles, Orson
Trial, The

Werker, Alfred
Adventures of Sherlock Holmes, The
Shock

West, Roland
Monster, The

Weston, Eric
Evilspeak

Whale, James
Frankenstein

Wiederhorn, Ken
Eyes of a Stranger

Wiene, Robert
Cabinet of Dr. Caligari, The

Wilcox, Fred McLeod
Forbidden Planet

Wilder, Gene
Adventure of Sherlock Holmes' Smarter Brother, The

Willis, Gordon
Windows

Wilson, James L.
Screams of a Winter Night

Wise, Robert
Andromeda Strain, The
Body Snatcher, The
Curse of the Cat People, The
Day the Earth Stood Still, The
Star Trek—The Motion Picture

Wood Jr., Edward D.
Bride of the Monster
Glen or Glenda?
Plan 9 from Outer Space

Woods, Jack
Equinox

Worsley, Wallace
Hunchback of Notre Dame, The
Penalty, The

Wyler, William
Collector, The

Wynn, Bob
Resurrection of Zachary Wheeler, The

Yabushita, Taiji
Panda and the Magic Serpent

Yarbrough, Jean
Hillbillys in a Haunted House
Jack and the Beanstalk
King of the Zombies

Yeaworth Jr., Irwin S.
Blob, The

Young, Terence
Dr. No
From Russia With Love
Thunderball
Wait Until Dark

Younkins, Jerry
Demon Lover, The

Zacharias, Alfredo
Bees, The

Zarchi, Meir
I Spit on Your Grave

Zeman, Karel
Fabulous World of Jules Verne, The

Ziehm, Howard
Flesh Gordon

Zimmerman, Vernon
Fade to Black

Zito, Joseph
Prowler, The

Zurli, Guido
Mad Butcher, The

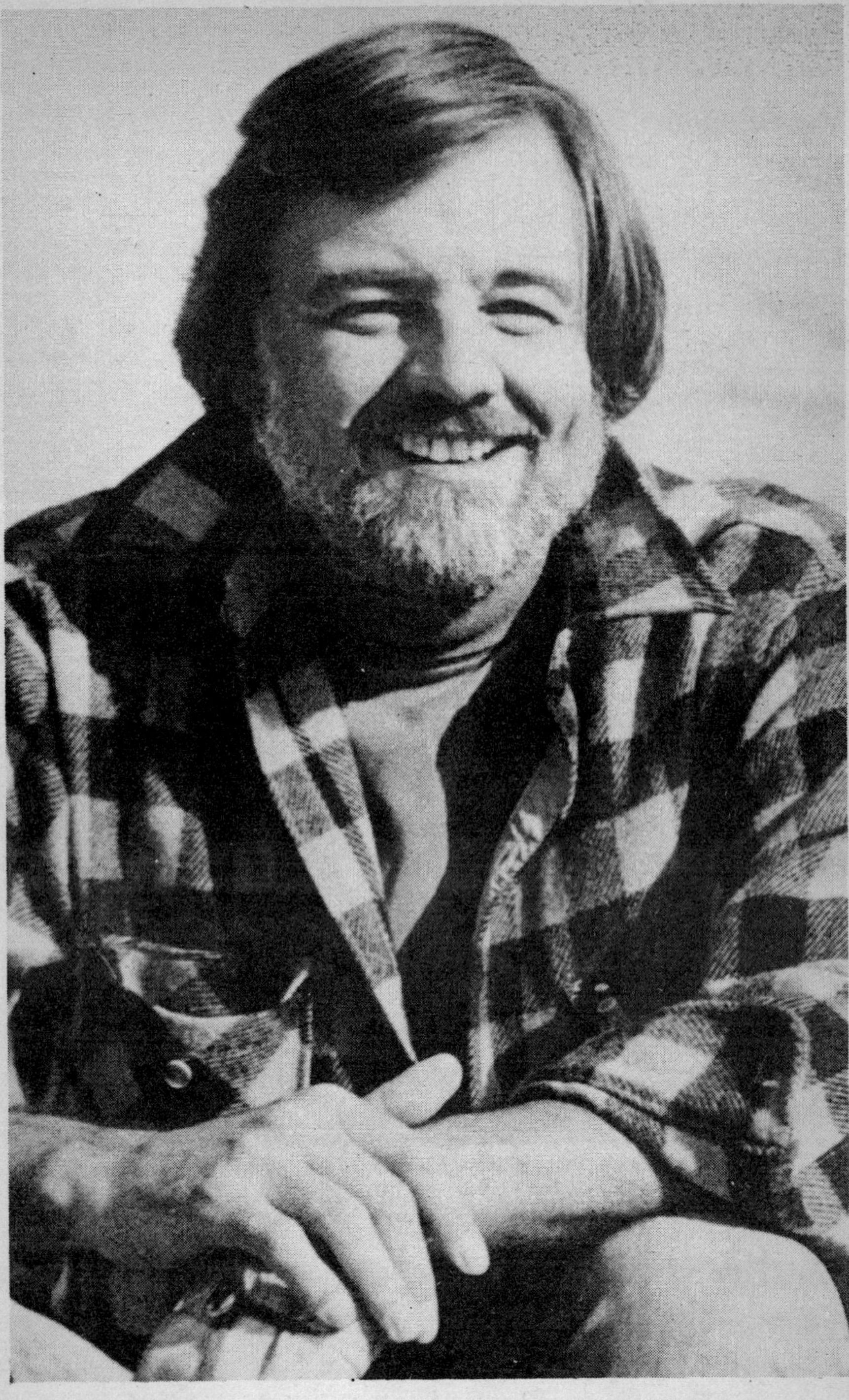

George A. Romero

Acknowledgements

Grateful acknowledgement is made to the following video and film production companies for the photographs that appear in this book: Blackhawk Films, Columbia Pictures Home Entertainment, CBS/Fox Video, Electric Video, Inc., Embassy Home Entertainment, Family Home Entertainment, William M. Gaines, Hammer Films, Ladd Co., Lucasfilms Ltd., MCA Videocassette and Disc, Media Home Entertainment, MGM/UA Home Video, Nostalgia Merchant, Paragon Video Productions, Paramount Home Video, RCA Selectavision (VideoDisc), Video Communications, Inc., Video Dimensions, Video Gems, Walt Disney Home Video, Warner Home Video, Wizard/Cult Video.

also available from

FantaCo Enterprises, Inc.

In 1963 he released a film so excruciatingly violent it caused mass panic among filmgoers and reviewers.

No in-depth information is known or has ever been published on him.

He initiated the violent horror genre which is so popular today.

Many negatives and promotional materials for his films have been presumed lost since the early '70s.

Posters, stills and other memorabilia from his films are so rare that, when available, they sell for astronomical sums.

Today, most of his films are banned from television (even cable!).

He is the most violent, gruesome, disturbing filmmaker in motion picture history.

THE AMAZING HERSCHELL GORDON LEWIS

Now, the whole story can be told...

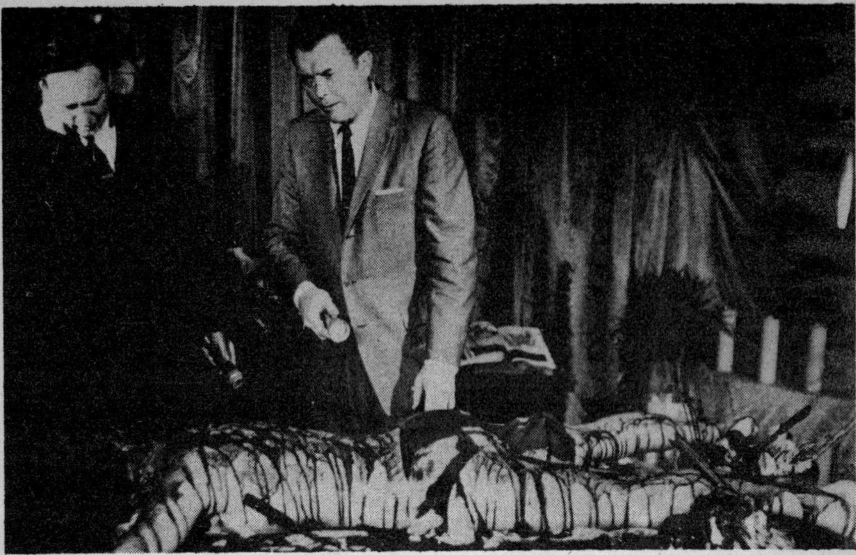

Blood Feast (1963) Directed by Herschell Gordon Lewis

THE AMAZING HERSCHELL GORDON LEWIS

by DANIEL KROGH

(Lewis' assistant cameraman and chief sound person)

with JOHN McCARTY

(author of *Splatter Movies* and *Video Screams*)

with full cooperation from

HERSCHELL GORDON LEWIS

including a lengthy preface and exclusive interview.

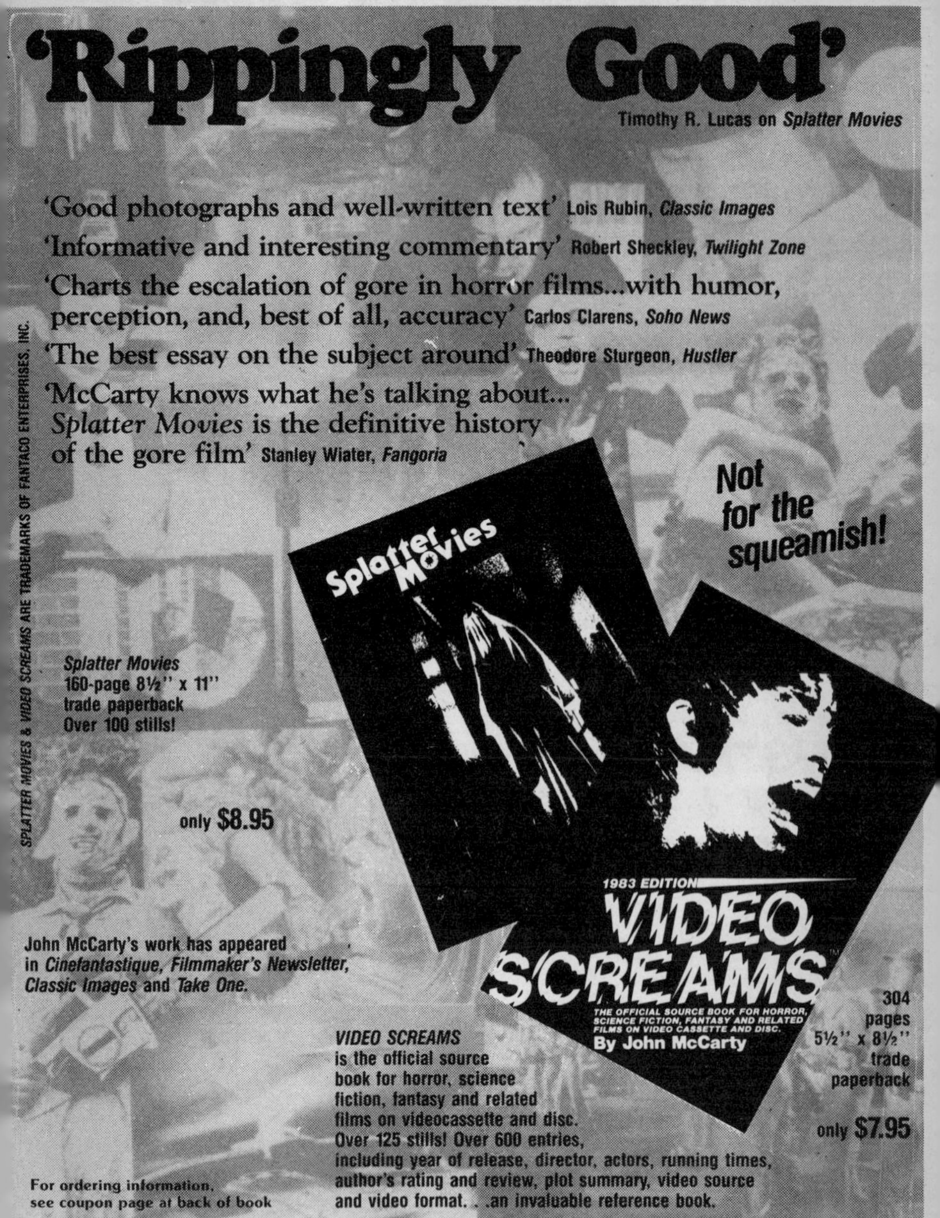
'Rippingly Good'
Timothy R. Lucas on Splatter Movies
'Good photographs and well-written text' Lois Rubin, Classic Images
'Informative and interesting commentary' Robert Sheckley, Twilight Zone
'Charts the escalation of gore in horror films...with humor, perception, and, best of all, accuracy' Carlos Clarens, Soho News
'The best essay on the subject around' Theodore Sturgeon, Hustler
'McCarty knows what he's talking about... Splatter Movies is the definitive history of the gore film' Stanley Wiater, Fangoria
Not for the squeamish!
Splatter Movies
Splatter Movies
160-page 8½" x 11"
trade paperback
Over 100 stills!
only $8.95
1983 EDITION
VIDEO SCREAMS
THE OFFICIAL SOURCE BOOK FOR HORROR, SCIENCE FICTION, FANTASY AND RELATED FILMS ON VIDEO CASSETTE AND DISC.
By John McCarty
John McCarty's work has appeared in Cinefantastique, Filmmaker's Newsletter, Classic Images and Take One.
304 pages 5½" x 8½" trade paperback
only $7.95
VIDEO SCREAMS is the official source book for horror, science fiction, fantasy and related films on videocassette and disc. Over 125 stills! Over 600 entries, including year of release, director, actors, running times, author's rating and review, plot summary, video source and video format. . .an invaluable reference book.
For ordering information, see coupon page at back of book
SPLATTER MOVIES & VIDEO SCREAMS ARE TRADEMARKS OF FANTACO ENTERPRISES, INC.

ORDERING INFORMATION

All of the unique publications described in the preceding pages are available directly from the publisher.

1 Phone orders accepted for MASTERCARD and VISA customers. Call **1-518-463-3667** to place your order.

2 To order by mail use the coupon below or a facsimile.

Please send me:

________copies of **VIDEO SCREAMS 1983** at $7.95 each

________copies of **DEMONIQUE #4** at $2.25 each

________copies of **SPLATTER MOVIES** at $8.95 each

________copies of **THE AMAZING HERSCHELL GORDON LEWIS** at $14.95 each

U.S. customers add $2.00 to total order for shipping.
Outside U.S. add $4.00 to total order for shipping.
Payment must be in U.S. funds. Make payment by money order or check.
Do not send cash!

Please fill out for MasterCard and Visa orders:

MC/VISA # ______________________________

SIGNATURE ____________________ EXP. DATE __________

Name ______________________________

Street Address ______________________________

City, State, Zip ______________________________

Country ______________________________

TOTAL AMOUNT ENCLOSED

$ __________

Send all orders to:

FantaCo Enterprises, Inc.
21 Central Avenue · Albany, New York 12210 · (518) 463-1400
Publishing · Mail Order · Retail

DEALERS: INQUIRE ABOUT WHOLESALE RATES